1987
YEAR BOOK OF
NEUROLOGY AND
NEUROSURGERY®

The 1987 Year Book Series

Anesthesia: Drs. Miller, Kirby, Ostheimer, Roizen, and Stoelting

Cancer: Drs. Hickey, Saunders, Clark, and Cumley

Cardiology: Drs. Schlant, Collins, Engle, Frye, Gifford, and O'Rourke

Critical Care Medicine: Drs. Rogers, Allo, Dean, Gioia, McPherson, Michael, Miller, and Traystman

Dentistry: Drs. Cohen, Hendler, Johnson, Jordan, Moyers, Robinson, and Silverman

Dermatology: Drs. Sober and Fitzpatrick

Diagnostic Radiology: Drs. Bragg, Keats, Kieffer, Kirkpatrick, Koehler, Miller, and Sorenson

Digestive Diseases: Drs. Greenberger and Moody

Drug Therapy: Drs. Hollister and Lasagna

Emergency Medicine: Dr. Wagner

Endocrinology: Drs. Bagdade, Ryan, Molitch, Braverman, Robertson, Halter, Kornel, Horton, Korenman, Morley, Rogol, Burger, and Metz

Family Practice: Drs. Rakel, Couchman, Driscoll, Avant, and Prichard

Hand Surgery: Drs. Dobyns, Chase, and Amadio

Hematology: Drs. Spivak, Bell, Ness, Quesenberry, and Wiernik

Infectious Diseases: Drs. Wolff, Tally, Keusch, Klempner, and Snydman

Medicine: Drs. Rogers, Des Prez, Cline, Braunwald, Greenberger, Wilson, Epstein, and Malawista

Neonatal/Perinatal Medicine: Drs. Klaus and Fanaroff

Neurology and Neurosurgery: Drs. DeJong, Currier, and Crowell

Nuclear Medicine: Drs. Hoffer, Gore, Gottschalk, Sostman, and Zaret

Obstetrics and Gynecology: Drs. Mishell, Kirschbaum, and Morrow

Ophthalmology: Drs. Ernest and Deutsch

Orthopedics: Dr. Coventry

Otolaryngology—Head and Neck Surgery: Drs. Paparella and Bailey

Pathology and Clinical Pathology: Drs. Brinkhous, Dalldorf, Grisham, Langdell, and McLendon

Pediatrics: Drs. Oski and Stockman

Plastic and Reconstructive Surgery: Drs. McCoy, Brauer, Haynes, Hoehn, Miller, and Whitaker

Podiatric Medicine and Surgery: Dr. Jay

Psychiatry and Applied Mental Health: Drs. Freedman, Lourie, Meltzer, Nemiah, Talbott, and Weiner

Pulmonary Disease: Drs. Green, Ball, Menkes, Michael, Peters, Terry, Tockman, and Wise

Rehabilitation: Drs. Kaplan and Szumski

Sports Medicine: Drs. Krakauer, Shephard, and Torg, Col. Anderson, and Mr. George

Surgery: Drs. Schwartz, Jonasson, Peacock, Shires, Spencer, and Thompson

Urology: Drs. Gillenwater and Howards

Vascular Surgery: Drs. Bergan and Yao

1987

The Year Book of NEUROLOGY AND NEUROSURGERY®

"Published without interruption since 1902"

Neurology

Editors

Russell N. DeJong, M.D.
Professor Emeritus of Neurology,
The University of Michigan Medical School

Robert D. Currier, M.D.
Professor and Chairman, Department of Neurology, University of Mississippi
Medical Center, Jackson

Neurosurgery

Editor

Robert M. Crowell, M.D.
Professor and Head, Department of Neurosurgery, University of Illinois,
College of Medicine at Chicago

Year Book Medical Publishers, Inc.
Chicago • London

The editor for this book was Steven Berman, and the production manager was H. E. Nielsen. The Editor-in-Chief for the YEAR BOOK series is Nancy Gorham.

Table of Contents

Journals Represented

Acta Chirurgica Scandinavica
Acta Medica Scandinavica
Acta Neurochirurgica
Acta Neurologica Scandinavica
Age and Ageing
American Journal of Diseases of Children
American Journal of Epidemiology
American Journal of Medicine
American Journal of Neuroradiology
American Journal of Obstetrics and Gynecology
American Journal of Roentgenology
American Journal of Surgery
Anesthesia and Analgesia
Annales de Chirurgie de la Main
Annals of Emergency Medicine
Annals of Internal Medicine
Annals of Neurology
Annals of Otology, Rhinology and Laryngology
Annals of Rheumatic Diseases
Annals of Surgery
Archives of Emergency Medicine
Archives of General Psychiatry
Archives of Neurology
Archives of Otolaryngology
Archives of Pathology and Laboratory Medicine
Archives of Surgery
Australian and New Zealand Journal of Medicine
Brain
British Medical Journal
Canadian Journal of Neurological Sciences
Canadian Medical Association Journal
Cancer
Clinical Endocrinology
Clinical Orthopaedics and Related Research
Clinical Physiology
Deutsche Medizinische Wochenschrift
Diagnostic Microbiology and Infectious Disease
Epilepsia
European Neurology
Experimental Neurology
Head and Neck Surgery
Headache
Injury
Intensive Care Medicine
International Orthopaedics
Investigative Radiology
Journal of the American Medical Association
Journal of Bone and Joint Surgery (American volume)
Journal of Cell Biology
Journal of Clinical Endocrinology and Metabolism
Journal of Clinical Investigation

Journal of Clinical Neuro-Ophthalmology
Journal of Computer Assisted Tomography
Journal of Neurological Sciences
Journal of Neurology
Journal of Neurology, Neurosurgery and Psychiatry
Journal of Neuropathology and Experimental Neurology
Journal of Neuroscience
Journal of Neurosurgery
Journal of Nuclear Medicine
Journal of Pediatrics
Journal of Surgical Research
Journal of Trauma
Journal of Urology
Journal of Vascular Surgery
Lancet
Laryngoscope
Magnetic Resonance Imaging
Mayo Clinic Proceedings
Muscle and Nerve
Nervenarzt
Neurochirurgie
Neurology
Neuroradiology
Neurosurgery
New England Journal of Medicine
Ophthalmology
Otolaryngology–Head and Neck Surgery
Pain
Pediatric Neurology
Pediatrics
Plastic and Reconstructive Surgery
Postgraduate Medicine
Presse Medicale
Quarterly Journal of Medicine
Radiology
Revue de Chirurgie Orthopédique et Réparatrice de l'Appareil Moteur
Revue Neurologique
Science
Southern Medicine Journal
Spine
Stroke
Surgical Neurology

NEUROLOGY

RUSSELL N. DeJONG, M.D.
ROBERT D. CURRIER, M.D.

Introductory Remarks

Medical literature, specifically that dealing with neurology and diseases of the nervous system, appears principally in the form of published books and in periodically published magazines or medical journals. Historically, books preceded journals by many years.

The first American book dealing with neurology was *Medical Inquiries and Observations Upon the Diseases of the Mind* by Benjamin Rush, published in 1812. Rush, a Philadelphia physician and psychiatrist, was also a signer of the Declaration of Independence. The book, which primarily concerned mental disease, went through many editions and for several decades served as the primary textbook and standard reference work for American practitioners and students of the subject. It did, however, also discuss injuries to the brain, tumors, apoplexy, and epilepsy.

Amariah Brigham, also a psychiatrist, published *An Inquiry Concerning the Diseases and Functions of the Brain, Spinal Cord, and Nerves* in 1840. Although most of the clinical portions of the book deal with mental diseases, he did discuss inflammation of the brain, apoplexy, epilepsy, tinnitis, chorea, delirium tremens, and tic douloureux. He was one of the founders of what is now the American Psychiatric Association and in 1844 founded and became the first editor of the *American Journal of Insanity*, now the *American Journal of Psychiatry*.

Charles Edouard Brown-Séquard, a peripatetic neurologist and neurophysiologist, in 1860 published his *Course of Lectures on the Physiology and Pathology of the Central Nervous System*. The lectures had been delivered before the Royal College of Surgeons in London in 1858. Brown-Séquard held appointments at the Medical College of Virginia in 1854 and at Harvard Medical School from 1864 to 1867.

Silas Weir Mitchell, who has been called one of the founders of American neurology, co-authored his epoch-making *Gunshot Wounds and Other Injuries of Nerves* with G. R. Morehouse and W. W. Keen in 1864. In 1872 Mitchell published, with the assistance of the same collaborators, a more extensive study, *Injuries of Nerves and Their Consequences*. Many other books and articles dealing with all aspects of neurology followed.

The first American textbook of neurology, *A Treatise on Diseases of the Nervous System*, was published in 1871 by William A. Hammond, a contemporary, close friend, and one-time collaborator of Mitchell's. This book went through seven editions in ten years and was followed by many other books by Hammond dealing with various aspects of neurology and psychiatry.

Following the publication of these books, others dealing with neurology and the neurologic sciences began appearing with increasing frequency throughout the years, and an immense neurologic literature has accumulated. At the present time so many books, many of which are of fundamental importance to both clinical and basic neurology, are appearing each year that it is becoming difficult to keep up with them.

A journal dealing with neurologic material first appeared in the United States in 1874 when the *Chicago Journal of Nervous and Mental Disease* was published, with James S. Jewell as editor and Henry M. Bannister as assistant editor. Two years later, its title was changed to the *Journal of Nervous and Mental Disease*. Shortly after the founding of the American Neurological Association in 1875, the *Journal* became the official publication of the Association. It still appears monthly, but in recent years it has become predominantly, if not entirely, a psychiatric publication and no longer serves as a forum for the publication of neurologic papers.

Brain, the major British neurologic journal, began publication in 1879, and *Revue Neurologique*, the major French journal, was first published in 1893.

In 1917 the Board of Trustees of the American Medical Association established a monthly journal, the *Archives of Neurology and Psychiatry*, with the understanding that it would replace the *Journal of Nervous and Mental Disease* as the official organ of the American Neurological Association. The first issue appeared in January 1919. In 1959 the Board of Trustees of the American Medical Association decided to have separate journals for neurology and psychiatry and established the *Archives of Neurology* and the *Archives of General Psychiatry*. The first issue of the *Archives of Neurology* appeared in July 1959, and its current editor-in-chief is Robert J. Joynt of Rochester, New York.

One of the first ventures of the American Academy of Neurology, after its establishment in 1948, was the founding of a journal, *Neurology*, devoted specifically to the specialty. The first issue appeared in January 1951, and the current editor-in-chief is Robert B. Daroff of Cleveland, Ohio. The *Annals of Neurology*, now the official journal of both the American Neurological Association and the Child Neurology Society, began publication in January 1977. Its current editor-in-chief is Arthur K. Asbury of Philadelphia, Pennsylvania.

Other important neurologic journals are the *Journal of Neurology, Neurosurgery and Psychiatry* (published in England); *Encephale* (France), *Acta Neurologica Scandinavica, Canadian Journal of the Neurological Sciences, European Neurology, Journal of Neurology, Zeitschrift für Neurologie, Der Nervenarzt*, and *Developmental Medicine and Child Neurology*.

In addition, there are many journals within the neurology subspecialties and the basic sciences related to neurology. The *Journal of Comparative Neurology* was established in 1891 and still appears regularly. It might, however, more appropriately bear the title Journal of Comparative Neuroanatomy. *Electroencephalography and Clinical Neurophysiology* is the official organ of the International Federation of Societies for Electroencephalography and Clinical Neurophysiology. *Epilepsia* is the journal of the International League Against Epilepsy. *Stroke: A Journal of Cerebral Circulation* was established by the American Heart Association. The *Journal of Neurophysiology* was founded by the American Physiology Society. The *Journal of Neuropathology and Experimental Neurology* was established by the American Association of Neuropathologists. The *Journal of Neurosurgery* was established by the Harvey Cushing Society, which later became the American Association of Neurological Surgeons. The *Journal of the Neurological Sciences* was established by the World Federation of

Neurology. The *American Journal of Neuroradiology* is the official journal of the American Society of Neuroradiology.

Other subspecialty journals include *Pain, Journal of Neurochemistry, Journal of Neuroscience, Muscle Nerve, Surgical Neurology, Journal of Neuroimaging,* and *Experimental Neurology.*

The EC/IC Bypass Study

There has been much controversy, especially among neurosurgeons, about the results of an eight-year international surgical study (*Stroke* 16:394–406, 1985). The 71-center study, of which Sydney J. Peerless, professor of neurosurgery at the University of Western Ontario (London), was principal neurosurgical investigator, was carried out to compare the results of surgery (an anastomosis of the superficial temporal artery to the middle cerebral artery) with those of chemotherapy (the use of aspirin and antihypertensive drugs) in preventing strokes, preserving function, and decreasing the mortality rate in symptomatic patients with stenosis of the internal carotid or middle cerebral artery.

A total of 1,377 patients were studied with preoperative and postoperative angiographic evaluations and all were followed up. The study showed that there was no difference between the two groups of patients and that there was no benefit associated with the surgical procedure (*N. Engl. J. Med.* 313:1191–1200).

In 1985, the results of this study were presented to the International Congress of Neurosurgery in Toronto, and they were discussed more fully at a special symposium at the meeting of the American Association of Neurological Surgeons in Denver in April 1986. The Association has formed a committee to review the bypass study, especially its data base, and to decide whether to accept or challenge its conclusions (*JAMA* 256:165–167, 1986; *J. Neurol.* 233:129–130, 1986).

Russell N. DeJong, M.D.

Introductory Remarks

Carola Eisenberg of the Harvard Medical School has said something that needs to be said these days (*N. Engl. J. Med.* 314:1113–1114, April 24, 1986). As Dean of Student Affairs, she has been hearing from students about their fears and their worries about medicine as a career. She summarizes the situation accurately, in my opinion, and finally says, "Our students need to know about the problems facing medicine. But those problems need to be seen in perspective. Medical education does not exist to provide doctors with an opportunity to earn a living, but to improve the health of the public. Let us enlist our students in the campaign for equity and quality in medical care. If that campaign is to succeed, it will need the efforts of the best and the brightest . . . What we do as doctors, most of the time, is deeply gratifying, whatever the mix of patient care, research, and teaching in our individual careers. I cannot imagine a more satisfying calling. Let us make sure our students hear that message from us."

Kurtzke et al. (*Neurology* 36:383–388, March 1986) are predicting a need in a United States population of 243.5 million for 16,500 neurologists, a prevalence rate of 6.76 per 100,000 population. Every prediction for the need for neurologists in the United States has seemed excessive to me over the years, and I have been proved wrong repeatedly. Again, this seems excessive unless, indeed, we do begin to take over the treatment of low-back pain, dizziness, headaches, and pain and numbness in general.

A recent comment in *Medicine* by Whitcomb and Caswell (*N. Engl. J. Med.* 314:710–712, Mar. 13, 1986) encourages us not to rely on free market economic forces in determining the numbers of trainees in any specialty area, since these forces are said not to apply. They make the point that most medical students choosing a field do not put the market forces very high on the list of factors influencing their choice. Therefore, they recommend that we allow the government to intercede and to "use the powers of the government to improve the delivery of health care."

Free market forces, however, do apply, and, although there are some trainees who will go into a field because of an intense interest no matter how overcrowded the field, most will attend to these forces, and one suspects that it will not be necessary for the government to dictate numbers for various fields of residency training in the United States. There is one thing that will have to be true if neurologists are to care for the most common diseases and compete effectively with other health care providers: our rates will have to be competitive.

The most entertaining and outrageous thing I have come across this year for once is not in *The Lancet*—it's in the *British Medical Journal* (292:947–948, Apr. 5, 1986)—and is by George Dunea, FRCP, of Cook County Hospital, Chicago. A short article on the state of medicine in the United States, it is difficult to abstract or summarize. He does mention that "for a less violent solution to the liability crisis, some economists want to . . . (export) our surplus of lawyers. . . . They could teach burglars to sue their clients for having unsafe lodgings (and) drunken drivers to sue telephone companies for putting obstructing booths in their way. . . ." You'll have to read it yourself.

Sarnat and Netsky (*Can. J. Neurol. Sci.* 12:296–302, November 1985) have in a very fascinating and useful way analyzed the brain of the planarian, said to be the simplest living animal with a body plan of bilateral symmetry and cephalization. The brain is bilobed and has a cortex and nerve fibers, some of which decussate; reflexes and neurotransmitters are also evident. The final paragraph of their contribution is lovely: "If another mass extinction should occur on Earth, life for humans probably would end as it did for the dinosaurs some 65 million years ago. The resilient planarian would likely survive as it has survived each of the several previous mass extinctions of life known from the fossil record. The plasticity of its primordial brain is extraordinary. Might another billion years of planarian evolution yield an intelligent dinosaur, an intelligent primate, or another yet unknown intelligent species?"

Lisman (*Proc. Natl. Acad. Sci. USA* 82:3055–3057, May 1985) has proposed a molecular switch for memory that can be turned on by an external stimulus and is not reset by protein turnover. The brain sounds more and more like a transistorized engine the more we learn about it.

Coscina et al. (*Life Sciences* 38:1789–1794, May 1986) find that rats learn better when fed a soybean oil diet. I wonder if saturated fats interfere with learning.

The significance of carotid bruits and indeed carotid stenosis is again unclear and one or more American studies of surgery for carotid disease may soon be mounted.

The World Health Organization has come in with the results of the European Collaborative Trial of Multifactorial Prevention of Coronary Heart Disease. After 6 years in the study, the group who followed guidelines on a cholesterol-lowering diet, control of smoking, reduction of weight and blood pressure, and regular exercise were improved in terms of coronary heart disease occurrences and deaths, and the benefit was related to the extent of risk factor change. The good people of the Massachusetts Department of Public Health have begun an "aggressive state wide program to reduce heart disease, cancer and stroke by the reduction of risk factors." They predict that within five years their publicity program will save 2,000 lives annually. They recommend similar efforts by public health agencies and practitioners throughout the country.

Four people who were dear to me have died. Elizabeth Hartman was not a neurologist but as a training program administrator with the National Institute of Neurological and Communicative Disorders and Stroke was mother to a complete generation of neurologists. At a time when training programs were small, young, and weak she, representing the hand of the government, provided friendship, support, and understanding to all of us.

Maurice Van Allen, Professor of Neurology at the University of Iowa was a friend of mine for more than 25 years, during which I grew to appreciate his kindly wit, accepting philosophy, and pungent insights.

I was not acquainted personally with Dr. John David Spillane (University Hospital of Wales, Cardiff), but was familiar with and appreciative of his contributions and particularly enjoyed a speech several years ago at the American Neurological Association annual meeting in which he detailed his trip in the 1930s with a friend through America in an old Ford. He divided his acquaintances into two groups—those who had seen the Grand Canyon and those who had not. His love for this country was evident and heart-warming.

Finally, I got to know and admire André Barbeau, who was Professor of Neurology at the Université de Montréal, when I worked with him on ataxia. His work on ataxia alone would cause him to be long remembered, but he did so many other things in other fields. He was not always right but his philosophy of forging ahead—causing turmoil and consternation on the way—was exciting and good for research.

Robert D. Currier, M.D.

1 Neurology of Aging

Neurologic Signs in Senescence
Lawrence R. Jenkyn, Alexander G. Reeves, Thomas Warren, R. Keith Whiting, Richard J. Clayton, Walter W. Moore, Alessandro Rizzo, Illhan M. Tuzun, John C. Bonnett, and Burford W. Culpepper (Dartmouth Univ. and Du Pont de Nemours, Wilmington, Del.)
Arch. Neurol. 42:1154–1157, December 1985   1–1

This study examined the changes in incidence of abnormal neurologic findings for nine clinical tests in 2,029 normal volunteers 50–93 years of age; 38 subjects were 80 years of age or older. The neurologic tests were the nuchocephalic reflex, glabellar blink, snout reflex, paratonia, upward and downward vertical gaze, visual pursuit, reverse spelling, and memory recall. These tests increased the average physical examination time by 3 minutes.

An increased frequency of abnormal responses with increasing age was observed for all signs; this trend was most apparent after 70 years of age. Several signs were associated as pairs, including upward and downward gaze, snout and glabellar reflexes, the nuchocephalic reflex and paratonia, and others. These may represent common sites of neurologic dysfunction. Subjects younger than 70 years of age may have up to three abnormal responses expected, while patients older than 70 years of age may have an increasing frequency of abnormal responses. An excessive number of abnormal responses may indicate coincidental pathologic processes such as Alzheimer's disease or Parkinson's disease.

This neurologic test battery may prove useful in screening for early diffuse cerebral dysfunction. A minimum number of abnormal responses allowable by age group on this screening battery is defined.

▶ This looks like a useful study since they give the normal values for each 5-year period for all nine of their simple tests.

Macdonald Critchley, who started writing about aging in the central nervous system 58 years ago, wrote a vivid article in the *Archives of Neurology* about language function in the elderly (41:1135–1139, Nov. 1984). C. Miller Fisher (*The Lancet* 173: January 19, 1985) points out that as couples age, the wife's memory for names is consistently better than the husband's and believes that this is a benign form of selective forgetting restricted mainly to males. In a follow-up letter Lennox (*The Lancet* 343; February 9, 1985) says that we should name it Fisher's syndrome. Since there are other Fisher's syndromes regarding which my memory already has me in trouble, I am not sure that we should do that. I am grateful to Drs. Fisher and Lennox for letting me off the hook in the way the latter suggests "I am terribly sorry I have forgotten your name, I've got Fisher's syndrome, you know."

Nicholas et al. (*J. Speech Hear Res.* 28:405–410, September 1985) point out that the speech problems of Alzheimer's disease and fluent aphasia are different, the former producing more empty phrases and conjunctions and the latter more neologisms and paraphasias. The difference they suggest may help us distinguish the two groups.—Robert D. Currier, M.D.

Autonomic Responses to Glucose Ingestion in Elderly Subjects With Orthostatic Hypotension
Brian J. Robinson, Ralph H. Johnson, David G. Lambie, and Karen T. Palmer (Wellington Hosp., New Zealand)
Age Ageing 14:168–173, May 1985   1–2

Cardiovascular and plasma catecholamine responses to oral glucose were investigated in five elderly subjects with orthostatic hypotension and 5 normal elderly subjects. All 10 had blood samples, blood pressure, and heart rate taken at intervals up to 3 hours after ingestion of glucose.

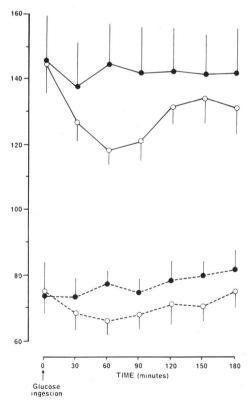

Fig 1–1.—Systolic *(continuous lines)* and diastolic *(broken lines)* blood pressures in subjects with *(open circles)* and without *(closed circles)* orthostatic hypotension before and after ingestion of glucose. Results are plotted as mean ± SE values. (Courtesy of Robinson, B.J., et al.: Age Ageing 14:168–173, May 1985.)

Subjects with orthostatic hypotension had significant reductions in blood pressure after receiving oral glucose, compared with control subjects (Fig 1–1). Levels of plasma norepinephrine and epinephrine increased also, as did heart rate, but no significant differences were seen between controls and subjects with orthostatic hypotension at any time for these three parameters.

The fall in blood pressure that was seen in subjects with orthostatic hypotension after receiving glucose demonstrated that this phenomenon is due to a generalized disorder of blood pressure control. Reduced baroreceptor sensitivity or peripheral sympathetic denervation can be primary causes of reductions in blood pressure. These data suggest that abnormal pathology of the venous system is responsible for orthostatic and postprandial hypotension in the elderly. In addition, cerebral autoregulation may fail in subjects with orthostatic hypotension. Because cerebrovascular accidents are common after large meals, elderly subjects with orthostatic hypotension may be at particular risk.

▶ It is hard to find a hole in this neat study. Mother always said that we should lie down after meals. Maybe there is something to it after all.—Robert D. Currier, M.D.

2 Amyotrophic Lateral Sclerosis

Controlled Trial of Thyrotropin Releasing Hormone in Amyotrophic Lateral Sclerosis
Michael H. Brooke, Julaine M. Florence, Scott L. Heller, K. K. Kaiser, Daniel Phillips, Allen Gruber, Debbie Babcock, and J. Philip Miller (Washington Univ.)
Neurology 36:146–151, February 1986   2–1

A double-blind controlled trial of the daily administration of 150 mg of intramuscular thyrotropin-releasing hormone (TRH) was conducted in 30 patients (10 women and 20 men) with classic amyotrophic lateral sclerosis (ALS). All patients had wasting and weakness in at least three of four limbs, with associated laboratory and clinical signs of denervation. All patients had obvious fasciculations. All had difficulty with speech or swallowing or signs of upper motor neuron involvement in the limbs. Signs indicating upper motor neuron damage included pathologically brisk reflexes, increased tone, or extensor plantar responses. No patient had any sensory abnormality or involvement of extraocular muscles; no patient had been treated with any other agent; and none had received TRH before the study. The drug/placebo was administered for 2 months, followed by a 2-month "wash-out." Five patients were in wheelchairs and 25 were ambulatory. The placebo was saline. Five patients failed to complete the study.

Side effects occurred in 13 of the 14 patients receiving TRH. These side effects were reported on all visits and were directly related to the injection of the drug. The most common effect was intense shivering, lasting 10–40 minutes, often with a sense of bladder or rectal fullness and sweating. Eight of the 14 patients also reported nausea at the time of the injection.

Other effects reported sporadically were rhinorrhea in 3 patients, excessive yawning in 2, and headache in 3. There was no significant difference between TRH and placebo group in individual muscles or in average muscle-strength scores (Fig 2–1). There were significant differences when proximal muscles were analyzed at weeks 2, 3, 8, 14, and 16 (Fig 2–2).

Results of this study showed that there was a small but definite increase in muscle strength associated with TRH administration, but none of the patients receiving TRH wished to continue the drug beyond the 2-month period. It is also important to point out that this study demonstrated that the administration of TRH had no clinical useful effect, although it was associated with some increase in strength.

▶ This article was accompanied by two other papers on exactly the same sub-

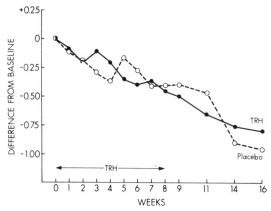

Fig 2–1.—Average muscle strength scores for both groups of patients. The average muscle strength is plotted as the difference of the group values from the baseline value at the time intervals as indicated. There was no statistically significant difference between the groups at any particular time point. Both groups showed a significant decline over the length of the trial. (Courtesy of Brooke, M.H., et al.: Neurology 36:146–151, February 1986.)

ject. The other two were by Mitsumoto et al. (*Neurology* 36:152–159, 1986) and by Caroscio et al. (Neurology 36:141–145, 1986). The choice of which one to abstract was more or less random, so I apologize to the other two groups. The three together pretty well lay to rest the thought that TRH is useful in the treatment of ALS. It is encouraging to know that there are several groups willing to engage in such labors that benefit us all.

The symptom of pathologic emotional lability in ALS has been successfully treated with amitriptyline (Caroscio, et al.: *N. Engl. J. Med.* 313:1478, Dec. 5,

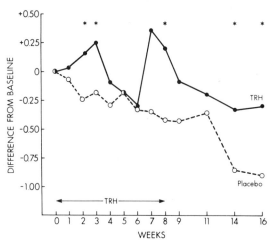

Fig 2–2.—This is the same type of graph as in Figure 2–1, illustrating the average strength of the proximal muscles (see text). The treatment group was significantly better ($P < .05$) at the time points indicated by the asterisks. (Courtesy of Brooke, M.H., et al.: Neurology 36:146–151, February 1986.)

1985). It would seem unlikely that a patient with ALS would write a benign, even optimistic comment on his experience with the disease, but this has been done by J. D. V. Woodcock (*N.Z. Med. J.* 98:1043–1045, Dec. 11, 1985) in a warm and wonderful way. He lists some good things about having motor neuron disease: "(1) as a general premise there is no pain; (2) intelligence is retained; (3) you get to find out how wonderful family, friends and neighbors can be; (4) very soon you appreciate how good our medical system really is; (5) there is time to put your affairs in order; (6) there is time to say thanks and goodbyes to loved ones; (7) daily living suddenly has a new dimension."— Robert D. Currier, M.D.

Intrathecal Thyrotropin Releasing Hormone Therapy of Amyotrophic Lateral Sclerosis
T. Stober, K. Schimrigk, S. Dietzsch, and T. Thielen (Univ. of Saarland, Federal Republic of Germany)
J. Neurol. 232:13–14, March 1985   2–2

Improved function has been described in patients with amyotrophic lateral sclerosis (ALS) given extremely high doses of thyrotropin releasing hormone (TRH) intravenously. Intrathecal treatment was evaluated in six patients who had typical clinical and electromyographic signs of ALS. Initial patients were given dosages up to 4,000, µg a dosage that was discontinued when postpuncture syndrome was observed. The average single dosage ranged from 1,000 to 2,500 µg, given weekly for 2 months and then every 2 weeks.

No patient had change in the progressive course of illness during TRH therapy for 2 to 6 months. Atrophy, paralysis, and disability scores increased. No reproducible increase in muscle strength could be demonstrated. One patient reported improved articulation, and 1 with chronic lung disease had an increase in tidal volume after TRH injection. Body temperature rose by 0.5 to 1 C after injection, and blood pressure rose by up to 40% above baseline. One patient had sudden convulsions starting an hour after TRH injection. Three patients felt tired and yawned several hours after injection, whereas 2 others reported severe unrest and sleeplessness.

Injections of TRH for up to 6 months failed to halt the progress of ALS in these patients. A decreased TRH concentration in the anterior horn region presumably is a secondary finding resulting from a reduced number of cells. It remains to be shown whether long-term subcutaneous, intravenous, or oral administration of a long-lasting TRH analogue could provide a substantial therapeutic effect.

▶ These results confirm what many other investigators have shown. Thyrotropin-releasing hormones, even when given intrathecally, are ineffective in the treatment of ALS.—Russell N. DeJong, M.D.

Detection of Picornavirus Sequences in Nervous Tissue of Amyotrophic Lateral Sclerosis and Control Patients

M. Brahic, R. A. Smith, C. J. Gibbs, Jr., R. M. Garruto, W. W. Tourtellotte, and E. Cash (Institut Pasteur, Paris; Ctr. for Neurologic Study, San Diego; Natl. Insts. of Health, Bethesda, Md; VA Wadsworth Med. Ctr. and Reed Neurological Research Inst., Los Angeles)

Ann. Neurol. 18:337–343, September 1985   2–3

Persistent viral infection of the CNS frequently is associated with chronic degenerative disorders, and some of these disorders, including amyotrophic lateral sclerosis (ALS), are thought to be possibly caused by slow viral infections. Limited viral expression is characteristic of most persistent infections of the CNS.

In situ hybridization was used in an attempt to identify picornavirus RNA sequences in frozen sections of CNS tissue from patients with ALS and control patients. Reconstruction experiments indicated that 30 copies of viral RNA per cell can be detected with the assay. Probes of CNS tissues were performed with tritiated (^{3}H) complementary DNA (cDNA) synthesized against the RNA of poliovirus or Theiler's virus.

Ribonucleic acid that hybridized to DNAs that were complementary to both poliovirus and Theiler's virus was identified at several levels of the CNS in two patients, one with ALS and one control. In transverse sections of the spinal cord these sequences predominated in cells of the anterior horns (Fig 2–3). Hybridization was not found with heterologous visna virus cDNA probes and it was abolished by pretreatment of sections with ribonuclease. The results were reproduced in three independent experiments. Chemographic artifacts were excluded.

Molecules of RNA, possibly from a picornavirus that has sequences in

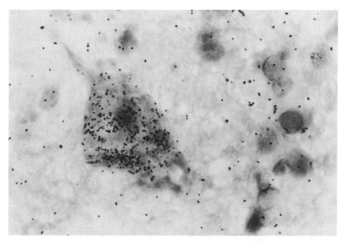

Fig 2–3.—In situ hybridization on frozen sections of spinal cord from patients with amyotrophic lateral sclerosis. Sections were hybridized with poliovirus type 1 (^{3}H)cDNA. Exposure time was 4 weeks. This is an example of large neurons in the ventral horn containing RNA sequences that hybridized to poliovirus cDNA. (×840 before 10% reduction.) (Courtesy of Brahic, M., et al.: Ann. Neurol. 18:337–343, September 1985.)

common with poliovirus and Theiler's virus, were found in tissue of the CNS in two patients in this study, and it might have been found more often with shorter autolysis times. There is now good evidence that genomes of common viruses can persist in the human CNS.

However, the finding of a viral genome in both disease and control tissue does not rule out a viral cause of neurologic illness, as is evident from measles and herpesviruses. Pathologic viral effects may be triggered by host factors such as immunogenetic background or by mutation in viral genes.

► I hope that efforts such as those described in this article will continue. Of all the theories of ALS, the viral theory seems the most likely.—Robert D. Currier, M.D.

Heavy Metal Concentrations in Blood Cells in Patients With Amyotropic Lateral Sclerosis
Hiroshi Nagata, Satoru Miyata, Shigenobu Nakamura Masakuni Kameyama, and Yoshikazu Katsui (Kyoto Univ., Kyoto, and Mie Univ., Mie, Japan)
J. Neurol. Sci. 67:173–178, February 1985   2–4

Epidemiologic studies suggest a causative role for manganese (Mn), selenium (Se), and several other metals in amyotropic lateral sclerosis

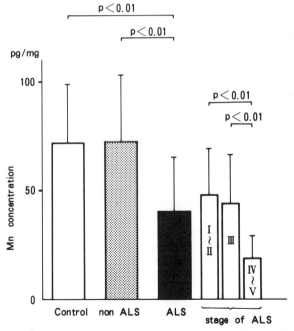

Fig 2–4.—Concentrations of manganese in blood cells from patients with ALS and other neurologic diseases (non-ALS) and control subjects. (Courtesy of Nagata, H., et al.: J. Neurol. Sci. 67:173–178, February 1985.)

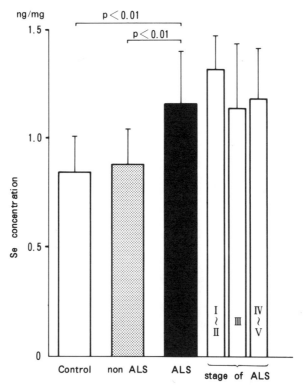

Fig 2–5.—Concentrations of selenium in blood cells from patients with ALS and other neurologic diseases (non-ALS) and control subjects. (Courtesy of Nagata, H., et al.: J. Neurol. Sci. 67:173–178, February 1985.)

(ALS). Data were examined from 40 patients with ALS, 25 control subjects, and 37 patients with other neurologic diseases, including Parkinson's disease, senile dementia, and spinocerebellar degeneration. Concentrations of Mn, Se, Zinc (Zn), rubidium (Rb), and bromine (Br) in blood cells were measured.

Mean concentration of Mn in blood cells of patients with ALS was significantly lower than that of control subjects or patients with other neurologic diseases. These relationships are depicted in Figure 2–4, along with mean concentrations of Mn in patients at various stages during the progress of ALS. Mean concentration of Mn in blood cells decreased as the severity of the deficit increased. Mean concentrations of Se in blood cells of study patients are represented in Figure 2–5. In contrast to the levels of Mn, levels of Se in patients with ALS were higher than in control subjects or in patients with other neurologic diseases. Mean concentrations of Se did not vary with the clinical stage of ALS. Mean concentrations of Br, Zn, Rb, and Fe in blood cells were similar in patients with ALS and the other two groups.

Those results demonstrate that a simple mechanism such as Mn intoxication is not a likely explanation for the pathogenesis of ALS, because other researchers have shown increased levels of Mn in neuronal tissue. The differences in Se levels between patients with ALS and control subjects suggest that systemic disturbances of Se metabolism may also be present in patients with ALS.

▶ What selenium has to do with ALS is a mystery. Quite possibly, nothing. On the other hand, I had thought the false sago palm seed had nothing to do with Guamanian ALS, and now thirty years later it appears that there is another toxin, D,L-BMAA, in the seed that when given to monkeys produces an ALS-like picture (Spencer et al.: *Lancet* 1:965, April 26, 1986). Tandan and Bradley (*Ann. Neurol.* 18:271–280, September 1985; 18:419–431, October 1985) have produced a two-part comprehensive statement on ALS which is thorough and reasonable. Recommended reading.—Robert D. Currier, M.D.

Amyotrophic Lateral Sclerosis: Part 2: Etiopathogenesis
Rup Tandan and Walter G. Bradley (Univ. of Vermont)
Ann. Neurol. 18:419–431, October 1985   2–5

The pathogenesis of amyotrophic lateral sclerosis (ALS) remains unproved. Any unifying hypothesis must explain diverse geographic occurrence of the disease and varying clinical presentation and course. Recognition of autosomal dominant inheritance in familial adult-onset ALS, of autosomal dominant and recessive inheritance in familial juvenile-onset cases, and of ALS in both members of twin pairs implicates a genetic predisposition in some patients.

The concept of "premature aging" underlies many progressive neuronal degenerations but is poorly understood. Exposure to lead, mercury, and aluminum has been implicated in some cases of ALS. There also is some evidence that manganese may be involved. Increased levels of calcium in the brain and spinal cord have been described.

Several progressive neurologic disorders are caused by chronic persistent or slow viral infections. Selective degeneration of motor neurons is present in both ALS and poliomyelitis. Positive viral isolates have not yet been confirmed in ALS tissues. An increased frequency of histocompatibility antigen (HLA)-A3 in classic ALS may correlate with rapid progression. Circulating immune complexes have been reported in patients with sporadic and Guamanian ALS. Little is known about the altered chemistry of motor neurons in ALS. An ALS-like syndrome has been associated with a deficiency of hexosaminidase A.

Many reports have suggested the possibility of abnormal neurotransmitter function in ALS. Defects in membrane structure or function have been implicated in several neuromuscular disorders. The question of an increased incidence of malignancies in ALS remains to be answered. Axonal transport may be altered in ALS. Both trauma and previous surgery have been found to be more frequent in patients who develop ALS, but the possible significance of these findings is unknown.

▶ Viruses, metals, endogenous toxins, immune dysfunction, endocrine abnormalities, impaired DNA repair, altered axonal transport, and trauma have all been linked etiologically with amyotrophic lateral sclerosis, but convincing research evidence of a causative role for any of these has yet to be demonstrated. Unfortunately, no animal model reproduces all of the salient features of ALS.—Russell N. DeJong, M.D.

3 Acquired Immunodeficiency Syndrome

Central Nervous System Involvement in Patients With Acquired Immune Deficiency Syndrome (AIDS)
Barbara S. Koppel, Gary P. Wormser, Alan J. Tuchman, Shlomo Maayan, Dial Hewlett, Jr., and Michael Daras (New York Med. College)
Acta Neurol. Scand. 71:337–353, May 1985   3–1

Review of 121 cases of AIDS seen at three centers revealed 25 patients with proved or presumed CNS infection and 3 with primary cerebral lymphoma. Twenty-two patients (78.5%) died. Intravenous drug abuse alone was identified in nearly two thirds of the cases of CNS involvement. The average age was 38.5 years. Neurologic features were the chief reason for hospitalization in 57% of the cases; in 10 cases, neurologic symptoms were the initial manifestation of AIDS.

Toxoplasmosis was diagnosed in 9 patients, most of whom had progressive headache or focal deficits such as partial seizures, without prominent meningeal signs. Computed tomography (CT) showed circumscribed, ring-enhancing lesions (Fig 3–1). Multiple *Candida* brain abscesses were found at autopsy in 1 patient. One had mycobacterial infection. Seven patients had a subacute progressive encephalopathy, and there was 1 with suspected progressive multifocal leukoencephalopathy. Cryptococcal meningitis was diagnosed in 7 patients, 2 of whom had possible cryptococcoma. Three patients had a biopsy or autopsy diagnosis of non-Hodgkin's malignant lymphoma. All these patients died before radiotherapy could be administered or completed.

The CNS is commonly involved in AIDS, as in other disorders that promote opportunistic infection and neoplasia. *Toxoplasma gondii* was the most frequent cause of infection in this series; cryptococcal meningitis was the next most common infection. Any neurologic symptoms in an immunocompromised patient require an aggressive diagnostic approach. Primary lymphoma of the brain and metastatic Kaposi's sarcoma may occur. Anti-*Toxoplasma* treatment may be given empirically if CT evidence of infection is obtained. Brain biopsy is performed if there is no improvement in 2 weeks. The cerebrospinal fluid should be analyzed for evidence of cryptococcal or mycobacterial meningitis.

▶ It is becoming increasingly apparent that CNS involvement plays a major role in AIDS. In this study, 28 of 121 patients with AIDS had such involvement.

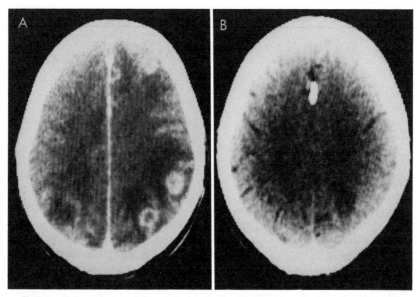

Fig 3–1.—Computed tomographic scans of brain after administration of iodinated contrast material showing multiple ring-enhancing *T. gondii* abscesses in right parietal lobe with surrounding edema (**A**) and disappearance of lesions 6 months later after treatment (**B**). (Courtesy of Koppel, B.S., et al.: Acta Neurol. Scand. 71:337–353, May 1985.)

The current literature emphatically confirms this (Snider W.D., et al.: *Ann. Neurol.* 14:403–418, 1983). The nervous system involvement included primary lymphomas of the brain as well as opportunistic infections. Those patients with focal neurologic features usually had toxoplasmosis. Progressive headache and meningeal signs occurred with cryptococcus. Progressive subacute dementia occurred with cytomegalovirus. Other infections included atypical mycobacteria, candida, and herpes zoster virus. Progressive multifocal leukoencephalopathy also occurred. A major risk factor in this AIDS population was intravenous drug use.—Russell N. DeJong, M.D.

Isolation of HTLV-III From Cerebrospinal Fluid and Neural Tissues of Patients With Neurologic Syndromes Related to the Acquired Immunodeficiency Syndrome

David D. Ho, Teresa R. Rota, Robert T. Schooley, Joan C. Kaplan, J. Davis Allan, Jerome E. Groopman, Lionel Resnick, Donna Felsenstein, Charla A. Andrews, and Martin S. Hirsch (Massachusetts Gen. Hosp., Harvard Univ., New England Deaconess Hosp., Boston; and Mount Sinai Med. Ctr., Miami Beach)
N. Engl. J. Med. 313:1493–1497, Dec. 12, 1985   3–2

Infection and neoplasia of the CNS are frequent complications of acquired immunodeficiency syndrome (AIDS). Subacute encephalitis, vacuolar degeneration of the spinal cord, chronic meningitis, and peripheral neuropathy all have been described. Attempts were made to isolate human T cell lymphotropic virus Type III (HTLV-III) from cerebrospinal fluid (CSF) brain, spinal cord, and peripheral nerve in 45 patients with AIDS or AIDS-related complex to determine whether the virus is directly involved in the pathogenesis of these disorders. A total of 56 specimens were analyzed, including 37 CSF samples and 15 brain tissue specimens. Twenty-nine subjects had AIDS, 7 had AIDS-related complex, and 9 were previously healthy men. Forty-one patients were seropositive for HTLV-III initially, and 2 seroconverted during acute meningitis; 1 patient was not evaluated.

Thirty-three patients had AIDS-related neurologic disorders, and 24 of them were positive for HTLV-III in at least one CNS site. None of 12 patients with unrelated neurologic deficits or no deficit had HTLV-III in the CSF or brain. Virus was isolated from the CSF during acute aseptic meningitis associated with HTLV-III seroconversion. HTLV-III also was isolated from CSF in 6 of 7 patients with AIDS or AIDS-related complex who had unexplained chronic meningitis. Ten of 16 patients with AIDS-related dementia had positive cultures in CSF and/or brain tissue. Virus was isolated from the spinal cord in a patient with myelopathy and from the sural nerve in one with peripheral neuropathy.

These findings support the neurotropic nature of HTLV-III and a role for the virus in both acute and chronic meningitis and dementia in patients with AIDS and AIDS-related complex. HTLV-III also may be the cause of spinal cord degeneration and peripheral neuropathy in these patients. Several of the present patients had neurologic problems associated with HTLV-III despite a lack of clinical immunodeficiency.

▶ This study and the one following it in the *New England Journal of Medicine* by Resnick et al. (313:1498–1504) describes AIDS dementia as a real entity. An editorial in the same issue by Black (313:1538–1539) produces more questions than answers about this type of encephalitis.—Robert D. Currier, M.D.

The Psychosocial and Neuropsychiatric Sequelae of the Acquired Immunodeficiency Syndrome and Related Disorders
Jimmie C. Holland and Susan Tross (Mem. Sloan-Kettering Cancer Ctr., New York)
Ann. Intern. Med. 103:760–764, November 1985   3–3

The social problems that result from AIDS, including greater homophobia and concerns by health care workers, have increased the psychosocial and neuropsychiatric sequelae of the disease. The diagnosis of AIDS is a catastrophic event because of the poor prognosis. The stigma associated with the contagious aspect of the disease can lead to avoidance of physical and social contact. Patients are vulnerable to rejection and to guilt feelings. Widespread discrimination is an important problem for these patients.

Most neuropsychiatric symptoms relate to anxiety or depression, with the latter associated with guilt, low self-esteem, and anticipatory grief.

With AIDS the complications in the CNS may include an encephalopathy (which in its early stages can resemble depression) and dementia that is associated with cerebral atrophy.

The attitude and responses of the medical staff are very important to AIDS patients. Fear of contagion is best dealt with by providing current information about appropriate safety precautions. Psychiatric consultation should always be considered, especially for patients with psychiatric symptoms. Those who care for patients with AIDS must be aware of their feelings about sexual matters and homosexuality in particular. Fears of progression of disease should be discussed with patients. They should be encouraged to explore feelings about sexual practices and about contagion, as well as feelings of anger about discriminatory behavior. Patients with related conditions have similar neuropsychiatric problems. Persons in risk groups and others not at risk but who are suggestible may have to deal with the fear of contracting AIDS.

▶ Since the summer of 1981 AIDS and its related conditions have become a public health problem of unprecedented proportions. The psychologic and social implications of the syndrome may cause psychiatric and social symptoms, including anxiety, depression, and delirium. Neurologic symptoms are frequent. Guidelines are needed for the management of the psychologic problems of AIDS and its related conditions.—Russell N. DeJong, M.D.

4 Behavioral Neurology and Cortical Function

Cerebral Lateralization: Biological Mechanisms, Associations, and Pathology: III. A Hypothesis and a Program for Research
Norman Geschwind and Albert M. Galaburda (Harvard Univ., Beth Israel Hosp., and Boston Univ., Boston; and Massachusetts Inst. of Technology, Cambridge, Mass.)
Arch. Neurol. 42:634–654, July 1985   4–1

Immune disorders have special importance in the anomalous dominance (AD) population. Disorders involving the gastrointestinal tract or thyroid are especially prevalent. Specific genes favoring immune attack on a specific system may be a factor, as may injury that exposes immunologically "privileged" regions such as the CNS to antigen. Similar factors may explain why many congenital lesions are not clinically manifest until late in adult life. Factors such as temperature and sympathetic innervation could help explain lateralized immune responses. Little is known about whether those with AD have a higher rate of immune complications or complications of drugs or diseases. Laterality is a prominent aspect of such brain disorders as epilepsy, dementia, and other progressive conditions. Psychiatric disorders may also exhibit lateralizing phenomena.

Chemical and pharmacologic asymmetries can explain why a drug action may be identical in terms of molecular events but different at various sites, depending on the side predominantly stimulated. Functional asymmetry of a given area could result from larger size, greater binding of neurotransmitters, or both. Asymmetric external forces can help explain the occurrence of asymmetry in symmetric organisms. Asymmetry in the single cell might be structural, chemical, or both. Linked asymmetry connotes an asymmetry that is induced in a given structure as the result of the appearance or modification of asymmetry in another structure. Dominance is now known not to be an exclusive property of humans. Both biology and physics may be required for understanding of the ultimate origins of asymmetry.

▶ This article by D. Geschwind, published posthumously, is one of a series of articles leading to his hypothesis and proposed program for research on cerebral lateralization. The entire series of articles, when published together, will be a significant contribution to neurologic knowledge.—Russell N. DeJong, M.D.

Lesions of Premotor Cortex in Man

Hans-Joachim Freund and Horst Hummelsheim (Univ. of Düsseldorf, Federal Republic of Germany)

Brain 108:697–733, September 1985   4–2

Eleven patients with frontal lobe lesions and weakness of the contra-lateral shoulder and hip muscles and a limb-kinetic apraxia were encoun-tered. The hemispheric lesion was restricted to frontal lobe structures that spared the precentral gyrus and its descending fibers. Nine lesions were due to infarction and 2 were due to tumor. A battery of manual dexterity tests was administered to the patients and to age-matched control subjects.

Computed tomography scans showed the posterior border of the lesions to be anterior to the precentral gyrus (Fig 4–1) and to involve the premotor but not the primary motor cortex. One patient had a purely subcortical lesion. All hip and shoulder muscles that were involved in abduction and elevation of the arm were primarily affected. Some patients reported a lack of skill and clumsiness of hand movements. Movement disorder was apparent when a temporal sequence of activities of the proximal muscles on both sides was necessary for movement. The gait typically was normal.

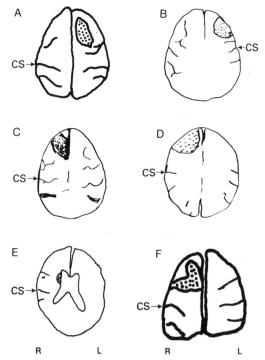

Fig 4–1.—Outlines of lesions seen at computed tomography in six cases of motor dysfunction. **A,** scan plane 2; **B,** scan plane 2; **C,** scan plane 3; **D,** scan plane 3; **E,** scan plane 5; **F,** scan plane 1. R, right hemisphere; L, left hemisphere; CS, central sulcus. (Courtesy of Freund, H.-J., and Hummelsheim, H.: Brain 108:697–733, September 1985.)

Limb-kinetic apraxia was most evident when a patient was lying on his back and was asked to make a bicycling motion with both legs. Preactivation of the proximal arm muscles on rapid arm movement was delayed on electromyographic evaluation. Two other patients with small lesions in the precentral gyrus and proximal hemiparesis had no limb-kinetic apraxia.

These neurologic deficits appear to result from damage that is anterior to the precentral gyrus and involve the premotor rather than the primary motor cortex. Temporal sequencing of muscle activation is disordered in these cases, suggesting that the nonprimary motor fields are relevant to the temporal aspects of motor programming.

This is in accord with a general concept of the significance of the frontal lobes for temporal organization. The premotor cortex may participate at a general level in establishing coordination between the eyes and extremities, between different extremities, and between different muscular task groups in one extremity.

► This is just what one would expect from lesions anterior to the precentral gyrus—some weakness on the other side with difficulty in programming motor activity. This is a fine example of a study correlating CT with neurologic findings. We should see more of these in the future.

Canavan et al. (*J. Neurol. Neurosurg. Psychiatry* 48:1049–1053, 1985) raise the question of whether Luria's frontal lobe syndrome is really strictly frontal lobe and, on the basis of a single case report, point out that the psychologic-behavioral syndrome, although occurring with frontal lobe damage, always occurs in association with other more widespread brain disease.—Robert D. Currier, M.D.

Quantitative Cytoarchitectural Studies of the Cerebral Cortex of Schizophrenics
Francine M. Benes, Jessica Davidson, and Edward D. Bird (Harvard Univ. and McLean Hosp., Belmont, Mass.)
Arch. Gen. Psychiatry 43:31–35, January 1986   4–3

Early histopathologic studies of the brains of schizophrenics gave mixed results, but recent computed tomographic studies have shown structural changes such as grossly visible volume losses. In the present study neuronal and glial density, neuron-glia ratios, and neuron size in the prefrontal and anterior cingulate cortex and in the primary motor cortex were quantified. Brains from 10 patients diagnosed as having schizophrenia by Feighner criteria under blind conditions were studied along with 10 control specimens. Potential confounding factors were controlled for by stepwise multiple regression and multiple classification analyses.

Neuronal density was significantly lower in layer VI of the prefrontal cortex, layer V of the cingulate cortex, and layer III of the motor cortex in schizophrenic brains. There was a trend toward fewer neurons in most layers of the prefrontal and motor cortices. Glial density also tended to be lower in most layers of all cortical regions. There were no differences between the schizophrenic and control groups in neuron-glia ratios or neuronal size.

These findings fail to indicate neuronal degeneration, as conventionally described, in the schizophrenic cortex, but cytoarchitectural variations in cortical structure may exist in some schizophrenics. The significance of decreased numbers of both neurons and glia occurring in associative and other cortical regions is unclear.

▶ The authors, after a careful study of brains of ten schizophrenics, conclude that the findings of decreased neuronal density in layer V of the cingulate cortex and III in the motor cortex and layer VI in the prefrontal cortex may be more developmental than acquired.

Bankier (*Br. J. Psychiatry* 147:241–245, 1985) reported that the third ventricular size was unrelated to the severity of schizophrenia, whereas Reveley (*Br. J. Psychiatry* 147:233–240, 1985) found that the lateral ventricles are enlarged. DeLisi et al. (*Arch. Gen. Psychiatry.* 43:148–153, February 1986) studied the lateral ventricles of schizophrenics as compared with normal controls in the same family and find that there is a familial tendency toward enlarged ventricles in schizophrenics. Is the situation beginning to make sense?

Kirch et al. (*Biol. Psychiatry* 20:1039–1046, 1985) studied the spinal fluid, albumin, and immunoglobulins of schizophrenics as compared with those of controls and found that there may be a defect in the blood-brain barrier in about 30% of those with this disorder and that the same percentage may have an elevated endogenous IgG production in cerebrospinal fluid.

It's too bad each of us has only one lifetime. If I were given two more I'd consider schizophrenia research from the clinical-pathological aspect.—Robert D. Currier, M.D.

Structural Abnormalities in the Frontal System in Schizophrenia: A Magnetic Resonance Imaging Study
Nancy Andreasen, Henry A. Nasrallah, Val Dunn, Stephen C. Olson, William M. Grove, James C. Ehrhardt, Jeffrey A. Coffman, and Judith H. W. Crossett (Univ of Iowa Hosps. and Clinics, and Ohio State Univ.)
Arch. Gen. Psychiatry 43:136–144, February 1986   4–4

The hypothesis that patients suffering from schizophrenia have structural abnormalities in the frontal system that can be observed with the use of magnetic resonance imaging (MRI) was investigated. These findings were examined within the context of an overall change in brain structure, as manifested by cerebral and cranial size.

Thirty-eight schizophrenics (mean age, 33.18 ± 8.6 years) and 49 normal controls (mean age, 27.65 ± 4.89 years) underwent MRI. The inversion recovery sequence with a 0.5 Tesla magnet gives a high degree of anatomic resolution.

Midline sagittal cuts indicated that the schizophrenics had significantly smaller frontal lobes, as well as smaller cerebrums and craniums. The findings are consistent with some type of early developmental abnormality that might retard brain growth and therefore skull growth. This could be due to such factors as genetics, maternal nutrition, maternal alcohol consumption, difficulties during delivery, or environmental factors (e.g., nutrition and infections) during the first year of life. As with the frontal findings, the cerebral and cranial findings appear to be relatively consistent and highly significant. It is not clear whether the decreased cerebral size is due to a relative decrease in frontal size or represents an overall atrophy or dysgenesis. A significant decrease in cranial area was noted on coronal section among the schizophrenic male patients, and there was also a trend toward decreased cerebral area. Decreased cerebral and cranial size are associated with prominent negative symptoms, although decreased frontal size is not. Decreased cranial and cerebral size was also associated with impairment on some cognitive tests. These data are consistent with the hypothesis that some schizophrenics may have a type of early developmental abnormality associated with prominent negative symptoms and cognitive impairment. Further, the results suggest that schizophrenics may have a type of structural frontal system impairment. Thus, they provide anatomic evidence for the "hypofrontality hypothesis."

Physiologic Dysfunction of Dorsolateral Prefrontal Cortex in Schizophrenia. I. Regional Cerebral Blood Flow Evidence
Daniel R. Weinberger, Karen Faith Berman, and Ronald F. Zec (Natl. Inst. of Mental Health)
Arch. Gen. Psychiatry 43:114–124, 126–134, February 1986   4–5

To evaluate dorsolateral prefronal cortex (DLPFC) physiology and function simultaneously, 20 medication-free patients with chronic schizophrenia and 25 normal controls underwent three separate xenon Xe 133 inhalation procedures for determination of regional cerebral blood flow (rCBF): first at rest, then while performing an automated version of the Wisconsin Card Sort (WCS), a DLPFC-specific cognitive test, and while performing a simple number-matching (NM) test. In rCBF topographic mapping, each blood flow procedure resulted in rCBF values for 32 cortical regions.

During rest, patients had significantly reduced relative, but not absolute, rCBF to DLPFC. During NM, no specific region differentiated patients from controls. During WCS, however, both absolute and relative rCBF to DLPFC significantly distinguished patients from controls. Controls showed a clear increase in DLPFC, whereas patients did not. The changes were regionally specific, involving only DLPFC. Also, in patients, DLPFC rCBF correlated positively with WCS cognitive performance, suggesting that the better DLPFC was able to function, the better patients could perform. Autonomic arousal measures, the pattern of WCS errors, and results of complementary studies suggest that the DLPFC finding is linked to regionally specific cognitive function and is not a nonspecific epiphenomenon.

Physiologic Dysfunction of Dorsolateral Prefrontal Cortex in Schizophrenia. II. Role of Neuroleptic Treatment, Attention, and Mental Effort
Karen Faith Berman, Ronald F. Zec, and Daniel R. Weinberger (Natl. Inst. of Mental Health)
Arch. Gen. Psychiatry 43:126–134, February 1986   4–6

Two xenon Xe 133 inhalation rCBF studies were conducted to clarify earlier findings of DLPFC dysfunction in mediation-free patients with chronic schizophrenia. In the first study, 24 neuroleptic-treated patients and 25 normal controls underwent three rCBF procedures, first while at rest, then during the WCS, which tests DLPFC cognitive function, and during a NM task that controlled for aspects of WCS-rCBF experience not specifically related to DLPFC. The results were qualitatively identical to those previously done for medication-free patients. In the second study, rCBF was estimated while 18 medication-free patients and 17 control subjects each performed two versions of a visual continuous performance task (CPT). No differences in DLPFC blood flow between the two groups were found during either CPT condition. These findings suggest that DLPFC dysfunction in schizophrenia is independent of medication status and not determined simply by such state factors as attention, mental effort, or severity of psychotic symptoms. Dysfunction of DLPFC appears to be a cognitively linked physiologic deficit in this illness.

It is concluded that the results of this two-part study, though preliminary, are consistent with the following three points: (1) The DLPFC, a cortical region selectively activated in normal individuals performing the WCS, is not activated in schizophrenic patients under similar circumstances. The degree to which patients successfully perform the test is linked to the degree of increase in metabolism in the DLPFC. (2) The findings do not appear to be epiphenomena of medication state, level of autonomic arousal, inattention, effort, or simply failing to perform well. (3) The DLPFC pathophysiologic changes appear to be linked to regionally specific cognitive function and may be an important neurobiologic aspect of schizophrenia.

▶ Psychiatrists, neuropsychiatrists, and neuropathologists (Alzheimer, Kraepelin, Bleuler, Greisinger, Cobb, etc.) have all researched for a structural basis for schizophrenia over the years; this is true also for mood disorders. Recent investigators have found neurochemical abnormalities and neurotransmitter alterations in the brains of patients with mental disease, but little in the nature of anatomic disorders. These two articles (Digests 4–5, 4–7) postulate the presence of cortical dysfunction in schizophrenia. The dysfunction is independent of medication status and is not influenced by such factors as tension, mental effort, or severity of psychotic symptoms. The dysfunction is a cognitively linked physiologic deficit. These studies suggest that schizophrenics have a type of structural frontal system impairment, and the authors provide anatomic evidence for what they term the *hypofrontality hypothesis.—*Russell N. DeJong, M.D.

Loss of Topographic Familiarity: an Environmental Agnosia

Theodor Landis, Jeffrey L. Cummings, D. Frank Benson, and E. Prather Palmer (Univ. Hosp., Zurich, Switzerland; West Los Angeles VA Med. Ctr.; Univ. of California at Los Angeles; and Lahey Clinic, Boston)
Arch. Neurol. 43:132–136, February 1986   4–7

In 1874, Hughlings Jackson discussed the "duality" of the cerebral hemispheres and suggested that a defect in the rear of the right hemisphere might impair the ability to find one's way about the environment. Sixteen cases of loss of environmental familiarity were reviewed. None of the patients was demented or acutely confused, or had evidence of amnesia, primary visual defect, or visual object agnosia.

Man, 61 years old, ambidextrous, awakened with a feeling of heat over the left side of the body and difficulty moving the left limbs. A complete left homonymous hemianopsia was noted, with mild left hemiparesis and hemisensory loss. Language and verbal memory were normal, but copy and delayed recall of the Rey-Osterrieth figure were impaired, and there was difficulty with maze learning and picture arrangement. The patient repeatedly got lost on the ward, and it never became familiar to him. Computed tomography showed changes consistent with infarction in the right temporo-occipital area and right lenticular nucleus. There was intermittent EEG slowing over the right posterior temporal area. The hemiparesis and hemisensory loss improved in the next months but environmental unfamiliarity and the hemianopsia were unchanged.

These patients are unable to recognize familiar environments despite seemingly normal general intellect and memory. A right posteromedial hemispheric lesion was a constant finding. Eleven patients had vascular occlusions in the distribution of the right posterior cerebral artery, with medial temporo-occipital infarction. The most frequent associated defects were prosopagnosia, impaired nonverbal learning, and constructional deficits.

Environmental unfamiliarity appears to represent an agnosia producing an impaired ability to integrate intact percepts with completely or partially preserved visuospatial memories. It is this ability that lends a sense of meaning and familiarity to a previously experienced environment. The deficit indicates a lesion in the medial temporo-occipital region of the right hemisphere.

▶ The patients described in this interesting article have an inability to recognize familiar surroundings despite relatively intact verbal memory, cognition, and perception. Radiologic studies reveal that all patients had a right medial, temporo-occipital lesion, and, in most cases, an infarction. These investigators express the belief that this syndrome is a specific variety of agnosia similar to prosopagnosia.—Russell N. DeJong, M.D.

A Contribution to the Anatomical Basis of Thalamic Amnesia

D. Y. von Cramon, N. Hebel, and U. Schuri (Max-Planck Inst. for Psychiatry, Munich, Federal Republic of Germany)
Brain 108:993–1008, 1985   4–8

Memory dysfunction that was caused by damage to diencephalic structures is described in 6 of the authors' patients and in 5 cases that have been reported in the literature. Computed tomography scans that were done in the chronic stage of the evolution of the stroke were used to delineate thalamic lesions.

Four of the present cases had chronic amnesia with no additional deficit. Two patients had no memory dysfunction but had some persistent neurologic deficits. In all 5 cases from the literature there was chronic memory dysfunction.

The overlap areas for most amnesic patients are shown in Figure 4–2. Involvement includes mainly the mamillothalamic tract (MTT) and the internal medullary lamina (IML). These areas are served by the polar artery and the paramedian thalamic arteries, which course primarily through

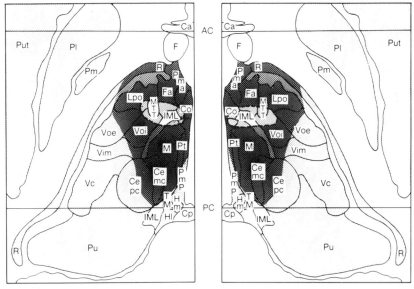

Fig 4–2.—The dark gray lesion area represents the vascular territory supplied by the polar and paramedian arteries. The overlap areas of the available infarctions of the patients with an amnesic syndrome are delineated by broken lines. Overlap area at the lower thalamic level (2.7 mm above AC-PC line) is shown in drawing. AC-PC interval is 25 mm. Ca, anterior commissure; Ce mc, N. centralis magnocellularis; Ce pc, N. centralis parvocellularis; Co, commissural nuclei; Cp, posterior commissure; F, fornix; Hl, N. habenularis laberalis; Hm, N. habenularis medialis; IML, internal medullary lamina; Fa, N. fascicularis; Lpo, N. lateropolaris; M, N. dorsomedialis; Pl, lateral pallidum; Pm, medial pallidum; Pma, N. paramedianus anterior; Pmp, N. paramedianus posterior; Pt, N. parataenialis; Pu, pulvinar; Put, putamen; R, reticular nuclei; TM, tract of Meynert; MTT, mamillothalamic tract; Vc, N. ventro-caudalis; Vim, N. ventro-oralis intermedius; Voe, N. ventro-oralis externus; Voi, N. ventro-oralis internus. (Courtesy of von Cramon, D.Y., et al.: Brain 108:993–1008, 1985.)

intrathalamic white matter. No significant differences in severity of learning deficits were seen between bilateral or left-sided thalamic lesions.

In most cases of diencephalic amnesia that are due to vascular lesions an infarction in the region of the thalamus that is supplied by the polar artery is responsible. Two patients with "pure" paramedian thalamic infarcts had no memory dysfunction. However, patients without adequate circulation of the polar artery may have significant irrigation by the paramedian thalamic arteries in the polar area; infarction in the paramedian thalamic arteries in these cases would lead to memory dysfunction.

The authors suggest that interruption of the Papez circuit in the MTT, combined with disruption of amygdalothalamic projections which traverse the IML, may be responsible for the "disconnection" syndrome of thalamic amnesia.

▶ This study narrows down the thalamic points necessarily involved for amnesia, namely, the mamillothalamic tract and the internal medullary lamina. The authors point out that the circulation of this region is from two separate arterial supplies. Involvement of two circuits, the Papez circuit in the MTT and the amygdalothalamic projections in the IML, may be necessary.

Duyckaerts et al. (*Ann. Neurol.* 18:314–319, 1985) have reported a curious case of a young man with Hodgkin's disease who had had a pure amnesic syndrome and who at autopsy showed a symmetrical neuronal loss without inflammatory changes bilaterally in the hippocampus and amygdaloid bodies.

Finally, Olesen and Jorgensen (*Acta Neurol. Scand.* 73:219–220, 1986) have postulated that transient global amnesia that so far does not fit well with either an epileptic or ischemic etiology may be an example of the spreading depression of Leao in the hippocampus triggered off by etiology.—Robert D. Currier, M.D.

Developmental Dyslexia: Four Consecutive Patients With Cortical Anomalies
Albert M. Galaburda, Gordon F. Sherman, Glenn D. Rosen, Francisco Aboitiz, and Norman Geschwind (Beth Israel Hosp. and Harvard Univ.)
Ann. Neurol. 18:222–233, August 1985   4–9

Neurologic abnormalities have been described in association with developmental dyslexia, but definite alterations in brain structure have been considered unlikely. Developmental anomalies of the cerebral cortex were found in consecutively examined brains of four male patients (14–32 years of age) for whom developmental dyslexia had been diagnosed. Personal and family histories revealed nonright-handedness and several autoimmune and atopic disorders.

Man, 20 years old, left-handed, had died in a fall. There was a history of speech delay until after age 3 years and of specific reading disability that was noticed shortly after school entrance. Reading and writing had never reached beyond the 4th grade level despite special education until age 18 years. Nocturnal seizures had

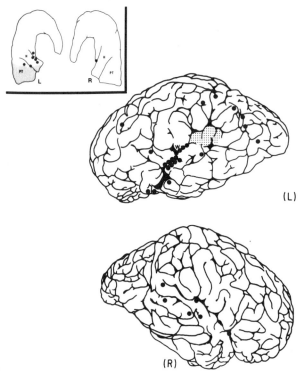

Fig 4–3.—Topography of ectopias and dysplasias *(closed circles),* brain wart *(w),* and micropolygyria *(stippled area)* in planum temporale *(inset)* and cortical convexities of left (L) and (R) hemispheres. Symmetry of plana and preponderance of anomalies in left hemisphere can be noted. PT, planum temporale; H, Heschl's gyrus. (Courtesy of Galaburda, A.M., et al.: Ann. Neurol. 18:222–233, August 1985.)

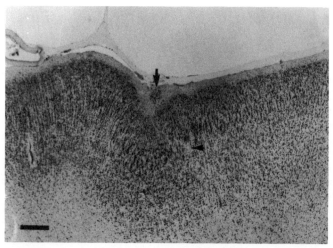

Fig 4–4.—Ectopia *(arrow)* and dysplasia *(arrowheads)* in the patient presented. *(Bar* = 500μ). (Courtesy of Galaburda, A.M., et al.: Ann. Neurol. 18:222–233, August 1985.)

developed at age 16 years, with a normal EEG. There was a family history of developmental dyslexia in several male members, as well as left-handedness and ambidexterity, rheumatoid arthritis, and migraine.

Anomalies predominated in the left hemisphere (Fig 4–3). Both architectonic dysplasias and neuronal ectopias were found in the cortex. The most severe form of dysplasia was micropolygyria in the region of the left planum temporale and posterior superior temporal gyrus. Ectopias were most frequent in layer I (Fig 4–4). Ectopic collections of neurons occasionally were seen in the white matter subjacent to the cortex.

Neuronal ectopias and architectonic dysplasias were chiefly in perisylvian regions of the left hemisphere in these cases. All the brains exhibited symmetry of the planum temporale, contrasting with the usual pattern of cerebral asymmetry. The same influences that lead to obvious defects of neuronal migration and asembly may also produce impairment of dendritic development in parts of the malformed cortex without obvious architectonic anomalies. Immune disorders may be directly involved in the production of cortical malformations. The male predominance of developmental dyslexia suggests that hormonal effects in utero may enhance the immune anomalies.

▶ This is probably an important contribution. The authors postulate that these cortical malformations may have an immune basis and that since they occur mainly in male patients, hormonal effects may also exert an influence.

Dyslexia of course is a defect that was unknown before the invention of the written word. If the inventors of writing had chosen color instead of forms for letters I, being color blind, would be dyslexic.

The necessary components for evolutionary survival in men may not include accurate color vision or accurate small form perception. They do now but obviously did not a million years ago. But they may be necessary in women.

Basso and Capitani (*J. Neurol. Neurosurg. Psychiatry* 48:407–412, May 1985) have reported the case of a conductor in Milan who from a stroke became aphasic and right hemiparetic but whose musical skills were essentially intact, evidently residing in the right hemisphere. Witelson *(Science* 229:665–668, Aug. 16, 1985) has remarked that the corpus callosum is larger in left-handed persons because the brain halves are more equal in such persons. There is thus a need for better communication between the hemispheres. Finally, Allen (*N. Engl. J. Med.* 313:642, Sept. 5, 1985) has described an interesting case of a woman with otosclerotic deafness who was receiving large doses of aspirin for her rheumatoid arthritis and almost constantly "heard" music from the 1930s and 1940s. The discontinuation of the treatment with the salicylate solved the problem.—Robert D. Currier, M.D.

Aphasia After Stroke: Natural History and Associated Deficits
Derick T. Wade, Richard Langton Hewer, Rachel M. David, and Pamela M. Enderby (Frenchay Hosp, Bristol, England)
J. Neurol. Neurosurg. Psychiatry 49:11–16, January 1986   4–10

Up to one fourth of acute stroke patients are aphasic shortly after the event, and up to a third of immediate survivors may have aphasia. It is likely that 10%–18% of survivors retain significant aphasia. The natural course of aphasia was studied in an unselected community sample of 976 patients with acute stroke, collected in a 28-month period. A total of 545 patients were evaluated within a week of stroke.

Twenty-four percent of patients assessed within a week of stroke were aphasic, and 28% were not evaluable. At 3 weeks, when more than 90% of surviving patients were studied, one fifth of them were aphasic. Twelve percent of 6-month surviving patients had significant aphasia, although 44% of patients and 57% of carers thought that speech was abnormal. Aphasia persisted at 6 months in 40% of initially aphasic patients, and in 60% of those aphasic at 3 weeks. Aphasia was associated with more marked disability and with less recovery of social activities. A majority of aphasic patients had right-sided weakness. Carers of aphasic patients were not depressed significantly more often than carers of nonaphasic patients.

Aphasia occurred in about one fourth of this unselected population of patients with acute stroke, but many made an early recovery. The severity of initial loss was the chief determinant of the extent of recovery. Social recovery was restricted by aphasia, but carers themselves were not particularly affected. The association of aphasia with functional disability may limit the number of patients who will tolerate intensive speech therapy.

▶ The authors run a very busy stroke service and have analyzed aphasia in a series of nearly 1,000 patients. Interestingly, they found that persons caring for aphasic patients were not more likely to be depressed than those caring for nonaphasic stroke patients.

Robinson et al. (*J. Nerv. Ment. Dis.* 173:221–226, April 1985) found that the poststroke depression may be of two types—the one immediately after onset, which relates to the nature and situation of the lesion, and the one developing later, which is a response to severity of the impairment.

Wade and Hewer (*Q. J. Med.* 56:601–608, September 1985) analyzed the importance of urinary incontinence to outcome and found that patients who were incontinent acutely after the stroke were more likely to die and more likely to be permanently disabled if they lived.

Wade has recently written an article for general practitioners (*Practitioner* 230:133–136, February 1986) on the care in the home of the patient with acute stroke. However, what is right for one area may not be right for another. I have no argument with home care for such a patient in Bristol, England, but in Mississippi we recommend that every patient with a recent stroke be admitted to the hospital for diagnosis and treatment. For some of our patients such an admission may be their first thorough medical evaluation.—Robert D. Currier, M.D.

Aphasia and Handedness in Relation to Hemispheric Side, Age at Injury and Severity of Cerebral Lesion During Childhood

Faraneh Vargha-Khadem, A. M. O'Gorman, and G. V. Watters (McGill Univ. and Mtl. Children's Hosp., Montreal, and Univ. of London)
Brain 108:677–696, September 1985   4–11

The "plasticity" of the immature brain allows for less serious sequelae of cerebral lesions than in adult life, and the most striking example is recovery of language function after early damage to the left cerebral hemisphere. The representation of auditory language comprehension and naming ability was studied in 6- to 17-year-old children with congenital and acquired left hemispheric lesions, and both age at injury and severity of the lesion were related to handedness. Twenty-eight children with left and 25 with right hemispheric lesions and 15 normal subjects were studied. Acquired lesions resulted from stroke, infantile hemiplegia, low-grade tumor, cyst, or trauma. Neuropsychologic testing was performed at least 2 years after injury.

Language deficits were characteristic of all groups of patients with left-sided cerebral injury. Impairment was more marked, as assessed by tests of auditory verbal comprehension and object naming, when left hemispheric injury was acquired after age 5 years. Prenatal and early postnatal left-sided cerebral lesions consistently resulted in strong sinistrality. Left hemispheric lesions were correlated with computed tomographic ratings of the severity of cerebral damage that were less abnormal. A positive correlation was found between ratings of motor and somatosensory function for the left and the right hemisphere groups and for both groups combined.

The neuronal substrate for specialization of the left hemisphere for language function is present at birth and exhibits clear laterality. Gross language function and intellectual ability are spared by prenatal and early postnatal injuries, regardless of severity. Either bilateral or right hemispheric mediation of language ensues or language function is reorganized within intact regions of the left hemisphere. Subtle language deficits may persist, however, even when left hemisphere injury is acquired in utero.

▶ It is interesting that laterality, according to these investigators, is programmed in at birth. If the left hemisphere is injured, speech may be represented in the right hemisphere, become bilaterally represented, or persist in uninjured areas of the left hemisphere.

There seems to be not much doubt that magnetic resonance imaging (MRI) is the study of choice in neurologically impaired children. Recent articles by Zimmerman and Bilaniuk (*Magnetic Resonance Imaging* 4:11–24, 1986) and Pennock et al. (*Magnetic Resonance Imaging* 4:1–9, 1986) argue that the benefits of MRI outweigh the difficulties in performing the study in children.— Robert D. Currier, M.D.

MRI and the Study of Aphasia

L. D. DeWitt, A. J. Grek, F. S. Buonanno, D. N. Levine, and J. P. Kistler (Massachusetts Gen. Hosp., Boston)
Neurology 35:861–865, June 1985   4–12

Magnetic resonance imaging (MRI) provides excellent gray-white matter discrimination and good lesion delineation and should be able to elucidate neurobehavioral and aphasic disorders. Saturation recovery, inversion recovery, and spin echo pulse sequences have been used.

Woman, 22 years old, left-handed in most activities, awoke with right-sided weakness and difficulty speaking. It was noted that repetition, oral reading, naming, and comprehension were moderately impaired. Fluency improved gradually, but the patient continued to grope for some words. Writing was slightly impaired, and slight oral apraxia was evident. A right hemiparesis was present. Computed tomography (CT) showed decreased attenuation in the left caudate, internal capsule, and lenticular nucleus. Magnetic resonance imaging showed a large area of decreased image intensity in the entire frontoinsulotemporal cortex and subjacent white matter (Fig 4–5). It extended medially to involve the basal ganglia and internal capsule.

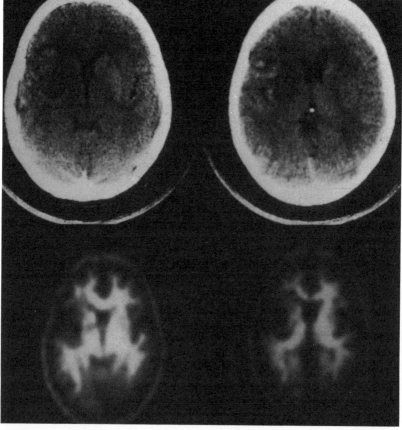

Fig 4–5.—Computed tomography scans (**top**) performed 24 hours after digital subtraction angiography clearly demonstrated a left subcortical midfrontal infarct, which is also seen on corresponding inversion recovery magnetic resonance images (**bottom**); latter, however, also show extensive involvement of the frontoinsulotemporal cortex. (TI = 400 msec, TR = 1 second, and data acquistion time = 39 minutes.) (Courtesy of DeWitt, L.D., et al.: Neurology 35:861–865, June 1985.)

Magnetic resonance imaging showed the extent of infarction in this patient better than did CT, as was also true in a patient with a middle cerebral artery infarct causing severe fluent aphasia. Inversion recovery images have been especially helpful. Magnetic resonance imaging is at least as sensitive in the detection of cerebral infarction as is CT. It is noninvasive and its three-dimensional imaging capability provides precise topographic relations of intracranial abnormalities. Coronal images aid in the visualization of the relation of a lesion to the opercular and perisylvian gyri. The three-dimensional capability of MRI also provides for volume measurements and estimation of how the volume of infarction influences the prognosis.

▶ Computed tomography may fail to show the extent of the cerebral lesions causing aphasia and neurobehavioral syndromes, whereas MRI may provide excellent gray-white matter discrimination and good lesion delineation, not only of subcortical areas, but also of the cortex as well.—Russell N. DeJong, M.D.

Spontaneous Recovery of Language in Patients With Aphasia Between 4 and 34 Weeks After Stroke

Wendy Lendrem and Nadina B. Lincoln (Nottingham Area Health Authority and Dept. of Health Care of the Elderly, Nottingham, England)
J. Neurol. Neurosurg. Psychiatry 48:743–748, August 1985   4–13

The course of speech recovery after stroke is an important aspect of rehabilitation. In a previous study, the language ability of aphasic stroke patients who received no speech therapy was shown to be comparable to that of such patients who received speech therapy twice weekly for 24

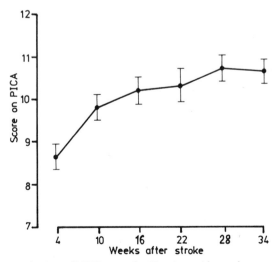

Fig 4–6.—Mean ± SEM overall PICA scores for 41 patients with complete assessments. (Courtesy of Lendrem, W., and Lincoln, N.B.: J. Neurol. Neurosurg. Psychiatry 48:743–748, August 1985.)

weeks from 10 weeks after stroke. Fifty-two of the stroke patients (mean age, 67 years; age range, 48–80 years) who received no speech therapy were evaluated in terms of spontaneous recovery. Wernicke, anomic, and Broca aphasias were most frequent. Assessments utilized the Porch Index of Communicative Ability (PICA), the Functional Communication Profile, and the Boston Diagnostic Aphasia Examination.

Improvement in language abilities over time was evident, independent of age, sex, and type of aphasia. Language ability 6 months after stroke was predictable from PICA scores at 4 weeks (Fig 4–6). The abilities of some patients, however, deteriorated, particularly at 22 to 34 weeks, and an increasing proportion deteriorated on PICA testing over time. The PICA gestural, graphic, and verbal scales all predicted final language level.

Most recovery of language ability occurs in the first 3 months after stroke, although some interpatient variation is observed. The amount of change that occurs appears to be relatively independent of age and sex. The level of language ability 6 months after stroke seems to depend chiefly on the severity of aphasia shortly after stroke. Speech assessment at 4 weeks is predictive of the level of function to be expected at 6 months. The PICA is a useful means of making this prediction.

▶ This paper describes spontaneous recovery of language abilities in stroke patients who were aphasic for more than four weeks after a cerebrovascular accident and received no supportive therapy. It was found that an aphasic patient's level of language ability at six months could be predicted on the basis of the test score on the Porch Index of Communicative Ability at four weeks. This brings up a question that has bothered investigators for as long as they have dealt with neurologic problems—how much does speech therapy actually contribute to recovery in aphasia?—Russell N. DeJong, M.D.

5 Cerebrovascular Disease

Various Consequences of Subcortical Stroke: Prospective Study of 16 Consecutive Cases
Davida Fromm, Audrey L. Holland, Carol S. Swindell, and Oscar M. Reinmuth (Western Psychiatric Inst. and Clinic and Univ. of Pittsburgh)
Arch. Neurol. 42:943–950, October 1985   5–1

Sixteen consecutive cases of subcortical stroke were assessed prospectively in the course of a larger study of language and cognitive recovery after stroke. The patients were observed from 1 to 3 days after the event until 2 months after discharge.

Considerable variation was found in cognitive, sensory, and motor symptoms. Only one patient, however, was asymptomatic at the outset. Three patients had only dysarthria. Linguistic and cognitive defects were most evident in patients with right-sided subcortical stroke, but the size of the lesion could not be closely related to these symptoms. Over time, impairments in oral and written language improved more rapidly than such cognitive deficits as confusion and inattention. Aphasia remained evident at discharge in half of the patients, but only one patient was aphasic on formal testing 2 months after discharge. Many patients, however, had such symptoms as deficits in reading and writing or they evidenced confusion.

Most language recovery in these patients occurred within a month after discharge. It may not be valid to compare behavior of patients immediately after ictus to that apparent some months later. Other problems in comparing observations arise from the probing of additional behaviors. The range of language and cognitive deficits associated with chiefly cortical lesions also can be observed after right- or left-sided subcortical stroke. Language deficits appear to recover more rapidly and more completely than do cognitive deficits in these cases.

Proposed mechanisms of the behavioral manifestations of subcortical stroke include compression of adjacent structures and/or widespread pressure effects; disordered corticosubcortical or reticulocortical connections; direct damage to deep structures; and general deterioration in neural function. Many of these mechanisms could interact to produce the observed effects of subcortical strokes.

▶ Since the introduction of computed tomography it has been possible to differentiate between strokes (cerebral hemorrhages and infarcts) that are limited to subcortical areas of the brain and those that are complicated by cortical extension. This study, part of a larger investigation of the true course of language and cognitive recovery from a stroke, shows that language skills recovered more rapidly and completely than did cognitive skills, especially during the first 6–8 weeks after onset.—Russell N. DeJong, M.D.

Arteriovenous Malformations of the Brain: Natural History in Unoperated Patients

P. M. Crawford, C. R. West, D. W. Chadwick, and M. D. M. Shaw (Liverpool)
J. Neurol. Neurosurg. Psychiatry 49:1–10, January 1986   5–2

The emphasis on surgical treatment for arteriovenous malformations has made it difficult to determine the natural history of the disorder. Before assessing the results of therapy, the natural history of the condition must be determined. In particular, the following questions need answers. (1) What is the risk of subsequent hemorrhage? (2) What is the likelihood of a late neurologic deficit developing? (3) What is the risk of de novo epilepsy developing? (4) What is the risk of death? (5) What factors influence these risks?

The authors report a retrospective survey of the natural history of 217 patients who did not undergo any form of surgery or irradiation from an unselected population of 343 (188 male and 155 female patients, aged 2 months–67 years) with arteriovenous malformations. The condition in over 59% of the patients was diagnosed before the age of 30 years. There was no difference in the rate of surgical treatment between the sexes (120 men and 97 women were managed conservatively). The mean follow-up was 10.4 years (range, 1–35 years). It is of interest that 1 in 4 women aged 20–29 years who had a hemorrhage were pregnant. In the third decade of life hemorrhage was commoner in women, a finding which suggests that pregnancy may increase the risk of hemorrhage. The majority of arteriovenous malformations were supratentorial (90%), the parietal lobe being the most frequently involved. The lobes of the brain involved in the arteriovenous malformation did not influence the mode of presentation. Twenty-four (7%) of the patients had aneurysms as well as an arteriovenous malformation. Five patients had multiple aneurysms, and in 18 (75%) the aneurysm was situated on the feeding blood vessel leading to the arteriovenous malformation. For patients presenting in the latter years of the study, those presenting with hemorrhage, were less likely to be managed conservatively. However, all patients with epilepsy who were diagnosed in the last 10 years of the study were managed conservatively. Although all the 217 patients were initially managed conservatively, 13 had surgical treatment at a later date: the arteriovenous malformations were excised in 9, 3 of whom postoperatively developed de novo epilepsy.

Life survival analyses revealed a 42% risk of hemorrhage, 29% risk of death, 18% risk of epilepsy, and 27% risk of a neurologic handicap by 20 years after diagnosis in patients not surgically treated. The risk of death in patients presenting with hemorrhage (Fig 5–1) was 32% by 20 years (18% at 10 years) compared with 28% (20% at 10 years) for patients who had never bled. Thus, the increased risk of rehemorrhage in patients

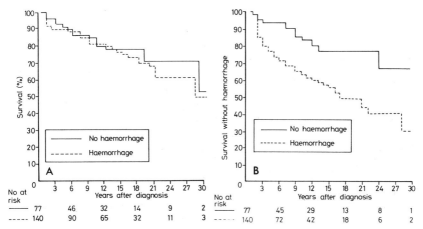

Fig 5–1.—A, risk of death from all causes in patients presenting with and without hemorrhage. B, risk of hemorrhage during follow-up in patients presenting with and without hemorrhage. (Courtesy of Crawford, P.M., et al.: J. Neurol. Neurosurg. Psychiatry 49:1–10, January 1986.)

presenting with initial hemorrhage does not reflect itself in an increased mortality over 20 years. The risk of death from all causes over the same period for other diagnostic symptoms was 21% for those with epilepsy (17% at 10 years), 27% for those in whom the arteriovenous malformation was a coincidental finding (27% at 10 years), and 22% among those with neurologic deficit (at 15 years). Patients with small lesions were more likely to present with hemorrhage as a major diagnostic symptom (82%). Neurologic disability may develop either as an immediate neurologic deficit resulting from an initial hemorrhage or as late progressive neurologic sequelae.

The natural history of patients suffering a hemorrhage from cerebral aneurysm is poor—it has been claimed that 60% will be dead at 2 months, and that 40% of those who survive the first 24 hours will also die within that time. In those surviving 6 months, the risk of rupture is 3%–4% per annum, with a mortality of 67%. The prognosis for patients with arteriovenous malformation is therefore much better.

▶ A 29% risk of death over a 10-year period is higher than I would have thought and indicates that those attempting various forms of treatment are probably doing the right thing. It is not a benign condition.—Robert D. Currier, M.D.

Volume Depletion and Natriuresis in Patients With a Ruptured Intracranial Aneurysm

E. F. M. Wijdicks, M. Vermeulen, J. A. ten Haaf, A. Hijdra, W. H. Bakker, and J. van Gijn (Univ. Hosp. Dijkzigt, Rotterdam; State Univ. of Utrecht; and Univ. Hosp. Amsterdam, the Netherlands)
Ann. Neurol. 18:211–216, August 1985

Hyponatremia is frequent in patients with aneurysmal subarachnoid bleeding. The roles of depletion and dilution were examined in a prospective study of 21 patients with subarachnoid hemorrhage who had computed tomographic evidence of blood in the basal cisterns. All were admitted within 48 hours of initial hemorrhage. Angiography showed an aneurysm in 18. Hyponatremia developed in 9 patients an average of 1 week after subarachnoid hemorrhage. The median serum sodium concentration in these patients was 131 mmole/L. The concentration became normal without treatment after an average of 4½ days.

Plasma volume fell by 10%–20% in 6 of the 9 patients with hyponatremia and in 5 of the 12 normonatremic patients. Eight hyponatremic patients initially had a negative sodium balance, as did 4 patients without hyponatremia. No patient was hyperglycemic. Arginine vasopressin concentrations were similar in patients with and those without hyponatremia. The clinical state of 10 patients deteriorated, 9 from rebleeding and 1 from cerebral infarction. In no patient was deterioration related to hyponatremia.

The findings in hyponatremic patients who have aneurysmal subarachnoid bleeding are consistent with a salt-wasting syndrome rather than inappropriate antidiuretic hormone secretion. Excessive loss of urinary sodium may result from inhibition of tubular sodium resorption with a concurrent loss of extracellular fluid, leading to a fall in plasma volume. Volume expansion is indicated in hyponatremic patients. When monitoring of salt balance shows negative sodium balance and volume depletion is present, hypertonic sodium solution or volume replacement seems to be warranted.

▶ It has always seemed strange to restrict fluids in a patient with a low level of serum sodium after an aneurysmal bleed. They always looked dry. Now we have some backing for giving them fluids and even some salt if the sodium balance is negative. Longstreth et al. (*Stroke* 16:377–385, May–June 1985), who reviewed the risk factors for subarachnoid hemorrhage, concluded that the only solid risk factor is hypertension—and the evidence even for that is not unambiguous. They recommended that risk factors such as oral contraceptives, cigarettes, and alcohol be studied further. Kikta et al. (*Stroke* 16:510–512, May–June 1985) described two patients with an intracranial hemorrhage, one of whom also had a subarachnoid hemorrhage secondary to the ingestion of diet pills containing phenypropanolamine. No one would argue with that as a risk factor.—Robert D. Currier, M.D.

Usefulness of Computed Tomography in Predicting Outcome After Aneurysmal Subarachnoid Hemorrhage: A Preliminary Report of the Cooperative Aneurysm Study
Harold P. Adams, Jr., Neal F. Kassell, and James C. Torner (Univ. of Iowa and Univ. of Virginia)
Neurology 35:1263–1267, September 1985   5–4

Computed tomography (CT) can be used to demonstrate subarachnoid blood and secondary intraventricular or intracerebral hemorrhage and also may show the aneurysm and complicating hydrocephalus. Its prognostic value was assessed in 1,778 patients seen with subarachnoid hemorrhage at 68 centers throughout the world. About half of the patients were alert when admitted, while 165 were comatose. Mortality was 11% in alert patients and 71% in those who were comatose. Mortality increased if orientation was impaired, and the quality of recovery declined.

Mortality after subarachnoid bleeding was higher in patients with CT evidence of blood. Both intraventricular and intracerebral bleeding had adverse effects on survival. Patients with localized, thick, or diffuse collections of subarachnoid blood had a worse outlook than those with a thin, localized clot. Hydrocephalus and a mass effect were other adverse findings. Mortality at 6 months was 2% for 124 alert patients without CT evidence of blood, 93% of whom made a good recovery. Mortality was 12% for 684 alert patients with intracranial blood, 73% of whom recovered well. Comatose patients with a thin, localized clot on CT scans had a better outcome than other comatose patients.

Computed tomography appears to be a useful adjunct to clinical evaluation in predicting the outcome after subarachnoid hemorrhage. The presence and amount of subarachnoid blood in an alert patient are predictive of an increased mortality risk. The outcome is related to hydrocephalus and, most important, to the presence of intraventricular hemorrhage.

▶ Computed tomography is useful as an adjunct to the clinical examination in predicting outcome after subarachnoid hemorrhage.—Russell N. DeJong, M.D.

Vertebrobasilar Insufficiency: A Review
James I. Ausman, Carl E. Shrontz, Jeffrey E. Pearce, Fernando G. Dias, and Jeffrey L. Crecelius (Henry Ford Hosp.)
Arch. Neurol. 42:803–808, August 1985   5–5

The limited value of anticoagulant therapy in patients with vertebrobasilar insufficiency (VBI) has prompted consideration of alternative approaches. Endarterectomy for intracranial vertebral artery stenosis was first reported in 1981. Percutaneous transluminal angioplasty has been used successfully to treat patients with vertebral-origin stenosis. It is uncertain why vertebrobasilar symptoms occur with proximal vertebral lesions when substantial distal collateral circulation in the vertebral artery seems to be present. Transient symptoms of VBI are difficult to understand on the basis of nonulcerated stenotic lesions unless changes in vertebrobasilar blood flow are involved. Emboli can lodge in the vertebrobasilar circulation, primarily at the basilar bifurcation. Vertebrobasilar flow may sometimes be compromised by proximal lesions amenable to surgery.

Transfemoral angiographic study of the vertebrobasilar system has been much safer than direct vertebral puncture or retrograde brachial studies. Much needs to be learned about the natural course of various vertebro-basilar lesions. Anticoagulant and antiplatelet measures have not been established to be effective. The entire vertebrobasilar system, however, is approachable surgically. Angiography including all the extracranial and intracranial circulation to the brain is warranted in patients with symptoms thought to be related to disease of the vertebrobasilar territory that are unexplained by other systemic causes. Longer follow-up is needed to eval-uate current surgical treatments for VBI.

▶ Neither medical nor surgical therapy has been found to be effective in pa-tients with vertebrobasilar artery insufficiency. The authors suggest "alternative methods of treatment" but really have no recommendations other than com-plete diagnostic investigations and thorough clinical observations of such pa-tients.—Russell N. DeJong, M.D.

Prognosis in Middle Cerebral Artery Occlusion
D. E. Moulin, R. Lo, J. Chiang, and H. J. M. Barnett (Univ. of Western On-tario, London)
Stroke 16:282–284, Mar.–Apr. 1985   5–6

The availability of extracranial to intracranial bypass surgery makes it necessary to know the natural course of middle cerebral artery (MCA) occlusion. Data were reviewed on 24 patients seen at a single unit with MCA trunk or branch occlusion between 1972 and 1982 who were fol-lowed up and did not have extracranial-intracranial bypass (mean age at presentation, 59 years). Seventeen patients had MCA trunk occlusions and 7 had branch occlusions. Five patients were seen with transient ischemic attacks and 19 with stroke. Eight stroke patients had major disability. Only 8 patients with stroke had had previous ischemic events. Two patients with branch occlusions were asymptomatic on the side of disease. Risk factors for vascular disease were prevalent.

Five of 11 patients with no substantial associated angiographic abnor-malities had evidence of cardioembolic disease. Eleven patients had sig-nificant ipsilateral proximal internal carotid disease, and 5 had significant contralateral proximal internal carotid involvement. Two patients had contralateral MCA stenosis. Five patients with MCA trunk occlusion died in the acute phase of stroke. The other patients were treated with anti-platelet agents and were followed up for a mean of 54 months. Two died of subsequent stroke, and 2 died of cardiac causes. Five other patients had further ischemic events. Nearly two thirds of patients surviving the initial ischemic event were completely functional.

Middle cerebral artery occlusion has a reasonably benign course with medical treatment only. Bypass surgery should be predicated on the pres-ence of potentially treatable disease at the origin of the ipsilateral internal carotid artery and in the heart and on the current state of the middle cerebral circulation.

► Occlusion of the middle cerebral artery does not necessarily carry a poor prognosis with medical treatment alone, and it is hoped that the role of bypass surgery in its treatment will be clarified by the results of an ongoing randomized clinical trial.—Russell N. DeJong, M.D.

Occipital Infarctions Associated With Hemiparesis

Tor Johansson (Södersjukhuset, Stockholm)
Eur. Neurol. 24:276–280, July–Aug. 1985   5–7

Occipital infarction sometimes may be associated with hemiparesis for reasons that are not clear. Data on 71 patients with computed tomographically (CT) confirmed infarction in the irrigation area of the posterior cerebral arteries were reviewed, along with 51 cases verified by radionuclide imaging. Twenty-two of the latter cases were normal on CT scans, but 8 of these CT studies were done within 24 hours of ictus. Twelve cases were abnormal on CT scans but normal on radionuclide imaging; 10 of these isotope studies were done within 10 days after ictus.

Sixteen of the 71 patients with unilateral occipital infarction confirmed by CT and 1 with CT-confirmed bilateral infarction had hemiparesis, without CT or radionuclide evidence of a lesion in the carotid territory. Symptoms of brain stem involvement were absent. Eight patients had permanent mild hemiparesis, 2 had a moderate motor deficit, and 2 had severe hemiparesis accompanied by hemisensory loss. Hemiparesis could not be related to the type of occipital infarction. Six patients had bilateral occipital infarction verified by CT. Nine of the 51 cases of occipital infarction that was verified by radionuclide imaging were associated with hemiparesis.

Hemiparesis in cases of occipital infarction may be explained by a simultaneous lesion in a small penetrating branch of the posterior cerebral artery. It has been reported that direct perforating branches and the terminal branches of the posterior cerebral artery often arise from the same part of the vessel.

► The author suggests that the cause of this mystery may be involvement of the perforating branches of the proximal posterior cerebral artery to the posterior portion of the internal capsule and thalamus. Since, as far as I know, there are no motor cells in the occipital cortex, the explanation seems likely. Speaking of unusual results of strokes, Price and Mesulam (*J. Nervous and Mental Disease* 173:610–614, 1985) have reminded us that infarctions of the right hemisphere, for some reason, are more likely to produce an acute psychotic state than are those of the left hemisphere. This observation is consistent with our experience and that of others. It took me a long time to accept the differences between hemispheres, and I suspect that it will take even longer for the notion that sanity or insanity is more likely to be lodged in one hemisphere to become acceptable.

Greenberg and Brown (*J. Nervous and Mental Disease* 173:434–436, 1985) have reported a case of mania resulting from a brain stem tumor that involved the right cerebral peduncle and the right thalamus and mentioned that lesions of the diencephalon had previously been reported as a cause of mania. They "favor the thesis that acquired mania is a nonspecific release phenomenon" related to the involvement of particular neurons running both ways in the brain stem.—Robert D. Currier, M.D.

The Clinical Manifestations of Pontine Hemorrhage
Michael J. Kushner and Susan B. Bressman (Univ. of Pennsylvania and Columbia Presbyterian Med. Ctr., New York)
Neurology 35:637–643, May 1985   5–8

The clinical spectrum of pontine hemorrhage is more varied than was previously thought. About 6% of all primary intraparenchymal bleeds involve the pons. Records of 27 patients who were seen between 1976 and 1981 with brain stem hemorrhage and no cerebellar involvement were reviewed. Ten had acute primary pontine hemorrhage (Fig 5–2).

Six patients had the classic picture of coma, quadriparesis, and death. Hemorrhages in these patients were centrally located and involved both sides of the midline. Four patients with a hemorrhage that was confined to either side of the midline had more benign courses. Hematoma involving the basis pontis and tegmentum was associated with hemiparesis, brain stem signs, and preservation of consciousness. Hemorrhage confined to the tegmentum was associated with gaze paresis, motor sparing, and preserved consciousness. Hemisensory loss and ipsilateral depression of facial sensation were consistent findings in the patients with unilateral hematoma. Three conscious patients had horizontal gaze paresis and sixth nerve palsy ipsilateral to the lesion. All 4 had ipsilateral seventh nerve palsy and dysarthria. All patients with hemipontine hemorrhage survived, whereas all those who were comatose died. Deficits resolved to a substantial degree in the survivors, and 2 of the 4 were independent in activities of daily living.

Early computed tomography can facilitate the diagnosis and manage-

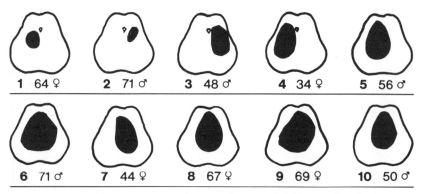

Fig 5–2.—Size and location on computed tomography scans of all 10 cases of pontine hematoma. (Courtesy of Kushner, M.J., and Bressman, S.B.: Neurology 35:637–643, May 1985.)

ment of pontine hemorrhage. Patients with brain stem stroke may be candidates for anticoagulation therapy, but not if fresh hemorrhage is present. Persons with preserved consciousness have a relatively favorable outlook and can benefit from vigorous supportive care. Impressive functional recovery has occurred in the patients in this study with unilateral pontine hematoma.

▶ Central intraponitive hemorrhage causes a picture of quadriparesis, coma, and death, but most patients with hemipantine hemorrhages survive. If there is no loss of consciousness at onset, there may be a significant degree of functional recovery in survivors.—Russell N. DeJong, M.D.

Occlusive Disease of the Middle Cerebral Artery
L. Caplan, V. Babikian, C. Helgason, D. B. Hier, D. DeWitt, D. Patel, and R. Stein (Michael Reese Hosp. and Univ. of Chicago, Massachusetts Gen. Hosp., and Harvard Univ.)
Neurology 35:975–982, July 1985   5–9

Twenty patients who had severe occlusive disease of the main middle cerebral artery (MCA) or its major branches were compared with 25 who had internal carotid artery disease. The MCA patients were younger and more often female and black. They had more evidence of previous coronary and peripheral vascular disease and more often had abnormal serum lipid concentrations. Transient ischemic attacks (TIAs) were much more frequent in the carotid group. All the patients with MCA disease had cerebral infarction, but 40% of the carotid group had TIAs only. Six patients had infarcts in the subcortical white matter or basal ganglia; five of these patients had MCA disease. Ten patients had wedge-shaped infarcts indicating occlusion of a major convex MCA branch. Six patients had border-zone infarcts.

Sixteen MCA patients were treated with anticoagulants, 2 of whom later underwent superior temporal-MCA bypass. Sixteen patients with carotid disease received antiplatelet agents, 7 received heparin or warfarin, and 11 underwent carotid endarterectomy. Three MCA patients had TIAs on follow-up for an average of 1 year, and 2 had new strokes because of disease of the contralateral MCA. One patient with carotid disease died of a massive contralateral cerebral infarct.

Patients with MCA occlusion in this study seldom had recurrent ischemia in the same vascular territory as their stroke. The incidence of subsequent cardiac death was low. The clinical, computed tomographic, and angiographic findings in patients with MCA disease are distinct from those in patients with carotid disease and lacunar infarcts.

▶ Occlusive disease of the middle cerebral artery usually affects the main stem of the artery or its superior division. Patients with middle cerebral artery disease seldom had recurrent ischemia in the same vascular territory as the stroke and had a low incidence of subsequent cardiac death.—Russell N. DeJong, M.D.

The Anterior Choroidal Artery Syndrome

J. P. Decroix, J. Cambier, and M. Masson (Hôpital Beaujon, Clichy, France)
Presse Med. 14:1085–1087, May 11, 1985   5–10

First described by Foix in 1925, this rare syndrome, when complete, includes hemiplegia, hemianesthesia, and homonymous lateral hemianopsia. Anatomical verification has shown an internal capsular lesion to be responsible for the hemiplegia in most instances. The sensory deficits are linked to involvement of the superior thalamic radiations situated in the thalamolenticular portion of the posterior limb of the internal capsule. The homonymous lateral hemianopsia may be the consequence of three different isolated or associated lesions, although frequently due to involvement of the optic radiations. Whereas hemiplegia is constant, incomplete forms of the syndrome have been described, without hemianopsia or sensory deficit.

Computerized tomography (CT) shows a low-density area suggesting an ischemic lesion located in the posterior limb of the internal capsule, sparing the thalamus medially but involving the tip of the pallidum externally (Fig 5–3) and corresponding to the territory of the anterior choroidal artery.

The syndrome may also be associated with neuropsychologic disorders, including left neglect syndrome in right-sided lesions and disorders of speech in left-sided lesions.

▶ This rare neurologic syndrome, which has puzzled physicians for many years, is shown by CT to be the result of an infarct affecting the anterior choroidal artery.—Russell N. DeJong, M.D.

Impact of Computed Tomography on Subdural Hematoma: A Population Study

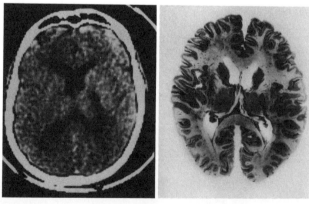

Fig 5–3.—Computerized tomography scans show the presence of a hypodensity in the posterior limb of the internal capsule, a territory attributed to the anterior choroidal artery. (Courtesy of Decroix, J.P., et al.: Presse Med. 14:1085–1087, May 11, 1985.)

Michael Garraway, Rolland Dickson, Jack Whisnant, and Teresa Turney
(Mayo Clinic)
JAMA 253:2378–2381, Apr. 26, 1985   5–11

The impact of computed tomography (CT) on the diagnosis, management, and outcome of subdural hematoma (SDH) was evaluated by reviewing records from the Mayo Clinic for Olmsted County, Minnesota, during 1965–1980. The 8 years before the introduction of CT in 1972 were compared with the subsequent 8 years.

The advent of CT did not alter the treatment, course, or prognosis of SDH, but it did markedly change the pattern of neurologic studies carried out. Nearly half of all cases of SDH were diagnosed within 2 days of presentation. The numbers of angiograms, echoencephalograms, and EEGs performed were all reduced. Angiography was performed in more than 60% of patients in 1969–1972 and in only 17% in 1977–1980. Computed tomography and angiography provided the highest levels of diagnostic confirmation, 86% and 87%, respectively. Only 2 noncontrast CT scans were normal in the presence of SDH. A 15% reduction in the cost of diagnosis of SDH was confirmed, at a time when the overall cost of health care in the United States increased by 87%. No differences in causes of death were apparent before and after the advent of CT. About half of survivors at all periods had residual neurologic deficits at 1 year.

Computed tomography has simplified the diagnosis of SDH and reduced its cost, helping to justify the introduction of this technology. It would be of interest to know the influence of CT on the costs of evaluating other neurologic disorders. Community-wide coverage of a new diagnostic procedure is desirable before attempts are made to assess its impact on the natural history of disease.

▶ The advent of CT has not altered the treatment of SDH or its course or prognosis. It has, however, reduced the time necessary for making the diagnosis, and has had a marked effect on the pattern of neurologic investigations used in the diagnosis of the disease. It has also resulted in marked reduction in the cost of confirming the diagnosis.—Russell N. DeJong, M.D.

Atheromatous Extracranial Carotid Arteries: CT Evaluation Correlated With Arteriography and Pathologic Examination

Mark D. Leeson, Edwin D. Cacayorin, Afif R. Iliya, Charles J. Hodge, Antonio Culebras, George H. Collins, and Stephen A. Kieffer (State Univ. of New York Upstate Med. Ctr., Syracuse)
Radiology 156:397–402, August 1985   5–12

Computed tomography (CT) demonstrates both the vessel lumen and its wall and might therefore be useful in the diagnosis of atheromatous extracranial carotid disease. Thin-section CT was used to study the common carotid bifurcation and the extracranial part of the internal carotid artery in 17 patients with a recent or remote cerebral ischemic episode involving the carotid territory and with angiographic evidence of extracranial carotid abnormality. Fifteen of the 13 men and 4 women aged 44–68 years had unilateral symptoms. Sixteen patients had conventional angiography and 1, intravenous digital subtraction angiography. Dynamic rapid-sequence CT of the neck was carried out.

Axial CT scans showed focal thickening of the wall of the distal common carotid and/or the proximal internal carotid artery in 19 vessels on the symptomatic side and 14 contralateral vessels. The degree of focal stenosis

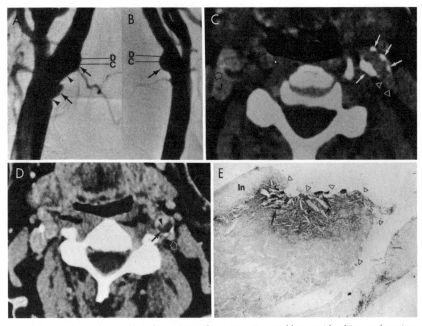

Fig 5–4.—Ulcerated, complex, atheromatous plaque in a 63-year-old man with a history of previous left hemispheric stroke who returned with a recent onset of decreased vision and ptosis on the left side. A, anteroposterior view from left common carotid arteriogram shows mild narrowing of the lateral margins of the distal common carotid and proximal internal carotid arteries *(arrowheads)*. Focal outpouchings of column of contrast material interpreted as ulceration within plaque can be seen *(arrows)*. Lines C and D indicate levels of CT scans illustrated in C and D, respectively. B, Lateral view from left common carotid arteriogram. The outpouching is more prominent on the posterior margin and appears more like diffuse bulge *(arrow)*. C, CT demonstrates posterolateral outpouching of opacified lumen at the bifurcation of the left common carotid artery consistent with large ulceration *(arrowheads)*. The adjacent calcifications of anterolateral and posteromedial walls of bifurcation can be noted *(closed arrows)*. The right common carotid artery shows a probable complex plaque posteriorly *(open arrow)*; J, internal jugular vein. D, CT scan at level 6 mm higher shows cephalad extension of the large ulceration *(open arrow)*. A large, markedly lucent posterolateral filling defect representing atheromatous plaque with associated calcification is seen *(closed arrow)*. Small ulceration extends into complex plaque *(arrowhead)*. E, cross-sectional photomicrograph of endarterectomy specimen from posterolateral wall of left internal carotid artery at a level corresponding to D. The plaque margin is composed primarily of proteinaceous precipitate with cholesterol clefts *(closed arrowheads)* and diffuse inflammatory cell infiltrates. Fibrin deposit and areas of old hemorrhage are present within plaque *(arrows)*. Open arrowheads indicate ulcerated intimal surface of plaque; in, intima. (Courtesy of Leeson M.D., et al.: Radiology 156:397–402, August 1985. Reproduced with permission of the Radiological Society of North America.)

correlated closely with the angiographic findings in 30 of 34 carotid arteries. In 4 instances, luminal narrowing was more marked on CT than on angiography. Ulceration (Fig 5–4) was evident in eight vessels on the symptomatic side and in one on the asymptomatic side. Dense calcification was somewhat more marked in areas of mural thickening on the symptomatic side. Reformatting of the CT scan data in paraxial or oblique planes yielded no further information. Marked lucency within plaques was associated with recent symptoms and with the presence of "complex" plaques. Isodense or slightly hypodense plaques represented intimal thickening and subintimal fibrosis.

Computed tomography has been useful in characterizing pathologic changes of the carotid arterial wall, although the therapeutic implications of a markedly lucent carotid plaque remain uncertain.

▶ Whereas arteriography provides information about the status of the lumens of arteries, CT demonstrates not only the lumens of the vessels but also their walls and the presence of pathologic changes such as ulcerations and atheromatous plaques. It offers accurate characterization of the extracranial carotid arteries in patients with symptoms of cerebral ischemia.—Russell N. DeJong, M.D.

Does Platelet Antiaggregant Therapy Lessen the Severity of Stroke?
James C. Grotta, Noreen A. Lemak, Howard Gary, William S. Fields, and Doralene Vital (Univ. of Texas, Houston)
Neurology 35:632–636, May 1985   5–13

Data from the Aspirin in Transient Ischemic Attack (AITIA) study, an ongoing study of two platelet antiaggregant drugs, and other reported trials were reviewed to determine whether patients with a history of transient ischemic attacks who subsequently have stroke have less disability if taking a platelet antiaggregant at the time of infarction. Patients in the AITIA study were randomized to receive 650 mg of aspirin twice daily or placebo. The ongoing study involves both aspirin and another active platelet antiaggregant.

Significantly fewer severe strokes occurred in patients in the AITIA study taking aspirin than in those taking placebo. Follow-ups were comparable in the two groups. No severe strokes have occurred in the ongoing study in patients taking either platelet antiaggregant. The Canadian Cooperative Study Group has failed to show a trend toward strokes of lesser severity in aspirin-treated patients. The Danish Cooperative Study indicated milder strokes in aspirin-treated patients but no reduction in the frequency of ischemic events.

It appears that if a patient is given platelet antiaggregant therapy and subsequently has a stroke, the stroke is less likely to be severe than if no treatment is given. Both the severity and the incidence of stroke should be considered in the evaluation of any platelet antiaggregant regimen. Platelet antiaggregant drugs seem to retard development of microemboli on atherosclerotic plaques or to impede formation of plaques themselves.

▶ Further studies to evaluate platelet antiaggregant therapy should include clinical assessment of the severity as well as the incidence of stroke.—Russell N. DeJong, M.D.

Anticoagulants and Cerebral Venous Thrombosis
J. P. Halpern, J. G. L. Morris, and G. L. Driscoll (Westmead Ctr., Australia)
Aust. N.Z. J. Med. 14:643–648, October 1985   5–14

Cerebral venous thrombosis (CVT) is an infrequent, often lethal disorder usually seen in later pregnancy or in the puerperium. The use of anticoagulants to prevent propagation of thrombus has been thought to be unwise because of the risk of cerebral hemorrhage. Experience with three cases suggests that anticoagulants can be used in certain circumstances.

Woman, 21 years old, had a seizure 3 weeks after section delivery. She had taken insulin for diabetes since the age of 6 years and thyroxine since Hashimoto's thyroiditis developed at age 13 years. Diabetic control had been difficult in the last trimester of pregnancy. The blood glucose concentration at admission was 3 mmole/L; the patient's husband, assuming that she was hypoglycemic, had given her honey. The patient did not obey commands and was incontinent. Computed tomography (CT) yielded normal findings, but carotid angiography showed features of sagittal sinus thrombosis (Fig 5–5). Frequent grand mal seizures continued despite anticonvulsant therapy, and irritability persisted. Intubation and althesin infusion were necessary. Marked improvement occurred on day 5. Warfarin and heparin were used, and the former was continued for 2 months.

Delayed oblique views and subtraction may be necessary to demonstrate occluded vessels in CVT. Computed tomography is probably more useful

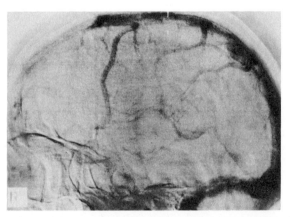

Fig 5–5.—Lateral view of the venous phase of the right carotid angiogram showing failure of filling of anterior portion of the superior sagittal sinus. (Courtesy of Halpern, J.P., et al.: Aust. N.Z. J. Med. 14:643–648, October 1985.)

in the guiding of treatment than in the confirmation of the diagnosis. Seizures can be controlled with anticonvulsants and the intracranial pressure with corticosteroids and mannitol. Anticoagulation may be considered if there is no clinical or CT evidence of cerebral hemorrhage or major infarction. Heparin therapy must be carefully monitored and preferably given as a continuous infusion until satisfactory oral anticoagulation is achieved. Antibiotic therapy is preferable to anticoagulation in cases of infective cerebral thrombophlebitis.

▶ It has always been unclear to me whether to treat presumed cerebral venous thrombosis with anticoagulants or not. These Australians have done it and suggest that it can be done safely if the CT scan shows no hemorrhage.

Wiebers (*Arch. Neurol.* 42:1106–1113, Nov. 1985) suggests that both arterial and venous occlusions are common during pregnancy, the former occurring during the second and third trimesters and the first week after delivery and the latter, one to four weeks after childbirth. He notes that "anticoagulant therapy with heparin for the (postpartum venous thrombosis) is controversial."—Robert D. Currier, M.D.

Digital Subtraction Angiography: Current Clinical Applications
David M. Pelz, Allan J. Fox, and Fernando Vinuela (Univ. of Western Ontario, London)
Stroke 16:528–536, May–June 1985   5–15

Intravenous digital subtraction angiography (DSA) carries less risk than conventional angiography and can be performed on an outpatient basis at reduced cost. The study is useful in the evaluation of patients for carotid artery disease in the neck, including postendarterectomy patients (Fig 5–6). The results compare favorably with those of conventional angiography in the detection of atherosclerotic disease at the carotid bifurcation. Decreased image sharpness and decreased spatial resolution are problems, and conventional angiography will retain a role in the evaluation of extracranial disease. Diagnostic intracranial images are obtained by intravenous DSA in up to two thirds of patients, but the quality is inferior to that of conventional angiography. The parasellar carotids can be assessed before transsphenoidal pituitary tumor operations. Venous sinus patency can be determined by DSA. The study may have a role in postoperative assessment of aneurysm clipping.

Arterial applications of DSA are becoming increasingly popular. Fine-contrast resolution by computer enhancement permits smaller volumes of dilute contrast to be used. Selective catheterization is often unnecessary. The study is completed more rapidly and is especially useful in older patients with tortuous vessels. Spatial resolution is adequate for nearly all clinical situations. There is a great saving in film cost. Arterial DSA has been highly useful in the rapid assessment of progress during interventions such as embolization. A portable digital unit allows intraoperative eval-

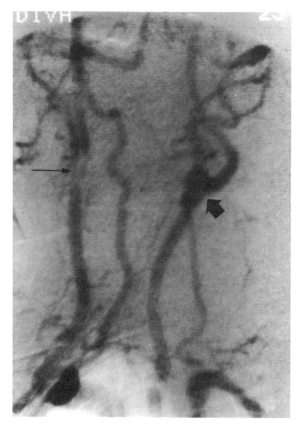

Fig 5–6.—Digital subtraction angiogram for a 63-year-old woman with a left carotid endarterectomy performed 3 months previously. Carotid bifurcation has normal postoperative appearance *(thick arrow)*. Severe stenosis of right carotid bifurcation on this oblique view can be noted *(thin arrow)*. (Courtesy of Pelz, D.M., et al.: Stroke 16:528–536, May—June 1985. By permission of the American Heart Association, Inc.)

uation of neurosurgical procedures. The need for postoperative angiography is eliminated in many instances.

▶ The future of DSA lies with intra-arterial contrast injections, since this technique substantially decreases the risks and costs of definitive cerebrovascular investigation. Intravenous DSA is still an accurate screening technique for extracranial carotid atherosclerosis, but intracranial imaging is less satisfying with intravenous injections.—Russell N. DeJong, M.D.

Persantine Aspirin Trial in Cerebral Ischemia. II. Endpoint Results
The American-Canadian Co-Operative Study Group
Stroke 16:406–415, May–June 1985   5–16

A cooperative trial was designed to determine whether patients with transient ischemic attacks (TIAs) have lower risks of stroke, retinal infarction, or death if taking both aspirin and dipyridamole (Persantine) rather than aspirin alone. A total of 890 subjects at 15 centers in the United States and Canada were randomized to receive 325 mg of aspirin plus either placebo or 75 mg of Persantine four times daily. All but 2% of subjects were followed up for at least 1 year (median follow-up, 25 months). The population consisted chiefly of white men (mean age, 64 years). More than half had had a single TIA before randomization.

Overall end point rates were nearly identical for the two treatment groups. Stroke end points clustered in the first month after randomization. No treatment differences were found in relation to age, sex, or history of previous TIAs. Comparable rates of myocardial infarction were found in the two groups at follow-up, and mortalities did not differ significantly.

These findings and those from the French study suggest that for TIA patients taking aspirin, the addition of Persantine is not significantly beneficial. Satisfactory compliance with assigned treatment was documented in this study. Neither stroke end points nor mortalities differed significantly between patients given aspirin only and those given aspirin with Persantine.

▶ This study shows that aspirin alone is just as effective as aspirin plus Persantine in the prophylaxis against transient ischemic attacks.—Russell N. DeJong, M.D.

Anticoagulant-Related Intracerebral Hemorrhage
Carlos S. Kase, R. Kent Robinson, Robert W. Stein, L. Dana DeWitt, Daniel B. Hier, Daryl L. Harp, J. Powell Williams, Louis R. Caplan, and J. P. Mohr (Univ. of South Alabama; Michael Reese Hosp., Chicago; Massachusetts Gen. Hosp., Boston; and Columbia-Presbyterian Med. Ctr., New York)
Neurology 35:943–948, July 1985   5–17

Intracranial bleeding is the most serious complication of anticoagulant therapy. Subdural, parenchymal, and subarachnoid bleeds are most frequent. Twenty-four cases of intracerebral hemorrhage (ICH) were encountered in a 6-year period at three centers in patients taking warfarin. The 13 men and 11 women had a median age of 62 years (age range, 23–90 years). Hypertension was present at admission in two thirds of the patients.

Fourteen patients had gradual progression of focal signs over several hours or days. The computed tomographic (CT) findings in 1 of these are shown in Figure 5–7. The most frequent sites of bleeding were the cerebellum, subcortical white matter, and basal ganglia. Nine patients had received anticoagulant therapy because of a previous infarct, but in only 1 did bleeding involve the previously affected area. Fourteen of the 23 evaluable bleeds occurred within 6 months of the start of oral anticoagulation therapy. In three fourths of cases the prothrombin time exceeded the "therapeutic" range. Eighteen cases of ICH were diagnosed by CT. Patients received vitamin K and fresh frozen plasma without effect on their

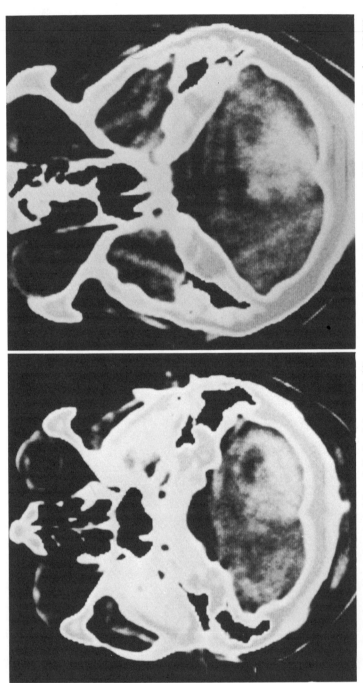

Fig 5–7.—Left, large hemorrhage in the left cerebellar hemisphere, with obliteration of the fourth ventricle. **Right,** extension of hemorrhage into the midline portions of the cerebellum. (Courtesy of Kase, C.S., et al.: Neurology 35:943–948, July 1985.)

neurologic status. Of 5 patients for whom surgical evacuation of cerebellar hematoma was attempted, 2 died and the rest were left with permanent disability. Overall mortality was 62.5%. Survivors generally had smaller hematomas.

Focal neurologic signs, even if slowly progressive, suggest possible ICH in a patient receiving oral anticoagulation therapy. Lack of systemic bleeding does not preclude the diagnosis in warfarin-treated patients. Close monitoring of the prothrombin time is necessary in the first year of anticoagulation; adherence to "conservative" levels of anticoagulation may minimize the risk of ICH.

▶ This carefully conducted study adequately emphasizes that intracranial bleeding is the most feared complication of anticoagulant therapy.—Russell N. DeJong, M.D.

Cardiovascular Regulation and Lesions of the Central Nervous System
William T. Talman (Univ. of Iowa)
Ann. Neurol. 18:1–12, July 1985   5–18

It is known that CNS disorders can influence cardiovascular function, and the role of central mechanisms in normal cardiovascular regulation is becoming increasingly apparent. The CNS can regulate arterial pressure, vasomotor tone, and cardiac output, rhythm, and metabolism through modulating excitatory and inhibitory influences on autonomic discharge. The CNS also indirectly affects the circulation through changes in fluid and electrolyte balance. The principal effector units of central cardiovascular regulation are the preganglionic sympathetic and parasympathetic neurons. These receive extensive connections from other central neurons, which themselves receive afferents from peripheral mechanoreceptors and chemoreceptors, and/or from other central nuclei.

Electrocardiographic evidence of myocardial damage accompanies CNS disease. A prolonged Q-T interval, S-T depression, flat or inverted T waves, and U waves are the most frequent findings and are associated with subarachnoid or intracerebral hemorrhage, ischemic cerebrovascular events, and head trauma. Experimental findings support a neurogenic origin for these changes. Catecholamines released with sympathetic stimulation or a central lesion may themselves be cardiotoxic. Arrhythmias associated with CNS disease also seem to be neurogenically mediated. Sudden death may be the result of a cardiac electric event rather than acute coronary occlusion, even if it occurs in the presence of coronary ischemia, and it might be triggered by the autonomic nervous system independent of intrinsic heart disease.

Lesions at any CNS site have the potential for producing an acute or fulminant rise in arterial blood pressure. Those at sites in the medulla and hypothalamus are most likely to have such an effect. Hypotension may also occur, especially with lesions of the rostral ventrolateral medulla or the fiber tracts from this region to the intermediolateral cell column of the spinal cord. Whether solitary CNS lesions can produce orthostatic hypotension is unclear.

▶ Chemical disturbances in the CNS that do not have associated structural lesions may be the cause of various cardiovascular disturbances such as hypertension, dyrhythmias, and even sudden death.—Russell N. DeJong, M.D.

The Causes of Stroke in the Young
David Hilton-Jones and Charles P. Warlow (Radcliffe Infirmary, Oxford, England)
J. Neurol. 232:137–143, July 1985   5–19

The causes of stroke were reviewed in a series of 75 patients younger than age 45 years seen between 1978 and 1982 with ischemic cerebral infarction (60 patients) or primary intracerebral hemorrhage (15). The age distribution is shown in Figure 5–8.

Thirteen patients had a history of trauma before stroke. The relationship with stroke was considered to be probable in 3 and possible in 10. Eight patients had a history of migraine, which for 7 of whom appeared to be the probable cause of stroke. Migrainous infarction was likely in 3 current users of oral contraceptives. Atheroma probably was responsible for stroke on angiographic grounds in 2 patients. One patient had a persistent, marked increase in blood cholesterol level. Two patients were known diabetics. Mitral leaflet problems were identified in 3 patients. Six patients in all were currently using combined oral contraceptive preparations. For 2 of the 8 patients in the series who were hypertensive, this was the only

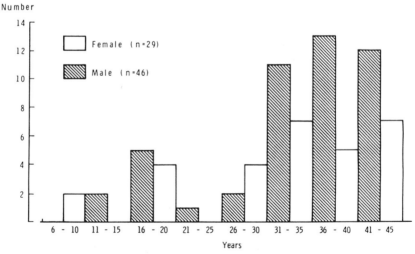

Fig 5–8.—Age distribution by sex of young stroke patients. (Courtesy of Hilton-Jones, D., and Warlow, C.P.: J. Neurol. 232:137–143, July 1985. Berlin-Heidelberg-New York: Springer.)

risk factor identified. One patient had primary thrombocythemia. One patient each had ulcerative colitis and vasculitis. No risk factors other than moderate unconfirmed lipid abnormalities were found in 23% of the patients in the series.

Trauma was the most frequent identifiable risk factor in this series of young adult stroke patients. At least one predisposing factor was identified in a majority of patients. Cerebral angiography is considered only if results of all studies including echocardiography are normal. Stroke in this setting is infrequently related to atherothrombosis and hypertension.

▶ Stroke in the younger age group (younger than 45 years) does not occur very frequently, but when it does is often due to identifiable and treatable disorders. Trauma and migraine are common predisposing factors and atheroma and hypertension, infrequent causes of stroke.—Russell N. DeJong, M.D.

Carotid Atherosclerosis in Familial Hypercholesterolemia
Alfredo Postiglione, Paolo Rubba, Biagio De Simone, Lidia Patti, Umberto Cicerano, and Mario Mancini (Univ. of Naples)
Stroke 16:658–661, July–Aug. 1985   5–20

Patients with familial hypercholesterolemia (FH) are at an increased risk for coronary heart disease, but little is known of extracoronary atherosclerosis in this disorder. The records of 15 patients of each sex with FH were reviewed. All had a plasma cholesterol level above 300 mg/dl and a low-density lipoprotein (LDL)-cholesterol level above 200 mg/dl, as well as tendon and cutaneous xanthomas or a pedigree with evidence of vertical transmission of hypercholesterolemia. The carotid vessels were assessed by a duplex device combining B-mode echography with pulsed Doppler ultrasound.

Fourteen patients (46%) had carotid lesions, but only 1 had a greater than 50% reduction in blood flow. Eight patients had more than 1 lesion. Both the severity and number of stenoses were related to age and to the level of hypercholesterolemia. Higher levels of LDL cholesterol and apolipoprotein B were associated with carotid lesions of greater severity. Levels of HDL cholesterol and plasma apolipoprotein A were highest in patients with normal findings on the echo-Doppler study. Marked hypercholesterolemia in patients younger than 32 years was associated with stenosis in 62% of carotid vessels.

Carotid atherosclerosis is a frequent finding in patients with FH. Noninvasive methods can be used to follow the course of atherosclerotic disease in these patients during lipid-lowering treatment. Carotid atherosclerosis in FH is related chiefly to patient age and the severity of hypercholesterolemia.

▶ These data indicate that the investigation of arterial districts other than those of the coronary arteries are useful in quantitative evaluation of atherosclerotic involvement.—Russell N. DeJong, M.D.

Delayed Cerebral Ischemia Following Arteriography

Mark Fisher, Rodney Sandler, and John M. Weiner (Univ. of Southern California)
Stroke 16:431–434, May–June 1985   5–21

Cerebral ischemia associated with arteriography in patients with occlusive cerebrovascular disease is usually ascribed to thrombus formation on the catheter tip or to dislodgment of plaque by the catheter. Other mechanisms may have been operative in 3 patients who had cerebral ischemic events starting 6–48 hours after arteriography. The possibility of sustained platelet activation was assessed in 8 patients who had angiography shortly after venipuncture (group I) and 8 who did not have angiography between samples (group II). Seven patients in each group had ischemic events within 2 weeks, and 1 in each group had a stable deficit. The platelet-specific protein β-thromboglobulin (BTG) was measured before and 24 hours after arteriography.

Seven of the 8 patients in group I had an increase in BTG concentration on the second day, compared with 2 of the 8 group II patients. The BTG increase on day 2 was significant in group I. Mean concentrations in group I were 19 ng/ml on day 1 and 22.5 ng/ml on day 2. No ecchymoses were seen at femoral puncture sites in group I. All but 2 of the patients had full heparin anticoagulation before and shortly after angiography or were taking aspirin. Patients taking neither medication had a mean increase in BTG concentration of 5 ng/ml.

Increased platelet activation is observed in some patients 24 hours after cerebral arteriography. Changes in BTG concentration could result from arterial thrombosis after femoral puncture or from platelet aggregation and thrombus formation on the catheter during arteriography. Contrast injection could also alter platelet function. Elevated BTG concentration might be a risk factor for stroke in patients with transient cerebral ischemia. Ischemic episodes occurring within 48 hours after arteriography may be considered possible complications of the procedure.

▶ There must be something wrong with arteriography in addition to the things that can happen immediately, such as the knocking off of plaques from the vessel wall, the obstruction of arteries with the catheter, osmotic changes, and blood-brain barrier problems. Whether the increase in BTG is significant remains to be seen.

Cerebral ischemic events associated with arteriography may occur on a delayed basis, and platelet activation manifested by increased BTG levels may contribute to this phenomenon.—Robert D. Currier, M.D., and Russell N. DeJong, M.D.

Subcortical Arteriosclerotic Encephalopathy (Binswanger's Disease): Computed Tomographic, Nuclear Magnetic Resonance, and Clinical Correlations

William R. Kinkel, Lawrence Jacobs, Ilydio Polachini, Vernice Bates, and Reid R. Heffner, Jr. (Millard Fillmore Hosp. and State Univ. of New York at Buffalo)

Arch. Neurol. 42:951–959, October 1985   5–22

By computed tomography (CT) study and nuclear magnetic resonance (NMR) imaging 23 elderly patients were found to have a consistent pattern of leukoencephalopathy. They represented 1.7% of all adults who had CT scans in a 5-month period. The leukoencephalopathy was idiopathic in all cases. Computed tomography showed areas of hypodensities of varying extent that symmetrically involved the periventricular white matter and centra semiovale, without contrast enhancement. In NMR imaging the involvement appeared dark on inversion recovery images and bright on spin-echo images. Ten patients had severe and 9 had moderate leukoencephalopathy.

The 15 women and 8 men in the series had a mean age of 72 years. Eight patients had no neurologic deficits. Five were hypertensive and 1 also had diabetes. The other 15 patients had dementia, motor deficits, urinary incontinence, or a combination of these abnormalities. Language function was normal in all but 2 severely demented patients. Seven patients presented with stroke that caused acute motor deficits. Five of them also were demented, and all were hypertensive. Five other patients presented with slowly evolving dementia, subacute motor deficits, and incontinence of 1–2 years' duration. All of them had severe leukoencephalopathy. Three patients had slowly progressive dementias of 1½–2 years' duration at presentation. The leukoencephalopathy generally was more severe in symptomatic patients than in those without neurologic signs.

This leukoencephalopathy appears to be a relatively common disorder that usually occurs in elderly persons. The term subcortical arteriosclerotic encephalopathy can be used to include asymptomatic patients whose condition is diagnosed from typical findings on CT scans and NMR images.

▶ There has been some controversy over the years as to whether so-called Binswanger's disease (subcortical arteriosclerotic encephalopathy), which probably occurs more frequently than has been recognized in the past, is an actual disease entity. It is not generally accepted as such. This article summarizes the variable symptoms and signs, as well as CT, NMR, and clinical correlations of this disease.—Russell N. DeJong, M.D.

Hemorrhagic Complications of Long-Term Anticoagulant Therapy for Ischemic Cerebral Vascular Disease

Mark Levine and Jack Hirsh (McMaster Univ. and Ontario Cancer Found. Hamilton Clinic)

Stroke 17:111–116, January–February 1986   5–23

The main complication of anticoagulant therapy is bleeding. Although the use of long-term oral anticoagulants in patients with transient cerebral ischemia and/or minor stroke is controversial, anticoagulants are still used in some instances.

The authors reviewed the literature on the risk of bleeding during long-term oral anticoagulant therapy in patients with cerebral vascular disease to determine the rate of bleeding and the clinical and laboratory risk factors that predispose patients to bleeding.

The risk of bleeding was substantial, with major bleeding episodes ranging from 2% to 22% per year and fatal hemorrhages from 2% to 9% per year. Only hypertension emerged as an identifiable risk factor, and its presence increased the relative risk of bleeding to more than twofold. Major bleeding was almost always intracranial, possibly because of associated hypertension or because of cerebrovascular disease per se. A relationship could not be detected between hemorrhage and the intensity of anticoagulant therapy, although major hemorrhage occurred frequently, even with only moderately intense anticoagulant therapy. The net gain or loss in the efficacy rate of treating patients suffering from minor stroke with long-term oral anticoagulant therapy was examined, and it was concluded that for such treatment to be beneficial, a risk reduction of more than 50% in stroke rate and a major hemorrhage rate of less than 2% per year are needed.

Since it is unlikely that the risk reduction of anticoagulant therapy in the prevention of stroke or death in patients with transient cerebral ischemia is 50% and is much more likely to be no greater than 20%–30%, the present evidence does not support the use of long-term anticoagulant therapy in patients with transient cerebral ischemia or minor strokes.

▶ Nothing is simple and controversy about the anticoagulant therapy for strokes goes on. It seems to me that we were hearing the same arguments 35 years ago. Regarding treatment of recent strokes with anticoagulants, Hornig et al. (*Stroke* 17:179–184, 1986) found with repeated CT scans and lumbar punctures that 28 of 65 patients with recent ischemic cerebral infarction had hemorrhagic transformation of the infarction. Almost all occurred in the first two weeks. Yet Ramirez-Lassepas et al. (*Arch. Neurol.* 43:386–390, 1986) found that of 150 consecutive stroke patients treated acutely with intravenous heparin, only 6 suffered a hemorrhagic complication. If 43% undergo hemorrhagic changes without anticoagulation therapy, why do only 4% get into trouble with bleeding when they receive anticoagulants?—Robert D. Currier, M.D.

Complications of Intravenous Digital Subtraction Angiography
James B. Ball, Jr., Robert R. Lukin, Thomas A. Tomsick and A. Alan Chambers (Univ. of Cincinnati)
Arch. Neurol. 42:969–972, October 1985   5–24

In a prospective study that was conducted from November 1982 to April 1983, complications were compared in 500 consecutive patients who had intravenous digital subtraction angiography (DSA) and 150 consecutive patients who had standard angiography for evaluation of extracranial carotid occlusive disease. The age ranges were 8–89 years for DSA and 32–83 years for standard angiography.

For DSA nearly all intravenous injections were made into an antecubital vein. Bolus injections of 35–45 ml of diatrizoate meglumine and diatrizoate sodium (Hypaque 75) were followed by 25 ml of 5% dextrose. The average number of injections was 3.4, and average amount of contrast used was 148 ml. More than 90% of conventional studies were done by the transfemoral route. An average of 65 ml of Conray 60 was administered.

Complications occurred in 16.6% of the patients who had intravenous DSA studies and in 7.3% of the patients who had standard angiography. Hives, itching, periorbital edema, nasal stuffiness, and sneezing were most frequent in the DSA group. Chest pain occurred in 23 (4.6%) of these patients and acute shortness of breath in 8. Two patients fainted without explanation. Hemiparesis progressed after DSA in 1 case, and 1 patient had transient monocular loss of vision. One patient with a treated seizure disorder had a generalized seizure during injection of contrast material.

Hematoma at the site of insertion of the catheter was the most frequent complication of standard angiography. Two patients had chest pain, and 1 developed pulmonary edema. Hemiparesis developed in 1 patient, who responded to emergency carotid endarterectomy.

Rapid injection of high volumes of hypertonic contrast medium can lead to hemodynamic and cardiac electrophysiologic complications in intravenous DSA. Only neurologic complications that are related to catheterization and formation of hematoma are more frequent with conventional angiography. Thus, DSA may be more risky than conventional angiography in patients who are in poor clinical condition.

▶ Extracranial carotid artery occlusive disease can be evaluated with either standard angiography or intravenous DSA. Serious systemic and neurologic complications occurred in a larger number of patients with the latter technique. The rapid injection of high volumes of hypertonic contrast media and the resultant hemodynamic and cardiac electrophysiologic changes occur with a higher incidence of complications with intravenous DSA.—Russell N. DeJong, M.D.

Cardiac Disease in Patients With Reversible Cerebral Ischemic Events
Morten Scheibel, Per Soelberg Sørensen, Jens Møgelvang, Holder Pedersen, and John Godtfredsen (Copenhagen County Hosps., Gentofte and Glostrup, Denmark)
Acta Med. Scand. 217:417–421, 1985   5–25

Cerebral ischemic events have been associated with mitral valve prolapse (MVP) in several studies, and it is possible that emboli arise from thrombi formation on the surface of the diseased valve in the cul-de-sac that is formed by the valve and atrial wall. Noninvasive studies were done in 45 consecutive patients younger than 60 years of age who had transient ischemic attacks (TIAs) or reversible ischemic neurologic deficits (RINDs) that resolved within 72 hours. Only patients with focal carotid symptoms or well-defined vertebrobasilar symptoms were included. The 33 men and 12 women had a median age of 53 years (range, 40–60 years).

Twenty-eight patients had TIAs and 17 had RINDs. The episodes were recurrent for 19 of the patients. Twenty-eight had carotid episodes and 17 had vertebrobasilar episodes. Seven patients had a history of acute myocardial infarction and 2 had angina. Abnormalities were present on ECGs in 12 patients. In 7 patients, including 1 with definite MVP, abnormalities were found at echocardiographic study. Two other patients had possible MVP. Results of aortocervical arteriography were normal in 4 patients with abnormal findings at cardiac study, including the one with MVP.

Mitral valve prolapse was not a frequent finding in these patients with cerebral ischemic events. A thorough cardiac examination nevertheless is indicated in all such patients, because finding a possibly embologenic cardiac disorder can lead to appropriate antithrombotic treatment.

▶ These investigators express the belief that all patients with transient cerebral ischemic attacks should undergo thorough cardiac evaluation, including, if possible, echocardiography.—Russell N. DeJong, M.D.

Delayed Cerebral Ischemia After Aneurysmal Subarachnoid Hemorrhage: Clinicoanatomic Correlations

A. Hijdra, J. Van Gijn, S. Stefanko, K. J. Van Dongen, M. Vermeulen, and H. Van Crevel (Univ. Hosp. "Dijkzigt," Rotterdam; Academisch Medisch Centrum, Amsterdam; and State Univ., Utrecht, The Netherlands)
Neurology 36:329–333, March 1986   5–26

Delayed cerebral ischemia (DCI) after the rupture of an intracranial aneurysm is an important cause of secondary deterioration. A group of 176 prospectively studied patients with aneurysmal subarachnoid hemorrhage were admitted within 72 hours of the first clinical symptoms and were in stable condition. In 130 patients, the offending aneurysm was demonstrated by angiography or autopsy. The study period was 28 days or less if the patients underwent surgery or died.

Delayed cerebral ischemia occurred in 57 patients (19 of 130 patients with angiography and 38 of 46 without angiography). Five of these patients had a second clinical episode in which a new infarct was confirmed by computed tomography (CT) or autopsy. Only 2 patients rebled before DCI developed, and 6 rebled after DCI developed. Clinical features included hemispheric focal signs (13 patients), decrease in level of consciousness (14), or both (30), and mutism (15). In all patients, CT was performed after clinical deterioration. In 1 patient, artifacts made diagnosis impossible. Nine patients never had abnormalities, including 6 who died soon after deterioration. In the other 47 patients, there were single, multiple, or diffuse hypodense areas in one hemisphere or both (Fig 5–9). Autopsy was performed in 18 patients with DCI; the interval between the appearance of ischemic signs and death was 1–3 days in 7 patients, 4–6 days in

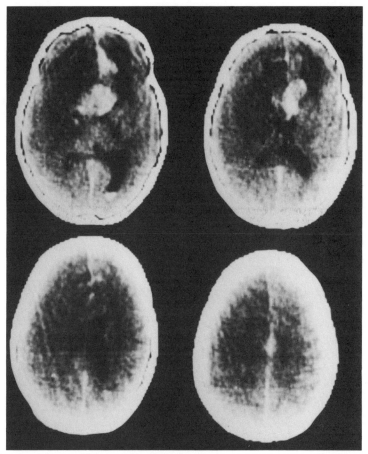

Fig 5–9.—A 52-year-old woman with an anterior communicating artery aneurysm became mute and developed a right hemiparesis 5 days after aneurysm rupture. The next day, CT showed diffuse decrease in attenuation of the left hemisphere with compression of the left lateral ventricle. She died the same day; at autopsy, vaguely demarcated ischemic neuronal changes were found in the left middle and distal left anterior cerebral artery territories, which were accompanied by extensive edema in both hemispheres. (Courtesy of Hijdra, A., et al.: Neurology 36:329–333, March 1986.)

3, and more than 6 days (8 days–6 months) in 8. Three patients had two separate episodes of DCI.

This clinical and pathologic picture differs from that of atherosclerotic brain infarcts. Although embolism and local thrombosis may play a role in some cases of DCI, the cerebral vessels remain patent in most patients. Some systemic factors might have contributed to the high incidence of multivascular and diffuse pathology in this series. Thirty-five (61%) of the 57 patients with and 53 (45%) of 119 without DCI were receiving antifibrinolytics. How antifibrinolytics contribute to cerebral ischemia is unknown. Since exposure of cerebral vessels to subarachnoid blood is an important factor in the pathogenesis of cerebral vasospasm, inhibition of lysis of cisternal blood clots might cause a higher incidence of vasospasm. Another explanation might be that, with impairment of flow in the microcirculation caused by vasospasm, the balance between fibrin formation and fibrinolysis changes in favor of fibrin formation when antifibrinolytics are given. The incidence of DCI increased in patients with hyponatremia, especially if they were treated with fluid restriction.

The clinical, CT, and pathologic features suggest that DCI after aneurysmal subarachnoid hemorrhage is a multivascular or diffuse process in most patients.

▶ The clinical as well as the CT and pathologic features of patients with delayed cerebral ischemia after aneurysmal subarachnoid hemorrhage are described. The findings suggest that such cerebral ischemia is a multivascular process in most patients. The authors express the belief that it is a diffuse brain disease leading to such nonlocalized features as lowering of consciousness, mutism, apathy, and confusion, and that these are signs of widespread brain dysfunction rather than of focal frontal lobe brain disease.—Russell N. DeJong, M.D.

6 Child Neurology

Safety of a Higher Loading Dose of Phenobarbital in the Term Newborn
Steven M. Donn, Thaddeus H. Grasela, and Gary W. Goldstein (Univ. of Michigan Med. Ctr.)
Pediatrics 75:1061–1064, June 1985   6–1

Some asphyxiated neonates continue to have seizures after a loading dose of phenobarbital. The safety of a higher loading dose of 30 mg/kg was examined in ten severely asphyxiated newborns with gestational ages of 37 weeks or more. Three infants had postasphyxial seizures; the others had a 5-minute Apgar score of 5 or less or required at least 1 minute of positive-pressure breathing for initiation of spontaneous breathing. The loading dose was given intravenously in 15 minutes and was followed by 2.5 mg/kg every 12 hours for maintenance.

There were no significant changes in cardiorespiratory variables after phenobarbital loading. Steadily increasing serum concentrations were found during the maintenance phase. Total clearance was lower than in previous studies, and the mean serum half-life of phenobarbital was longer. Of the three infants treated for seizures, one responded, whereas two required further treatment. All 3 had abnormal EEG findings after 1 week. None of the 7 infants treated for asphyxia developed clinical or EEG evidence of seizure activity.

Asphyxiated term neonates tolerate a loading dose of phenobarbital of 30 mg/kg given intravenously over 15 minutes without adverse short-term cardiorespiratory effects. A controlled trial is needed to determine the efficacy and long-term safety of phenobarbital in preventing seizures in asphyxiated infants.

▶ The conventional loading dose of phenobarbital for newborn infants with hypoxic-ischemic seizures often fails to control convulsive activity. These investigators have found that a higher loading dose is more effective and is not associated with adverse effects on cardiorespiratory function. This should be confirmed by other investigators.—Russell N. DeJong, M.D.

Alexander's Disease: A Disease of Astrocytes
Donald Borrett and Laurence E. Becker (Univ. of Toronto and Hosp. for Sick Children)
Brain 108:367–385, June 1985   6–2

The association of diffuse Rosenthal fiber formation with progressive neurologic deterioration in an infant with megalocephaly was first described in 1949. It has since been seen in various age groups with diverse symptoms; six cases were reported.

Boy, aged 14 months, had a grand mal seizure and, on evaluation 3 months later, was functioning at an 8- to 10-month developmental level and had generalized hypotonia. At age 2 years, he was able to walk if held and had better muscle tone, but marked deterioration ensued, with gross retardation and generalized hypotonia

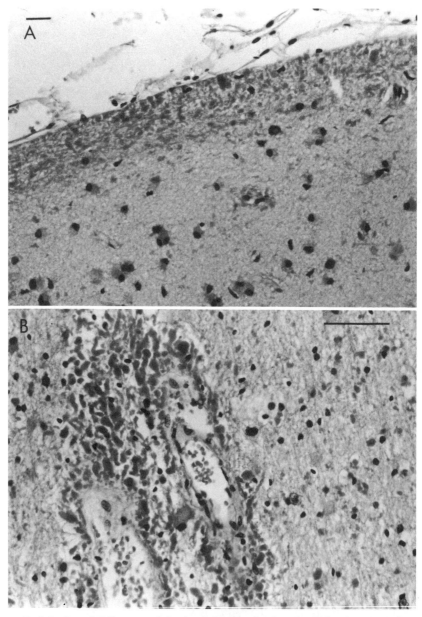

Fig 6–1.—Rosenthal fiber accumulation in subpial (A) and perivascular (B) locations. Bars indicate 100 μ luxol fast blue. (Courtesy of Borrett, D., and Becker, L.E.: Brain 108:367–385, June 1985.)

and hyperreflexia. Pneumoencephalography showed mild ventriculomegaly. The patient died at age 4 years of intercurrent infection.

The right frontal brain biopsy showed maximal Rosenthal fiber deposit in the subpial and perivascular regions (Fig 6–1) and reactive astrocytes in the gray and particularly the white matter. Moderate demyelination and axonal loss were seen. Autopsy showed an arachnoid cyst occupying the cerebellar vermis. Rosenthal fiber accumulation was also seen in the subependymal region. The white matter was more extensively involved than the cortex. Rosenthal fiber deposit was prominent in the brain stem and in the midbrain below the aqueduct. Involvement was maximal below the fourth ventricle in the pons and medulla. Both the gray and the white matter of the spinal cord were severely involved; demyelination was most marked in the anterior and lateral columns.

Alexander's disease occurs over a wide age range. Its pathologic hallmark is diffuse accumulation of Rosenthal fibers, especially in the subependymal, subpial, and perivascular regions. Demyelination is extensive in infantile cases, but neurons are relatively well preserved. The disorder is generally described as a leukodystrophy rather than as a primary, nonneoplastic disease of astrocytes, but accumulation of Rosenthal fibers is the most conspicuous abnormality.

▶ Although this disease is poorly understood, it appears to be a nonneoplastic disease of astrocytes. An accumulation of Rosenthal fibers is the most conspicuous pathologic abnormality. The disease is unique and the authors propose that its manifestations are related to astrocytic dysfunction.—Russell N. DeJong, M.D.

Subclinical Brain Swelling in Children During Treatment of Diabetic Ketoacidosis

Elliot J. Krane, Mark A. Rockoff, James K. Wallman, and Joseph I. Wolfsdorf (Children's Hosp. and Joslin Diabetes Ctr., Boston)
N. Engl. J. Med. 312:1147–1151, May 2, 1985   6–3

Fatal cerebral edema is an increasingly recognized complication of diabetic ketoacidosis in childhood. Its occurrence is sudden and unpredictable, but it takes place when the blood glucose concentration is falling and adequate circulation has been restored. Cranial computed tomography (CT) was performed during treatment of ketoacidosis in 6 boys to identify subclinical brain swelling. The children, aged 11–14 years, received standard fluid and low-dose insulin therapy. Normal saline or Ringer's lactate was given to correct clinical hypovolemia, followed by infusions of 0.45% saline. The goal was to replace half the fluid deficit in 8 hours and the rest in the next 16 hours, with current urine losses. Three patients were newly diagnosed diabetics.

Only one patient received sodium bicarbonate in initial resuscitation. The mean amount of crystalloid solution given before initial CT, performed 7–12 hours (mean, 9.8 hours) after the start of treatment, was 61 ml/kg. No patient had abnormal neurologic signs during treatment. No unusual

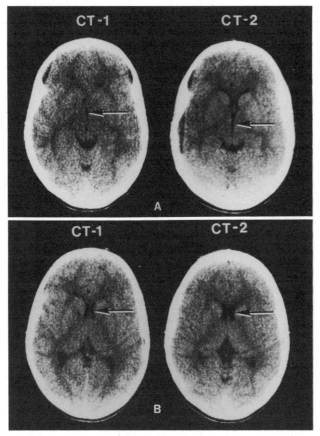

Fig 6–2.—Representative pairs of scans from one patient. Third ventricle (**A**, *arrows*) and lateral ventricles (**B**, *arrows*) are narrowed on earlier scans (*CT-1*). (Courtesy of Krane, E.J., et al.: N. Engl. J. Med. 312:1147–1151, May 2, 1985. Reprinted by permission of The New England Journal of Medicine.)

blood chemistry changes were found. Narrowing of the third and lateral ventricles was observed on initial CT, compared with repeat studies made after 3–6 days. The subarachnoid space appeared to be reduced. Representative findings are shown in Figure 6–2. The mean reductions in ventricular dimensions on early scans were 1.3 mm for the third ventricle and 3.7 mm for the intercaudate diameter of the lateral ventricles.

Mild brain swelling may be frequent in children treated for diabetic ketoacidosis. Cerebral edema and/or cerebral vasodilatation may explain the CT findings. If the changes are related to clinically significant cerebral edema, they might provide a means of evaluating modifications in current treatment.

▶ These data suggest that subclinical cerebral edema may be a common occurrence during the treatment of diabetic ketoacidosis in children. Computed tomographic scans of the brain may aid in diagnosing and preventing its development and in evaluating the results of therapy.—Russell N. DeJong, M.D.

Chloramphenicol Alone Versus Chloramphenicol Plus Penicillin for Bacterial Meningitis in Children
Frank Shann, Jane Barker, and Peter Poore (Goroka, Kundiawa, and Lae Hosps., Papua, New Guinea)
Lancet 2:681–683, Sept. 28, 1985   6–4

The use of penicillin in addition to chloramphenicol in treating childhood meningitis requires more staff time and cost and carries the risks of the overhydration and sepsis that are associated with intravenous fluid therapy. In a prospective multicenter trial the results of using combined intravenous antibiotic therapy were compared with those of giving only intramuscular chloramphenicol to children with findings in the cerebral spinal fluid (CSF) that were suggestive of bacterial meningitis.

A total of 367 children were admitted to the trial at three hospitals. The combined antibiotics were infused in dextrose-saline infusion. Chloramphenicol was given in a dose of 25 mg/kg every 6 hours, and benzylpenicillin was given in a weight-related dose at 3-hour intervals. Treatment continued for 2 weeks. Intramuscular injection of chloramphenicol was followed by oral treatment once clinical improvement began.

Sequential analysis of the results is shown in Figure 6–3. Mortality was 26% in 183 chloramphenicol-treated children and 27% in 184 who were given combined antibiotic therapy. Seventy percent of all patients were younger than age 1 year. The treatment groups were similar in age and sex distribution, presence of coma, and finding of bacteria on culture of the CSF. Surviving children were not more frequently permanently brain damaged if given chloramphenicol alone.

Intramuscular chloramphenicol therapy appears to be as effective as

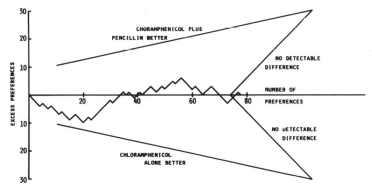

Fig 6–3.—Sequential analysis of effect of chloramphenicol alone vs. chloramphenicol plus penicillin. Repeated significance test plan: $2\alpha < 0.05$; $1-\beta > 0.95$; θ_1, 0.70, [9], 104. (Courtesy of Shann, F., et al.: Lancet 2:681–683, Sept. 28, 1985.)

intravenous chloramphenicol plus penicillin in treating children with bacterial meningitis. Intramuscular treatment for 2 or 3 days followed by oral treatment may be no more difficult than insertion of an intravenous cannula and restraint for several days. The intramuscular regimen is much less expensive, makes fewer demands on staff, and avoids complications of intravenous treatment.

▶ It's amazing how we accept dictums. What was this one based on, that chloramphenicol plus penicillin was better than either alone in treatment of bacterial meningitis? The authors note further that the intramuscular route seems to be just as effective as the intravenous. Congratulations to the authors for originating and carrying out this study.

Krober et al. (*AJDC* 139:889–892, Sept. 1985) very carefully studied the causes of fever in 182 consecutive sick infants in Honolulu. Only one had bacterial meningitis, 75 had a viral infection, and 27 a bacterial disease. Nonpolio enteral viruses were the most common pathogen and were isolated from 64 infants, 40 of whom had aseptic meningitis. Urinary tract infection was the most common bacterial infection.—Robert D. Currier, M.D.

Degenerative Neurologic Disease in Patients Formerly Treated With Human Growth Hormone
Committee on Growth Hormone Use of the Lawson Wilkins Pediatric Endocrine Society
J. Pediatr. 107:10–12, July 1985   6–5

Recent cases of Creutzfeldt-Jakob disease (CJD) have been reported in recipients of growth hormone (GH) prepared from human pituitary glands. Changes of a spongiform encephalopathy typical of CJD were confirmed in 2 patients; autopsy was not performed on a third. The precise nature of the infectious agent causing CJD is unknown. Iatrogenic transmission to humans has resulted from corneal transplantation and from the neurosurgical use of contaminated instruments. Oral transmission is also thought to take place. All 3 index patients received GH prepared before 1978, when relatively crude methods were used. Current methods are likely to exclude the CJD pathogen should it contaminate a pool of pituitary glands.

Up to 3 years will be required to test previous batches of pituitary GH to exclude contamination with the CJD pathogen. Growth hormone derived from pituitaries should not be given to previously untreated GH-deficient patients, and ongoing treatment should be discontinued. Deficient patients with hypoglycemia are treated on a compassionate need basis, but pituitary-derived GH should be avoided in patients not previously treated. Compassionate need protocols may be developed for GH-deficient patients with impending epiphyseal closure. Patients given pituitary GH in the past should be under long-term surveillance. Biosynthetic GH is effective in promoting growth, but it produces a higher incidence of GH antibodies than do pituitary GH preparations.

▶ This report is included in the Year Book to record its place in the literature for those who will need to refer to it over the next several years. The recommendations are quite specific, and if you have a patient who has received GHs derived from pituitary glands you would best have a copy of it available.— Robert D. Currier, M.D.

Management of Hydrocephalus in Infancy: Use of Acetazolamide and Furosemide to Avoid Cerebrospinal Fluid Shunts
Shlomo Shinnar, Karen Gammon, Eldo W. Bergman, Jr., Melvin Epstein, and John M. Freeman (Johns Hopkins Hosp., Baltimore)
J. Pediatr. 107:31–37, July 1985   6–6

Acetazolamide and furosemide can be used to reduce the rate of cerebrospinal fluid (CSF) production and prevent progressive ventricular enlargement in hydrocephalus. Such treatment was evaluated in 49 infants seen in 1977–1982 with progressive hydrocephalus who were candidates for CSF shunting. All were aged younger than 1 year and had a head circumference increasing substantially faster than normal for their age. The most frequent diagnoses were meylomeningocele and posthemorrhagic hydrocephalus. Acetazolamide was given in a maximal dose of 100 mg/kg daily, and furosemide in a dose of 1 or 3 mg/kg daily.

Shunts were avoided in at least 22 infants and in 57% of 30 infants having hydrocephalus not associated with spina bifida. Medication was started much later in life in patients who responded. The metabolic acidosis produced by the regimen used consistently necessitated prophylactic base therapy. No infant who responded has required hospitalization for problems related to hydrocephalus since the completion of medical therapy.

Medical treatment with acetazolamide and furosemide can be useful in infants with progressive hydrocephalus by reducing the rate of CSF production. Any infant with slowly progressive hydrocephalus can be treated, as can those with a transient insult who require only temporary treatment. The rate of increase in head circumference should be less than three times the upper limit for age in an infant older than 2 weeks old, and symptoms of acutely elevated intracranial pressure should be absent. Because medical treatment takes several days for its effect to be achieved, it is contraindicated for patients with symptoms of acute elevation of intracranial pressure or for those for whom the delay of a shunt by 1–2 weeks would be harmful.

▶ Intraventricular hemorrhage in the premature infant is often complicated by the development of hydrocephalus. A clinical problem is the management of hydrocephalus in small infants. The standard management has been the placement of a ventriculoperitoneal shunt. The authors point out the multiple complications associated with this procedure and present alternative medical therapy. The indications for this method of treatment, the complications, and diagnosis are discussed in detail.—Owen B. Evans, M.D.

Central Nervous System Hypoxia in Children Due to Near Drowning

Sarah J. Fitch, Barry Gerald, H. Lynn Magill, and Ina L. D. Tonkin (Univ. of Tennessee)

Radiology 156:647–650, September 1985   6–7

Cerebral computed tomography (CT) studies can be of help in evaluating children with acute, profound hypoxia. The CT findings were reviewed for nine boys and five girls who experienced acute, marked hypoxia of the CNS that was secondary to near drowning, aspiration, or respiratory arrest in a 3-year period. The 14 patients were aged 3 months to 7 years. Six were near-drowning victims, 4 had respiratory arrest after a seizure, and 4 had respiratory arrest from aspiration, epiglottitis, motor vehicle injury, or postoperative complications.

In the first 72 hours CT scans showed decreased gray-white matter differentiation, with effacement of sulci and cisterns by edema and decreased cortical attenuation. A hemorrhagic infarction of the basal ganglia was present in one of 3 patients who were studied after 4–6 days. Four studies that were done 7–13 days after the insult showed residual edema, and in 1 case there were bilateral putamenal infarctions. Ventriculomegaly and widened sulci and cisterns indicated global parenchymal loss at 14–28 days in 7 patients. Four had signs of hemorrhagic infarction at this time. Both patients who were followed up at 2–5 months had global parenchymal loss; 1 had leukoencephalomalacia. All EEGs showed background slowing that was consistent with encephalopathy.

Computed tomography is helpful in early detection of cerebral edema in children with marked acute hypoxia and also in subsequent determination of the extent of cerebral damage. The earlier findings indicate cerebral edema, whereas later studies show changes of cerebral infarction, and in surviving patients show the varying degrees of global parenchymal atrophy. These patients have a poor outlook. Half of the present patients died, and the survivors had severe neurologic deficits.

▶ The prognosis is very poor in children with hypoxia associated with near drowning. In a related article, S. B. Taylor et al. (*Radiology* 156:641–646, 1985) have stated that the prediction of the clinical outcome in these cases cannot be made on the basis of the initial CT findings alone.—Russell N. De-Jong, M.D.

7 Dementia

Progressive Dementia, Visual Deficits, Amyotrophy, and Microinfarcts
Jerry G. Kaplan, Robert Katzman, Dikran S. Horoupian, Paul A. Fuld, Richard Mayeux, and Arthur P. Hays (Albert Einstein College of Medicine and Columbia Presbyterian Med. Ctr., New York)
Neurology 35:789–796, June 1985   7–1

Brain biopsy in a patient with possible Jakob-Creutzfeldt disease showed multiple microscopic infarcts of the cerebral cortex.

Man, 46 years old, was admitted for brain and muscle biopsies after generalized atrophy and fasciculations were noted. At age 30 he had had a generalized seizure after several minutes of aphasia. An EEG then showed left temporal spikes, and seizures were subsequently controlled by phenytoin therapy. Memory loss and difficulty concentrating were progressing steadily at age 40, and computed tomography at age 45 showed a left frontal lucency and severe cortical atrophy. The patient had a history of acute rheumatic fever in childhood and systolic hypertension. Markedly impaired memory, language, and abstractions were evident. Weakness was confined to the arms and hands. Diffuse hyperreflexia was present. Muscle biopsy showed grouping of angulated fibers. Multifocal neuropsychologic dysfunction was documented; visually related skills and visuospatial reasoning were especially impaired, as was letter recognition. Insight and emotional reactivity were preserved better than higher cortical functions. Biopsy showed thickened and fibrotic leptomeningeal vessels containing organized thrombi; numerous microscopic infarcts in the cerebral cortex were also evident (Fig 7–1). The patient's condition deteriorated, and he died 6 years after the onset of dementia.

Innumerable stellate or wedge-shaped infarcts were present in the cerebral and cerebellar cortices at autopsy. Leptomeningeal arteries overlying the granular cortex showed fibrosis and partial recanalization. Bilateral pyramidal tract degeneration was present, and there was variable loss of motor neurons in the ventral horns of the spinal cord. The muscles showed severe neurogenic atrophy.

Review of data on three patients and of 22 previously reported cases, most of which were found in middle-aged men, suggested that cerebral microinfarction produces a recognizable clinical syndrome of stroke, followed by progressive dementia and, often, visual field defects, peripheral vascular disease, and signs of motor neuron dysfunction. Many patients have had valvular or ischemic heart disease. The role of cerebral emboli is unclear, but one of the three newly presented patients had mitral stenosis and embolic microinfarcts. No effective treatment of cerebral microinfarction is available.

▶ Data from this case and other previously reported cases suggest that cerebral microinfarction causes a recognizable clinical syndrome. The first symptom

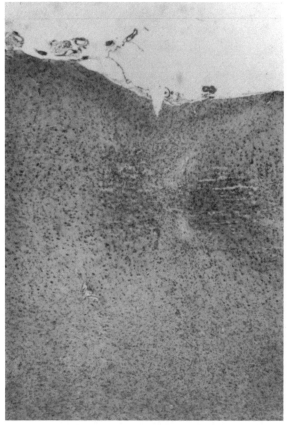

Fig 7–1.—Stellate infarct interrupting normal laminar pattern of cortex. Hematoxylin-eosin; original magnification × 10. (Courtesy of Kaplan, J.G., et al.: Neurology 35:789–796, June 1985.)

is a stroke, and this is folowed by progressive dementia, often associated with visual field defects, peripheral vascular disease, and symptoms of motor dysfunction.—Russell N. DeJong, M.D.

Survival in Alzheimer's Disease and Vascular Dementias

Laurie L. Barclay, Alexander Zemcov, John P. Blass, and Joseph Sansone (Cornell Univ. Med. Ctr., White Plains, N.Y.)
Neurology 35:834–840, June 1985   7–2

Longitudinal studies have suggested that life expectancy is increasing in both dementia of the Alzheimer type (DAT) and multi-infarct dementia (MID). Patients with mixed dementia (MIX) have features of both DAT and MID. A group of 199 patients with DAT were followed over 5 years,

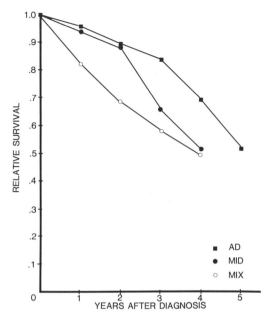

Fig 7–2.—Relative survival from initial evaluation. Relative survival rates were calculated for each group by dividing observed survival for group by survival of nondemented group matched for age, with survival rates taken from 1978 census data. The control group for DAT were aged 73 years, the control group for MID 76 years, and the control group for MIX 77 years. (Courtesy of Barclay, L.L., et al.: Neurology 35:834–840, June 1985.)

as were 69 with MID and 43 with MIX (mean follow-up, 22.6 months, 17.6 months, and 17.5 months, respectively.

Patients in all diagnostic groups had comparable rates of progression of behavioral and cognitive impairments. The need for home care or institutionalization at follow-up was also similar in the three groups. The 50% survival times from diagnosis were 3.4 years for DAT, 2.6 years for MID, and 2.5 years for MIX. Fifty percent survival times from the onset were 8.1, 6.7, and 6.2 years, respectively. Survival in DAT was consistently better than that in the vascular dementias, whether measured from the date of evaluation or from the estimated date of onset. The relative survival was lower in the vascular dementias when calculated by dividing the actual survival rate by the expected survival of age- and sex-matched white controls, using 1978 census data (Fig 7–2).

All of these forms of dementia clearly carry increased mortality, but despite comparable rates of behavioral progression, the vascular dementias are associated with higher mortality than is Alzheimer's dementia, presumably because of the associated morbidity from vascular disease.

▶ It is important to know that the duration of the dementia is longer and the mortality rate is lower in patients with DAT than in those with MID or the so-called mixed dementias.—Russell N. DeJong, M.D.

Decreased Cerebral Blood Flow Precedes Multi-Infarct Dementia, but Follows Senile Dementia of Alzheimer Type

Robert L. Rogers, John S. Meyer, Karl F. Mortel, Roderick K. Mahurin, and Brian W. Judd (VA Med. Ctr., Baylor College of Medicine, and Univ. of Houston, Houston)

Neurology 36:1–6, January 1986   7–3

Between 1940 and 1980, there has been an eightfold increase in the number of people over the age of 65 years and a similar increase in the number of patients with dementia. The two most common forms of dementia are senile dementia of the Alzheimer type (SDAT) and multi-infarct or vascular dementia (MID). The prevalence of dementia of all types has been estimated to be 5% in the United States at age 65, with an increase to around 20% at age 85. Senile dementia of the Alzheimer type accounts for about 50–60% of all cases of dementia that have been confirmed at autopsy, whereas MID accounts for about 18% of cases, and both forms may occur together. Cerebral blood flow (CBF) is lower in patients with SDAT and MID than in neurologically normal volunteers of a similar age. Several recent reports indicate that SDAT more symmetrically reduces CBF, whereas MID is associated with focal, patchy reductions.

Between 1976 and 1983, the authors prospectively followed two cohorts of 181 neurologically normal elderly volunteers aged 50–99 years, one cohort group of 93 subjects (mean age, 69.5 years) without risk factors for stroke and the other group of 88 subjects (mean age 72.1 years) with risk factors. The latter group included 30 individuals with hypertension, 3 with diabetes, 9 with hyperlipidemia, 5 with atherosclerotic heart disease, and 41 with a combination of these risk factors. Diagnosis of SDAT was made according to the following criteria: insidious onset of mental deterioration and memory impairment with a score of 23 or less on the Cognitive Capacity Screening Examination (CCSE), a score of 3 or less on Hachinski's Ischemic Index, loss of intellectual abilities, a score of 3, 4, or 5 on the Global Deterioration Scale; and exclusion of all other known causes of dementia. Diagnosis of MID was based on the following criteria: Hachinski's Ischemic Index score of 5 or more, a CCSE score of 23 or less, at least one identifiable low-density lesion on computed tomography or magnetic resonance imaging (MRI; compatible with ischemic infarction), and definite symptoms of bilateral focal neurologic abnormalities with stepwise progressive mental deterioration.

Results showed an incidence of 3.3%, or 0.47% new cases per year, for SDAT and 5.5%, or 0.78% new cases per year, for MID. The unusually high incidence of MID is considered to reflect preselection of a large percentage of volunteers (48.6%) with risk factors for, but without symptoms of, atherothrombotic stroke. Of the 88 subjects at risk of stroke, 11.4% developed MID within the 7-year period. In the MID patients, CBF values began to decline around 2 years before the onset of symptoms, whereas in the SDAT patients CBF levels remained normal until symptoms of dementia appeared; thereafter, CBF declined rapidly.

As in other studies, the present report revealed that hypertension was the most frequent risk factor among MID patients. In a previous study 87% of patients with MID secondary to subcortical atherosclerotic disease had hypertension. Another frequent risk factor that appeared predominantly among the present MID patients was heavy cigarette smoking, which has been linked to atherogenesis, risk of coronary heart disease, and reduced CBF. The normal age-related declines in CBF and metabolism after age 70 are significant risk factors, accelerating dementia from any cause, because both circulatory and neuronal metabolic reserves are progressively depleted.

▶ The message is quite clear in the title. It all makes sense. One wonders if the reason for the decreased perfusion prior to the onset of multi-infarct dementia is previous ischemia that is not obvious.

It may be that MRI may help to differentiate these two conditions, as Harrell et al. (*Neurology* 36 [Suppl. 1]:180, April 1986) reported at the recent American Academy of Neurology meeting in New Orleans: "this procedure should be employed on a routine basis in the evaluation of dementia."—Robert D. Currier, M.D.

Clinical Subtypes of Dementia of the Alzheimer Type

Helena Chang Chui, Evelyn Lee Teng, Victor W. Henderson, and Arthur C. Moy (Univ. of Southern California and Rancho Los Amigos Med. Ctr., Downey, Calif.)
Neurology 35:1544–1550, November 1985   7–4

It has been suggested that Alzheimer's disease represents several different biologic disorders, and age at onset has previously been used to distinguish between subtypes of dementia.

Other factors that may define clinical subtypes were studied in a series of 95 women and 51 men with Alzheimer's disease who were seen between November 1982 and May 1984 at university-affiliated clinics. The diagnosis was based on *Diagnostic and Statistical Manual of Mental Disorders* (DSM)-III criteria for primary degenerative dementia and the presence of symptoms for longer than 1 year. The mean age at onset of disease was 68 years, and the mean duration of symptoms was 4½ years.

The duration and severity of illness were significantly related. Forty-five percent of the total group had first-degree relatives with symptoms of dementia. Aphasia was present in 60% of the patients, and extrapyramidal signs were present in 44.5%. Earlier age at onset was related to greater disturbance in language. Relative familial risk could not be differentiated on the basis of age at onset of symptoms or aphasia. Both myoclonus and noniatrogenic extrapyramidal disorders were associated with more severe dementia, independent of the duration of illness.

These findings support the view that clinical subtypes of Alzheimer's disease exist, although cross-sectional studies may show large variations in expression of a degenerative disorder that do not necessarily reflect underlying biologic differences. Longitudinal follow-up is under way to confirm the findings and to seek distinct biologic and anatomical markers. A longitudinal study of patients with Alzheimer's disease has indicated that intellectual decline and impaired daily function are more marked in patients with myoclonus and extrapyramidal signs.

► Apparently there are clinical subtypes of Alzheimer's disease representing various aspects of the disease. This study shows that patients who have myoclonus and extrapyramidal signs have more severe dementia independent of the duration of the illness.—Russell N. DeJong, M.D.

The Concept of Subcortical and Cortical Dementia: Another Look
Peter J. Whitehouse (Johns Hopkins Univ.)
Ann. Neurol. 19:1–6, January 1986   7–5

Subcortical dementias such as Huntington's disease and Parkinson's disease are presumed to be characterized by slowed mentation and apathy, whereas symptoms such as aphasia, agnosia, and apraxia are thought to be more frequent in cortical dementias such as Alzheimer's disease. The distinction, however, is problematic because of vagueness of the terms used, difficulties in defining symptoms, and methodologic problems in currently available studies. Systematic controlled studies of subcortical dementias are rare, and there is little support for the validity of the specific defining features. Cognitive dysfunction in various disorders may change at different rates. Pathologic studies have shown both cortical and subcortical changes in most dementias. The dense interconnections between cortical and subcortical structures also diminishes the possible importance of the distinction.

A distinction between cortical and subcortical dementias remains to be established, but adequate comparative studies rejecting such a distinction also remain to be done. Positron emission tomography using drugs that bind to neurotransmitter receptors may improve the ability to define subtypes of dementia on the basis of neurotransmitter-specific dysfunction. Changes in neurotransmitter systems may reflect early pathophysiologic processes that could serve to categorize dementias. Such a classification also might permit predictions of responsiveness to various drug treatments. Cluster analysis could be used to determine whether different types of dementia can be discerned statistically. Autopsy programs will establish the diagnosis and show whether subtypes of dementia can be neuropathologically distinguished.

► In recent years, dementia has been classified as cortical dementia (Alzheimer's and Creutzfeldt-Jakob diseases, with aphasia, agnosia, apraxia, and other difficulties with language, perception, and praxis) and subcortical dementia (Huntington's, Parkinson's, and Wilson's diseases; progressive supranuclear palsy, normal-pressure hydrocephalus, and multi-infarct dementia, with slowness of intellectual function, apathy, and inertia [Albert, M. L., et al.: *J. Neurol. Neurosurg. Psychiatry* 37:121–130, 1974]). This author questions the validity of this classification on recent neuropathologic and neurochemical grounds and recommends further multidisciplinary studies that may contribute to the understanding of the causes of dementia and may help to develop new therapies for these disorders.—Russell N. DeJong, M.D.

General Comments

Chawluk et al. (*Ann. Neurol.* 19:68–74, January 1986) have commented on two patients with slowly progressive aphasia without generalized dementia for whom positron emission tomography scans showed clear-cut focal dysfunction of the dominant hemisphere. Magnetic resonance imaging and CT scans were normal, but arteriograms were not done. This disease remains something of a mystery.

Brun and Englund (*Ann. Neurol.* 19:253–272, March 1986) have reported a peculiar white matter degeneration associated with dementia, which, they say, is different from Binswanger's disease. One wonders, however, if they are giving us a very careful histologic analysis of a variant of that disorder.

On the subject of Alzheimer's disease, aluminosilicates have been in plaques found by workers in Newcastle with the use of energy-disbursive radiographic microanalysis. (*Lancet*, 1:354–356, Feb. 15, 1986). In a comment on this paper in *The Lancet* (1:681, Mar. 22, 1986) Yates and Mann of Manchester have pointed out that plaques tend to accumulate noxious substances rather than the noxious substances causing the plaques, but they agree that perhaps the substance in the plaque may "proceed to the neuron body and interrupt its metabolism." On the subject of silicates, some support for a causative effect has come from a recent report from Italy by Bianchi, et al. (*Ital. J. Neurol. Sci.* 7:145–151, February 1986), who found severe Alzheimer's lesions in the brain in ten patients with asbestosis-related malignant pleural mesothelioma. Five of the ten patients had "long-term psychiatric alterations." Typical clinical Alzheimer's disease may not have been present. Originally, I was quite dubious of the relationship between these substances and Alzheimer's disease, but this Italian report makes me wonder.—Robert D. Currier, M.D.

8 Epilepsy

Physiological Mechanisms of Focal Epileptogenesis
David A. Prince (Stanford Univ.)
Epilepsia 26(Suppl. 1):S3–S14, 1985   8–1

A key element in epileptogenesis appears to be the capacity of membranes in pacemaker neurons to develop intrinsic burst discharges. Events leading to intrinsic burst discharges in nonbursting neurons may make populations of cells more susceptible to epileptogenesis. Disinhibition is also a prominent factor, since postsynaptic inhibition is a powerful and widespread phenomenon in cortical structures, preventing synchronous epileptiform discharge. Excitatory synaptic circuitry is another critical element in epileptogenesis. Excitatory postsynaptic potentials trigger intrinsic membrane events in susceptible neurons. Propagation of impulses in excitatory synaptic circuits serves to synchronize the population by activation of excitatory postsynaptic potentials on groups of neurons. Synchronization of neuronal populations has been ascribed to a variety of mechanisms, including electronic coupling of neurons via gap junctions with low electric resistance.

Inhibitory interneurons may be more vulnerable to injury than are other neurons. For example, selective loss of glycinergic interneurons in the spinal cord is produced by hypoxic-ischemic injury. Acquired or inherited changes in intrinsic membrane properties may be associated with increased excitability under some circumstances. Additional excitatory synaptic contacts on cell somata may be present after injury when axonal sprouting provides new functional connections, and a marked increase in cell excitability could result. Impairment of the ability of glial cells to clear K^+ from the extracellular space could promote epileptogenesis. Accumulation of protons in some neurons decreases conductance of voltage-dependent K^+ channels and increases membrane excitability. Disorders of neurotransmitter metabolism might give rise to excessive amounts of excitatory modulators or to a reduction in inhibitory modulators.

▶ Different pathologic entities presumably produce epileptogenesis through different combinations of pathogenetic mechanisms.—Russell N. DeJong, M.D.

Focal Epilepsy in Diabetic Non-ketotic Hyperglycemia
Clare Grant and Charles Warlow (John Radcliffe Hosp., Oxford, England)
Br. Med. J. 290:1204–1205, Apr. 20, 1985   8–2

Hyperglycemia may be present without ketosis for some time before noninsulin-dependent diabetes is recognized. Five patients so affected, 4 not previously known to be diabetic, were seen with focal epilepsy resistant to anticonvulsants and were found on investigation to be hyperglycemic. No other cause of seizures was found, and treatment of diabetes with insulin or sulfonylurea drugs abolished them. No patient was ketotic. Most such patients are elderly and have mild noninsulin-dependent diabetes. They tend to have chronic disease and to be taking drugs, especially steroids and diuretics. For some patients, focal epilepsy may be the first indication of diabetes. Seizures are frequent and repeated and often leave a transient postictal paralysis. Hyperglycemia is generally not marked. Hyperosmolarity and impaired consciousness develop if the diabetes is untreated, and the seizures stop. Seizures are not seen as long as the diabetes is controlled.

Nonketotic hyperglycemia may be characterized by focal neurologic impairment, myoclonic twitching, nystagmus, or meningeal signs, as well as seizures. Experiments suggest that hypertonic solutions activate existing seizure foci, but most of the patients in this study had seizures when hyperglycemia was moderate, and the plasma osmolarity was normal or only slightly elevated. It has also been suggested that ketosis has an anticonvulsant effect. Focal epilepsy in an elderly patient with noninsulin-dependent diabetes may herald hyperosmolar coma and calls for control of diabetes. Anticonvulsants are ineffective, and phenytoin may aggravate hyperglycemia. The occurrence of frequent focal seizures with no apparent cause should suggest the possibility of diabetes.

▶ Focal convulsions that respond only to treatment of the diabetes and not to antiepileptic drugs may occur in diabetic patients with non-ketotic hyperglycemia.—Russell N. DeJong, M.D.

Incidence of Seizures With Tricyclic and Tetracyclic Antidepressants
Bahman Jabbari, George E. Bryan, Ellis E. Marsh, and Carl H. Gunderson (Uniformed Services Univ. of the Health Sciences, Bethesda, Md., and Walter Reed Army Med. Center, Washington, D.C.)
Arch. Neurol. 42:480–481, May 1985   8–3

Antidepressants have exhibited epileptogenic potential in animal studies, but the incidence of seizures in treated patients is unknown. Seizures were analyzed in 186 depressed psychiatric inpatients seen in 1982. Forty-five patients received tricyclic antidepressants, while 32 received maprotiline hydrochloride, a tetracyclic compound, and 20 received other medications. Eighty-nine patients received no drug treatment.

Five patients (15.6%) given maprotiline had generalized tonic-clonic seizures, as did 1 patient given tricyclics (2.2%). One of the maprotiline-treated patients may also have had two complex partial seizures. The affected patients had no history of seizures. Doses of maprotiline ranged from 75 to 300 mg. Four patients had their first seizure within 3 weeks after the start of maprotiline therapy. In all cases the seizure followed an increase in dosage by 6 days or less. All patients with seizures had normal neurologic, cerebral spinal fluid, and computed tomographic findings. An EEG obtained 2 days after a seizure showed diffuse spike-and-wave bursts; a follow-up study 3 months later was normal.

The tetracyclic antidepressant maprotiline may precipitate seizures in depressed patients, as it did in this series for about 16% of the patients. The epileptogenic potential of maprotiline may result from its strong lipophilic activity, high brain concentration, or selective blockade of norepinephrine re-uptake with little or no effect on serotonin metabolism.

▶ These studies show that tetracyclic antidepressants have an even higher epileptogenic potential than tricyclic antidepressants.—Russell N. DeJong, M.D.

Alcoholism and Epilepsy

Arthur W. K. Chan (Research Inst. on Alcoholism, Buffalo)
Epilepsia 26:323–333, July–Aug. 1985   8–4

Available data suggest that epilepsy is at least three times more prevalent among alcoholics than in the general population, and that alcoholism may be more prevalent among epileptic patients. There are conflicting reports on whether or not alcohol can directly provoke epileptic seizures other than alcohol withdrawal seizures. Alcohol abuse, compared with the intake of small amounts, does seem to increase the frequency of seizures in epileptic patients. Sleep deprivation may be a factor in triggering of seizures by alcohol intake. Persons who abuse alcohol tend to comply poorly with medication. Alcohol effects on serum anticonvulsant drug concentrations may be a factor. Metabolic effects of alcohol such as hypoglycemia, altered acid-base balance, electrolyte changes, hydration or dehydration, and vitamin deficiency may influence seizure control.

More detailed population-based epidemiologic studies are needed to ascertain the frequencies of epilepsy among alcoholics and of alcoholism among epileptics. Although moderate alcohol use may not increase the frequency of seizures in nonalcoholic epileptics, it probably is wise to caution patients about the possible adverse effects of drinking, particularly those with refractory forms of epilepsy. The evidence that alcohol can directly provoke seizures in those with no epileptic disposition is not strong. Patients with both alcoholism and epilepsy should be followed closely, particularly for status epilepticus. Most believe that anticonvulsants should not be prescribed for alcoholics who have seizures only during alcohol withdrawal.

▶ This is an excellent discussion of the relationship between alcoholism and epilepsy.—Russell N. DeJong, M.D.

The Risk of Seizure Disorders Among Relatives of Children With Febrile Convulsions

W. Allen Hauser, John F. Annegers, V. Elving Anderson, and Leonard T. Kurland (Columbia Univ., Univ. of Texas at Houston, Univ. of Minnesota, and Mayo Clinic)
Neurology 35:1268–1273, September 1985   8–5

Febrile convulsions (FC) are known to aggregate in families, but reports vary as to the risks to different classes of relatives. The extent of familial aggregation was studied in a series of 421 children who were residing in Rochester, Minn., between 1935 and 1964 when their first FC occurred. The mean age at initial FC was 1.3 years. A total of 1,046 siblings of the probands were followed up for 19,962 person-years. The probands also had 103 half-siblings, 178 children, 474 nieces and nephews, and 9 grand-children.

Febrile convulsions occurred in 84 (8%) of sibings of the FC probands. The relative risk of FC in siblings was 3.7. The risk for children of probands was 4.4, and for nieces or nephews, 2.7. Risk estimates were not significantly influenced by the proband's sex. The convulsions were known to have occurred in parents of 51 probands, and parental involvement was associated with a higher relative risk in siblings. The risk for FC in siblings increased with the number of FCs in probands and also with the presence of complex seizure patterns in probands. The relative risks of both FC and unprovoked seizures in siblings increased when afebrile seizures followed the first febrile seizure in the proband.

This study confirmed an increased risk of both FC and epilepsy in siblings of children with FC. The increase in risk for unprovoked seizures does not extend to nieces and nephews or to offspring of probands.

▶ The risk for both FC and epilepsy is greater in siblings of children with FC than it is in other family members.—Russell N. DeJong, M.D.

Comparison of Carbamazepine, Phenobarbital, Phenytoin, and Primidone in Partial and Secondarily Generalized Tonic-Clonic Seizures

Richard H. Mattson, Joyce A. Cramer, Joseph F. Collins, Dennis B. Smith, Antonio V. Delgado-Escueta, Thomas R. Browne, Peter D. Williamson, David M. Treiman, James O. McNamara, Charlotte B. McCutchen, Richard W. Homan, Wayne E. Crill, Michael F. Lubozynski, N. Paul Rosenthal, and Assa Mayersdorf (VA Med. Ctrs., VA Cooperative Studies Program Coordinating Ctr., West Haven, Conn., and American universities)
N. Engl. J. Med. 313:145–151, July 18, 1985   8–6

A ten-center double-blind trial was conducted to compare the efficacy and safety of four anticonvulsant drugs that were widely used in the management of 622 adults with partial and secondarily generalized tonic-clonic seizures. Patients were randomly assigned to receive carbamazepine, phenobarbital, phenytoin, or primidone. Initial doses were planned according

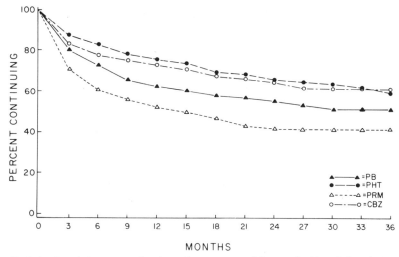

MONTHS

Fig 8–1.—Cumulative percent of patients who were successfully treated with each drug during 36 months of follow-up. PB, phenobarbital; PHT, phenytoin; PRM, primidone; and CBZ, carbamazepine. There were 275 patients at 12 months, 164 at 24 months, and 97 at 36 months. (Courtesy of Mattson, R.H., et al.: N. Engl. J. Med. 313:145–151, July 18, 1985. Reprinted by permission of the New England Journal of Medicine.)

to expected side effects and pharmacologic differences, and doses were increased to produce serum levels in the middle-to-high therapeutic range. Patients were followed up for at least 2 years or until seizures persisted or unacceptable side effects occurred.

Success with the four drug regimens is compared in Figure 8–1. Results at 3 years indicated that phenobarbital was as successful as carbamazepine and phenytoin for patients with tonic-clonic seizures but that primidone was less effective. Failures were most often due to lack of seizure control and toxicity and to side effects alone. Carbamazepine caused no side effects that were significantly worse than those associated with the other drugs. Potentially life-threatening side effects were infrequent, and no deaths were caused by use of a study drug. Partial seizures were completely controlled most often by carbamazepine.

Carbamazepine and phenytoin are recommended for initial single-drug therapy for adults with partial or generalized tonic-clonic seizures. Most patients for whom epilepsy is reasonably controlled must tolerate some side effects. Further efforts are needed to prevent epilepsy and to develop more effective and less toxic drugs and other approaches to treatment.

▶ This is a well-done study, that, among other things, demonstrates clearly that phenytoin and carbamazepine are the best drugs for partial seizures. The side effects of primidone were the greatest limiting factor in its use. This paper is a beginning answer to the comment by Chadwick and Turnbull (*J. Neurol. Neurosurg. Psychiatry* 48:1073–1077, November 1985) concerning the need for studies of the relative efficacy of antiepileptic drugs. The authors are to be congratulated for their combined efforts.—Robert D. Currier, M.D.

The Role of Antiepileptics in Sudden Death in Epilepsy

A. Lund and H. Gormsen (Inst. of Forensic Medicine, Copenhagen)
Acta Neurol. Scand. 72:444–446, 1985   8–7

Failure to take anticonvulsant medication probably is the most frequent cause of sudden unexpected death in epileptics, but drug overdose from self-poisoning is a factor in some cases. Study of 55 sudden deaths of epileptic persons taking phenobarbitone, phenytoin, or carbamazepine showed that half had subtherapeutic drug levels, while one third of them had lethal levels, chiefly of phenobarbitone. Subtherapeutic levels of all three drugs and of drug combinations were observed, but lethal concentrations were represented almost exclusively by phenobarbitone. In one fifth of cases therapeutic blood drug levels were present, but there was no autopsy evidence of other causes of death.

About half of these sudden deaths of epileptics were associated with subtherapeutic anticonvulsant levels in the blood, while one third of deaths were associated with lethal levels, especially of phenobarbitone, the only drug represented that is a hypnotic and a central depressant. A majority of the latter cases undoubtedly were suicides, but some might have been accidents, since drowsiness and fatigue from the medication may have resulted in an unintentional overdose. Therapeutic monitoring might be helpful. Although valproate is used more often at present, phenobarbitone still is used by about one fifth of epileptics.

▶ It's not news that overmedication with antiepileptics may be fatal. For a period of time this neurologist denied that epileptics use their medications to attempt suicide but I have since learned better. So both over- or underdosage may be fatal. Chadwick and Reynolds (*Br. Med. J.* 290:1885–1888, June 22, 1985) have discussed their experience and provided well-thought out recommendations on the initiation and discontinuation of treatment with medications. It is a good paper to have around since they neatly summarize the available knowledge.—Robert D. Currier, M.D.

Patterns of Seizure Activation After Withdrawal of Antiepileptic Medication

Maria Grazia Marciani, Jean Gotman, Frederick Andermann, and André Olivier (McGill Univ., Montreal, and Univ. of Rome)
Neurology 35:1537–1543, November 1985   8–8

The effects of reduction in dose or withdrawal of various anticonvulsant drugs on the temporal course and type of seizures were studied in 40 patients aged 19 to 45 years who had complex partial seizures. Thirty-four patients had developed secondary generalized tonic-clonic attacks on at least one occasion. Twenty-nine patients had a temporal lobectomy and 2 had a frontal lobectomy. Eight patients received single-drug therapy at admission, usually with carbamazepine. The others most frequently received carbamazepine and phenytoin. At least two drugs were withdrawn in 28 cases. Twenty patients were observed for an average of 2 weeks when they were not receiving any medication.

Rapid withdrawal of anticonvulsants triggered generalized seizures for a brief time or partial seizures for a longer period. The increases in frequency of seizures appeared to be related to a change in dosage rather than to the dosage itself, because these increases were largely confined to the early period after reduction in drug therapy. Several patients had rebound events in a "clustered" temporal pattern, although it was not always possible to formally define these events as a "withdrawal cluster."

About half of the patients in this study had what could be considered "withdrawal" seizures when anticonvulsants were reduced in dosage or no longer administered. Whether the mechanism is the same as that of seizures that occur after withdrawal of alcohol, barbiturates, or other drugs is uncertain. Partial recovery can occur in a few days. The time of vulnerability to partial seizures may exceed that of vulnerability to secondarily generalized seizures.

▶ Apparently the tendency to have partial seizures persists longer than the tendency to have generalized seizures following withdrawal or decrease in dosage of antiepileptic drugs.—Russell N. DeJong, M.D.

Exacerbation of Seizures in Children by Carbamazepine

O. Carter Snead, III, and Lynn C. Hosey (Univ. of Alabama)
N. Engl. J. Med. 313:916–921, Oct. 10, 1985   8–9

Carbamazepine is an effective anticonvulsant when used to treat children, but two reports of apparent exacerbation of seizures have appeared. Review was made of data on 861 children with seizures, 509 of whom had two or more types of classifiable epileptic seizures and a diagnosis of mixed seizure disorder. Carbamazepine was given to 122 of these patients. Eight girls and 7 boys (mean age, 6 years) had exacerbation of one or more types of seizures during carbamazepine therapy.

The mean daily dose of carbamazepine was 16.2 mg/kg daily, with a mean trough level of 7.15 µg/ml for a mean of 3 months. No significant changes in serum levels of other anticonvulsant drugs were noted. All patients but 2 were receiving other medications when carbamazepine therapy was begun. Video-EEG monitoring showed generalized paroxysmal abnormalities in all 15 cases. Generalized seizures increased in frequency in 4 patients, complex partial seizures increased in 2, and myoclonic seizures increased in 1. Eleven patients had a marked increase in atypical absence seizures. The increased activity of all types of seizures disappeared when carbamazepine therapy was discontinued. Patients with severe generalized seizures while taking carbamazepine had generalized bursts of high-voltage spikes and waves at 1–2 cps, and those with increased generalized absence seizures had bursts of bilaterally synchronous spikes and waves at 2.5–3 cps.

Carbamazepine should be used cautiously to treat a complex partial component of mixed seizure disorders in children. Those with generalized absence or atypical absence seizures are especially at risk of exacerbation. A pattern of generalized synchronous spike-wave discharges at 2.5–3 cps that is demonstrated on video-EEG study is predictive of carbamazepine-induced atypical absence, but a slower spike-wave burst seems to indicate a risk of worsened generalized seizures.

▶ Carbamazepine must be considered a possible precipitating factor in any child with increased frequency of seizures who is receiving this drug. It should be used with caution in treating children with a mixed seizure disorder or generalized or atypical absence seizures.—Russell N. DeJong, M.D.

Psychomotor Status

Joost Van Rossum, Alexandrina A. W. Groeneveld-Ockhuysen, and Rudolf J. H. M. Arts (Univ. of Leiden, The Netherlands)
Arch. Neurol. 42:989–993, October 1985   8–10

Psychomotor status is a continuous state of complex symptoms, ranging from mild lethargy to marked clouding of consciousness with behavioral and psychologic changes and automatisms. The patient is amnesic, and the EEG shows a temporal or bitemporal discharge or a secondary bilateral synchronous discharge from a temporal lobe focus. Four such cases were encountered within a 2-year period. Three others may have been affected, but the EEG was not recorded. One case is described below.

Woman, 43 years old, had had brief attacks of speech disturbance with distortion of words and anxiety for 8 years, which sometimes were followed by involuntary extension of the right arm. Focal epilepsy had been diagnosed, with postictal right-sided hemiparesis. The dosage of antiepileptic medication had been reduced a month before admission. Attacks of anxiety and visual hallucinations that lasted 10 to 30 seconds were frequent. In some instances a generalized tonic-clonic seizure followed. The patient was confused at admission and exhibited regressive childlike behavior. The neurologic findings otherwise were normal. Analysis of the cerebral spinal fluid produced negative results, and results of left carotid angiography were normal. The EEG showed bradyrhythmia with some slow aberrant activity over the left frontotemporal region. Bilaterally synchronous generalized spike-wave discharges were seen. The confusional state lasted 5 days. Seizures ceased after an infusion of diazepam, and the patient became alert and resumed normal behavior.

Thirty-five of these cases were reported through 1983. About one third of the patients have had signs of preexisting brain damage. All but 10 of 39 cases, including the present ones, occurred in known epileptics. Some patients were initially thought to be psychotic. Antidepressant drugs may precipitate the epileptic status. Neurologic evaluation and EEG study are necessary in all patients who present with apparently psychotic behavior and altered consciousness with no known intoxication.

▶ Contrary to the limited number of published case reports, the actual incidence of psychomotor status must be higher than suspected. In many incidences, the patients' conditions are mistakenly diagnosed as psychotic. Neurologic and EEG examinations are indicated in all patients with apparently psychotic behavior and an altered state of consciousness.—Russell N. DeJong, M.D.

Reproductive Endocrine Disorders in Women With Partial Seizures of Temporal Lobe Origin
Andrew G. Herzog, Machelle M. Seibel, Donald L. Schomer, Judith L. Vaitukaitis, and Norman Geschwind (Beth Israel Hosp., Harvard Univ., Boston City Hosp., and Boston Univ.)
Arch. Neurol. 43:341–346, April 1986   8–11

Reproductive dysfunction is unusually common in women with temporal lobe epilepsy (TLE). The level of reproductive hormones was assessed in 50 women aged 20 to 40 years with TLE to determine if menstrual problems in these patients were related to hormonal abnormalities. Eight normal women served as controls.

Menstrual disturbances included amenorrhea, oligomenorrhea, and prolonged or shortened menstrual cycles. Serum levels of serum leuteinizing hormone (LH), follicle-stimulating hormone (FSH), prolactin (PRL), total and free testosterone, estradiol, dehydroepiandrosterone sulfate, thyroxine, triiodothyronine, thyrotropin, and cortisone were measured.

Twenty-eight (56%) of the 50 women had menstrual dysfunction, and 19 (68%) of those 28 women (vs. 38% overall) had abnormal serum concentrations of reproductive hormones. The reproductive endocrine disorders included polycystic ovarian syndrome (PCO), hypogonadotropic hypogonadism (HH), premature menopause, and hyperprolactinemia. The incidence of these syndromes was significantly greater in the population with TLE than in the general female population. Although antiseizure medications may alter serum levels of hormones, this study demonstrated similar percentages of disorders among patients who used medication and those who did not. No relationship was found among the endocrine syndromes and the type or level of antiseizure medications used. Abnormal serum levels of LH was the most consistent endocrine finding.

Limbic seizure activity may disrupt normal limbic modulation of hypothalamic gonadotropin-releasing hormone (GnRH) regulation of the secretion of LH and thereby favor the development of PCO or HH. Epileptic discharge may influence the levels of dopamine, thus further altering levels of hormones.

Lateralization of EEG activity was significantly correlated with PCO and HH syndromes, as well as diminished sexual interest. Since right and left temporal lobes differ in structure and function, lateralization of TLE may determine whether levels of LH are increased or decreased, leading to PCO or HH, respectively. Reproductive disorders may favor the development of TLE and prenatal factors common to the development of both the brain and reproductive systems may be related to familial susceptibility to TLE.

▶ One of the interesting findings of this study was that half of the women with right-sided epileptiform abnormalities had diminished sexual interest but none of those with left-sided abnormalities did. Does this mean that sexual interest in women joins appreciation of the visual and auditory arts in being right brained?—Robert D. Currier, M.D.

Prolonged Focal Cerebral Edema Associated With Partial Status Epilepticus
Michele Sammaritano, Frederick Andermann, Denis Melanson, Hanna M. Pappius, Peter Camfield, Jean Aicardi, and Allan Sherwin (McGill Univ., Montreal; Izaak Walton Killam Hosp. for Children, Halifax, Nova Scotia; and Hôpital des Enfants Malades and Institut National de la Santé et de la Recherche Médicale, Paris)
Epilepsia 26:334–339, July–Aug. 1985   8–12

Status epilepticus has long been thought to lead to cerebral edema, but this has only rarely been documented in man. Three patients with partial status epilepticus had clinical and radiographic evidence of long-lasting focal cerebral edema.

Woman, 32 years old, had begun having partial complex seizures at age 13 years at a rate of up to 15 per day. Neurologic examination yielded normal findings, but the EEG showed a left inferomedial temporal spike focus. An episode of partial complex status at age 24 years lasted 18 hours, and the patient was amnesic for 4 days. Currently, partial complex status had been present for 5 days. Computed tomographic (CT) findings were normal (Fig 8–2), but a contrast-enhanced study 2 weeks after onset of status showed hyperdense cortex in the left temporoparietal region, surrounded by an area of hypodensity thought to represent edema. An-

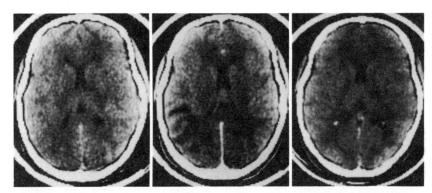

Fig 8–2.—**Left,** normal CT scan 2 days after onset of partial complex status. **Middle,** contrast-enhanced CT scan 2 weeks after onset of status shows a hyperemic cortex surrounded by an area of hypodensity corresponding with cerebral edema. **Right,** CT scan 12 weeks after status shows that the edema has resolved. (Courtesy of Sammaritano, M., et al.: Epilepsia 26:334–339, July–Aug. 1985.)

giography showed a capillary blush in the same region, and a ^{68}Ga ethylenediamine tetra-acetate positron emission tomographic (PET) study showed irregular focal uptake in the area of the supramarginal and angular gyri. The focal CT changes had resolved 12 weeks after status, and an angiogram and PET study were normal. Perfusion was moderately reduced in the left temporal region. Expressive dysphasia persisted. No evidence of tumor developed during 3 years of follow-up.

Vasogenic edema presumably was present in these patients, in association with abnormal, possibly leaky, blood vessels. Fluid in the extracellular space of the white matter results from breakdown of the blood-brain barrier. Changes were maximal in the area of peak epileptic discharge in all cases. Neurologic disability was long-lasting but completely reversible. Awareness that partial status epilepticus can be associated with focal cerebral edema will help avoid the misdiagnosis of cerebral tumor or infarction.

▶ The clinical, CT, and angiographic findings herein described suggest that partial status epilepticus can be associated with abnormal vascular permeability, leading to focal cerebral edema. Physicians should be aware of this clinical and radiologic entity.—Robert D. Currier, M.D.

Incidence of Seizures With Phenytoin Toxicity
Naemi Stilman and Joseph C. Masdeu (Montefiore Med. Ctr. and Albert Einstein College of Medicine, Bronx, N.Y.)
Neurology 35:1769–1772, December 1985   8–13

A paradoxical increase in seizure frequency, which can result from phenytoin toxicity, may be difficult to recognize. Review of 50 patients at three hospitals with phenytoin intoxication revealed 14 cases with seizures. Seizures were ascribed to poor control in 9 cases and to phenytoin toxicity in 5 (10%).

Toxicity occurred in the course of therapeutic use in 28 cases, resulted from accidental ingestion in 13 cases, and from deliberate overdose in 9 cases. Partial complex seizures were frequent in patients with seizures unrelated to toxicity. The median serum phenytoin level in patients with seizures due to toxicity was 49 μg/ml, compared with 34 μg/ml in patients without seizures, and 31 μg/ml in those with seizures unrelated to toxicity. Signs and symptoms of toxicity were similar in all groups; ataxia was the most frequent feature. Mental status findings were similar in the various groups. One of 5 subsequent patients with phenytoin toxicity had phenytoin-induced seizures.

Seizures were ascribed to phenytoin toxicity in 10% of the cases in this series. The only clinically significant association was with higher serum phenytoin levels. No increased susceptibility to seizures was found in relation to any other factor analyzed, and clinical features of toxicity were similar for all groups.

▶ The fact that excessive phenytoin levels can increase the frequency of seizures is probably not generally appreciated and in fact may be disbelieved by some. A fellow neurologist tipped me off on this years ago and it took a while for me to accept it. It probably really does occur.—Robert D. Currier, M.D.

Long-Term Follow-up of Seizures Associated With Cerebral Arteriovenous Malformations: Results of Therapy
Martin J. Murphy (Univ. of Iowa)
Arch. Neurol. 42:477–479, May 1985   8–14

Reported cases indicate that seizures associated with cerebral arteriovenous malformations (AVMs) rarely are incapacitating and usually are well controlled medically, but follow-up data are limited. Review was made of data on 115 patients with angiographically proved cerebral AVMs, seen in 1966–1979. Cases of dural or diplic malformations, capillary angioma, and Sturge-Weber syndrome were excluded. There were 111 malformations in supratentorial sites and 9 in the brain stem or cerebellum in this series.

The mean age at onset of symptom was 24 years and 29 years at angiographic diagnosis. Seizures occurred in 66 (57%) of the patients and were the initial manifestation in 36 (31%) of cases; the age of onset ranged from 6 to 60 years (mean, 23 years). Seizures developed within 30 days of hemorrhage or resection in 14 cases, and after a mean of 3½ years in 16 others. Simple partial seizures were most frequent. The clinical features of the seizures were unrelated to the site of malformation, except for hemifield visual phenomena in patients with occipital-lobe AVMs. A majority of patients had mild to moderate seizures; only 9 had severe or incapacitating seizures. Of 46 patients followed for a mean of 9 years, half were seizure free for at least 2 years when last evaluated. The outcome was similar in surgically and medically managed patients. Seizures starting soon after resection or hemorrhage had the best prognosis regardless of management.

Seizures developing within 30 days of surgery on cerebral AVM or hemorrhage have a relatively good prognosis. Although removal of the malformation itself is paramount, removal of the intervening neural tissue as well might improve the rate of remission of seizures.

▶ Evidently, surgery neither increases nor decreases the tendency to epilepsy in this disorder. Speaking of unusual causes of seizures a recent note in *The Lancet* (2:1294, December 7, 1985) mentions that in the United States, 12% of cocaine users suffer convulsions. It is strange that I am unaware of having seen such a patient if the use of cocaine is as widespread as it is said to be. Probably my sheltered environment.—Robert D. Currier, M.D.

Epidemiologic Features of Isolated Syncope: The Framingham Study
Daniel D. Savage, Lee Corwin, Daniel L. McGee, William B. Kannel, and

Philip A. Wolf (Framingham Heart Study, Natl. Heart, Lung and Blood Inst., and Boston Univ.)
Stroke 16:626–629, July–Aug. 1985   8–15

A recent study of patients with syncope showed increased mortality in those with underlying cardiovascular or other serious diseases but not in patients without other major illnesses. The prevalence and significance of isolated syncope, or transient loss of consciousness without evidence of cardiovascular or neurologic disease, were examined in the Framingham population, who were followed up for 26 years. The study included 2,336 men and 2,873 women aged 30–62 years at entry to the study in 1950.

At least one syncopal episode occurred in 3% of men and 3.5% of women in the study. Criteria for isolated syncope were met by 56 men and 89 women reporting syncope. Isolated syncope was not associated with excessive stroke, including transient ischemic attack, or myocardial infarction during follow-up, and no association with any excessive all-cause or cardiovascular mortality, including sudden death, was evident. No significant associations were found on age- and sex-specific comparisons.

Syncope not associated with past, or recurrent, cardiovascular or neurologic disorder carries no increased morbidity or mortality risk. The comparatively benign course of syncope in the Framingham population should not, however, obscure the possibility of a malignant course and the need for evaluation and appropriate therapy in individual cases.

▶ It's surprising how benign syncope in a healthy person seems to be. A recent note by Gilchrist (*Neurology* 35:1503–1505, October 1985) details a young man with episodes of cardiac asystole that were evidently precipitated by a left temporal lobe discharge. Demand ventricular pacing did not stop the seizures but carbamazepine did.

Teplinsky and Hall (*Arch. Intern. Med.* 146:801–802, April 1986) reported a case of postictal pulmonary edema following a grand mal seizure that responded to therapy. They point out that the neurogenic pulmonary edema secondary to massive CNS injury requires intensive support, but the postical variety may resolve rapidly within 24 hours.—Robert D. Currier, M.D.

9 Extrapyramidal Disorders

Combined Resting-Postural Tremors
William C. Koller and Frank A. Rubino (Loyola Univ., Maywood, Ill., and Hines VA Hosp., Hines, Ill.)
Arch. Neurol. 42:683–684, July 1985   9–1

Postural tremor occurs in patients with essential tremor, whereas resting tremor is characteristic of Parkinson's disease. Eight patients with prominent resting and postural tremors and no definitive diagnosis were encountered. The six men and two women had an average age of 60 years. Tremor had been present for 10½ years on average. Treatment, which was given alone for more than 3 months in a randomized manner, consisted of daily administration of either 10 mg of trihexyphenidyl, 500 to 1,000 mg of levodopa with carbidopa, or 160 to 320 mg of propranolol hydrochloride.

Two patients had a family history of essential tremor and 1 of possible Parkinson's disease. One patient had bilateral Babinski signs, but no other neurologic signs were evident, and parkinsonian features were not observed. The postural component of tremor was more marked. Tremors began unilaterally but became bilateral and asymmetric as they progressed. All patients had significant functional hand disability, as in eating and writing. All treatments failed to lessen the tremors, but one patient who drank alcohol reported that it improved his tremor.

Postural tremor predominated in these patients with combined resting-postural tremor. Lack of a family history and unresponsiveness to β-blockers are not infrequent in patients with essential tremor. Slight cogwheeling may be related to poor muscle relaxation. The limits of drug therapy in these patients must be recognized to avoid toxic drug effects. The existence of different subtypes of essential tremor may reflect various pathophysiologic mechanisms.

▶ Combined resting and postural tremors are usually classified as a subtype of essential tremor. Neither trihexyphenidyl hydrochloride, levodopa, nor propanolol hydrochloride was effective in reducing these tremors. The possibility of toxic drug effects must be borne in mind in attempting to treat patients with tremors of this type.—Russell N. DeJong, M.D.

Clonidine in Essential Tremor: Preliminary Observations From an Open Trial
M. R. Caccia and A. Mangoni (University of Milan and Ospedale "L. Sacco")
J. Neurol. 232:55–57, March 1985   9–2

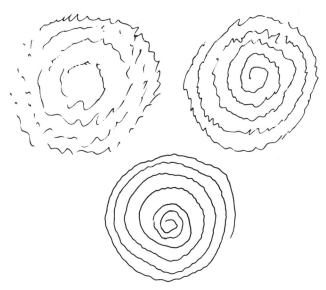

Fig 9–1.—Archimede's screw drawing, done by a 77-year-old woman. **Left,** before treatment. **Right,** after 15 days, **Center,** after 1 month of treatment. (Courtesy of Caccia, M.R., and Mangoni, A.: J. Neurol. 232:55–57, March 1985. Berlin-Heidelberg-New York: Springer.)

Clonidine is an α-adrenergic agent that has fewer side effects on the cardiorespiratory system than the β-blockers used to treat essential tremor. The drug was evaluated in 10 subjects aged 58–77 years, 8 of them women, with essential tremor of the upper limbs. The head and jaw also were affected in some cases. Drawing and writing tests were carried out before and during treatment with clonidine in oral doses of 0.1–0.9 mg daily, except for one patient, who received 0.15 mg daily intravenously. Control tremor recordings were obtained from other patients with essential tremor who were treated with levodopa, piribedil, or diazepam.

Representative drawings before and after clonidine therapy are shown in Figure 9–1. All patients showed objective and subjective improvement after 15–20 days of treatment. All affected muscles responded. The condition of a patient with severe generalized tremor responded dramatically to clonidine therapy, after years of treatment with levodopa and anticholinergic agents. Some patients reported less anxiety during treatment. Blood pressures remained normal. Mean tremor amplitude fell by 30% to 60% during treatment. Control subjects receiving other drugs showed no significant changes in tremor.

Clonidine consistently reduces the amplitude of essential tremor. A desynchronizing effect is apparent, with no change in frequency in most cases. Clonidine appears to inhibit the anticholinergic effect of levodopa and to restore upset dopamine-acetylcholine balance. It also may act on the acetylcholine-norepinephrine balance and exert an anxiolytic effect.

▶ The effectiveness of certain beta-blockers in the treatment of essential tremors has been known for several years, but the side effects of some of these drugs on autonomic function, especially heart rate and respiratory function in elderly patients, may contraindicate their use. These observers have demonstrated that clonidine, an α-adrenergic agent, was effective in treating essential tremor without causing side effects. This work should be confirmed by other investigators.—Russell N. DeJong, M.D.

Levodopa-Induced Dyskinesia: Clinical Observations
Andrzej Friedman (Medical School, Warsaw)
J. Neurol. 232:29–31, March 1985   9–3

The mechanism of the involuntary movements that sometimes develop during levodopa therapy for Parkinson's disease is uncertain. Levodopa-related dyskinesia was studied in a series of 144 patients treated with levodopa for Parkinson's disease over 2 to 14 years. The 76 men and 68 women had a mean age of 59.9 years at onset of illness (range, 35–83 years). The dosage of levodopa, used with carbidopa, ranged from 500 to 1,000 mg daily. Forty-one patients received an anticholinergic as well, usually trihexyphenidyl. Eleven patients received amantadine and 3 bromocriptine.

Dyskinesia was seen in 64% of the patients. Those who became ill earlier in life appeared to be most susceptible, but no association with the duration of levodopa therapy was apparent. Dyskinesia usually appeared in the first year of treatment and persisted throughout treatment. Patients with predominant bradykinesia and those with mixed forms of disease were more susceptible to dyskinesia than patients with predominant tremor. Concomitant treatment did not seem to be related to susceptibility to dyskinesia.

Levodopa-induced dyskinesia is most likely to develop in younger patients with predominant bradykinesia and rigidity. Delayed levodopa therapy may result in enhanced sensitivity of dopaminergic receptors and a greater susceptibility to dyskinesia. Delayed treatment can be recommended for patients with a longer history of parkinsonian symptoms who have not received the drug. Early levodopa treatment is indicated for patients with a short history of symptoms.

▶ Levodopa-induced dyskinesias in Polish patients with Parkinson's disease are similar to those that we observe in American patients.—Russell N. DeJong, M.D.

Dystonia and Calcification of the Basal Ganglia
T. Andreo Larsen, Henry G. Dunn, James E. Jan, and Donald B. Calne (Univ. of British Columbia)
Neurology 35:533–537, April 1985   9–4

Calcification of the basal ganglia without apparent abnormality of calcium metabolism may be a rare familial trait. A family spanning five

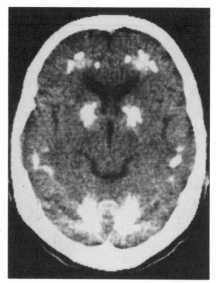

Fig 9–2.—Symmetric calcifications in the basal ganglia bilaterally, in the dentate nuclei, and in the frontal and parietal areas. (Courtesy of Larsen, T.A., et al.: Neurology 35:533–537, April 1985.)

generations was encountered with autosomal dominantly inherited intracerebral calcification and dystonia. The family, of English-Scottish ancestry, included 14 affected members. Intellectual impairment accompanied the dystonic movements. Either dysarthria and buccolingual dyskinesia or dystonic posturing of the limbs was seen; some subjects had both patterns of movement disorder. Intracranial calcification involved predominantly the basal ganglia. The computed tomographic findings for the mother of the propositus are shown in Figure 9–2. Dysarthria was a frequent but not constant finding. The IQ was below normal, but gross dementia was not a feature. Seizures and pyramidal signs were not observed.

Thirteen of the 37 members of this family who were examined had dystonia, predominantly affecting the voice, face, neck, and extremities. Intracranial calcification was seen in the putamen, pallidum, cerebral white matter, cerebral cortex, and cerebellar nuclei. Some patients had dystonia or calcifications alone. The abnormalities were inherited in an autosomal dominant manner. No abnormalities of calcium metabolism were found. The findings in one case suggested that anterior putaminopallidal pathologic changes correlate with dystonia predominating in the upper half of the body.

▶ The abnormalities in calcium metabolism are not evident in the serum but must be abnormal in the cells of the basal ganglia.

Spasmodic torticollis has been treated recently by injections of botulinum toxin (Tsui, J. K., et al.: *Can. J. Neurol. Sci.* 12:314–316, November 1985) and by nitrous oxide (Gillman, M. A., and Sandyk, R.: *Eur. Neurol.* 24:292–293, September/October 1985). Nitrous oxide treatment lasted for four days but the toxin treatment lasted up to three months.—Robert D. Currier, M.D.

Lisuride Infusion Pump: A Device for the Treatment of Motor Fluctuations in Parkinson's Disease

J. A. Obeso, M. R. Luquin, and J. M. Martínez-Lage (Univ. of Navarra, Pamplona, Spain)
Lancet 2:467–470, March 1, 1986 9–5

Daily fluctuations in motor performance, frequently accompanied by dyskinesias, are one of the most common problems in patients with Parkinson's disease after long-term treatment with levodopa. Initially, such changes in mobility are precisely related to the timing of levodopa administration ("wearing off" or "end-of-dose deterioration"), but as the duration of the disease and of levodopa therapy increase, patients may fail to respond to individual doses, and sudden, unpredictable changes in mobility ("on-off" phenomenon) occur. Pharmacokinetic factors controlling levodopa intracerebral availability seem to have an important role in the origin of motor fluctuations in Parkinson's disease, and intravenous levodopa infusions have been found to correct random on-off fluctuations.

Three patients (1 woman and 2 men) received continuous subcutaneous administration of lisuride, a potent dopamine agonist, by means of a portable mini-infusion pump, in addition to oral levodopa plus decarboxylase inhibitor. Dry lisuride (2–2.5 mg) was diluted in 3.2 ml of saline for continuous (24-hour) subcutaneous administration. Oral treatment with levodopa plus carbidopa or benserazide was maintained unchanged during the initial 2–4 weeks of treatment. All patients received oral domperidone (10 mg every 8 hours) to prevent nausea and vomiting. The disease was long-standing (20, 11, and 8 years), and all patients showed severe on-off fluctuations unresponsive to control with conventional treatment. The pattern of fluctuation of these patients was classified as "complicated end-of-dose deterioration" (patients 1 and 2) and "end-of-dose deterioration" with levodopa-resistant off periods (patient 3).

The three patients showed considerable improvement in mobility after starting treatment with subcutaneous lisuride infusion added to oral levodopa (Fig 9–3). "Off" periods were reduced or abolished. This response was maintained for 4–7 months without toxic side effects. All three patients were discharged and were able to live independently during the months on treatment; periods of immobility disappeared after a few days of treatment. Levodopa-resistant off periods were abolished and every dose of levodopa became effective under the new therapeutic regimen. However, stable motor function was not maintained throughout the day; there were brief periods of impaired mobility in patients 1 and 3 (Fig 9–3). Chorea was not noted in any of the 3 patients during the first 3–4 weeks of treatment but appeared in all during the second or third month. In patients 2 and 3, the dyskinesias were controlled by reduction of the total daily dose of levodopa (Fig 9–3).

Subcutaneous lisuride infusion in conjunction with oral levodopa can abolish off periods in patients with severe daily fluctuations of motor performance. The positive effect can be maintained over several months without loss of efficacy. Local and systemic tolerance was excellent. A

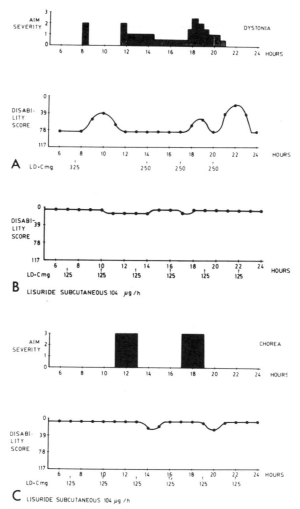

Fig. 9–3.—Disability scores and response to lisuride infusion. **A,** mean disability score (bottom) over the 7 days before initiation of treatment with subcutaneous lisuride. This patient (3) showed a fairly good response during the morning but a poorer one in the afternoon. Periods of immobility were accompanied by severe dystonia (*top*) mainly affecting the left limbs. **B,** response to subcutaneous lisuride infusion during the second week of treatment. Normal mobility was achieved most of the day, and dyskinesias were not present. **C,** 12 weeks after treatment with subcutaneous lisuride was started, mobility was normal most of the day, but brief periods of generalized chorea (*top*) were present, which was resolved by slight reduction in Madopar (levodopa-benserazide) doses (*black arrows*). AIM (abnormal involuntary movements) severity was graded from 0 (absent) to 3 (generalized, almost continuous movements interfering with purposeful motor tasks). (Courtesy of Obesco, J.A., et al.: Lancet 2:467–470, Mar. 1, 1986.)

drawback to the regimen could be the oral levodopa component, which may depend on lisuride's selective stimulation of D-2 receptors. This system could probably be improved with technical developments for the pump and/or by the use of some other water soluble dopamine agonist with even more potent anti-parkinsonian effects and better tolerance than lisuride has at present.

▶ C. J. Todes of England, a psychiatrist with parkinsonism tried the lisuride pump and found the psychiatric side effects "hazardous" (*The Lancet* 2:36–37, July 5, 1986). He suggests that a psychiatrist to monitor such effects should be a part of the treatment team. In spite of the side effects and its apparent cumbersome nature, the lisuride pump likely will become more popular.—Robert D. Currier, M. D.

Low Cancer Rates Among Patients With Parkinson's Disease
Birger Jansson and Joseph Jankovic (M. D. Anderson Hosp. and Tumor Inst. and Baylor College of Medicine, Houston)
Ann. Neurol. 17:505–509, May 1985   9–6

Since it was first suggested that cancer rates are low in in patients with Parkinson's disease reports have been inconclusive. Data were reviewed on 406 patients with Parkinson's disease who were followed up by a single investigator. Cancer rates were about one third those for the general population. The risk increased during the treatment period but remained significantly low. Malignant and benign thyroid tumors were significantly more frequent than expected in the patient group. The occurrence of two malignant melanomas among 20 cancers was also more than expected.

A relatively low risk of cancer was confirmed in this series of patients with Parkinson's disease. It has been reported that a high total body potassium concentration protects against cancer, and patients with Parkinson's disease have been found to have an elevated total body potassium concentration. Levodopa may increase potassium excretion and thereby increase the risk of cancer. This effect may help explain the different cancer rates reported when mortality and postmortem data are used. Levodopa also is a precursor in melanin biosynthesis, and its administration may increase the risk of malignant melanoma.

▶ The conclusion that levodopa may increase the risk of malignant melanoma is challenged by Rampen (*J. Neurol. Neurosurg. Psychiatry* 48:585–588, June 1985) who, while reporting three melanoma occurrences, in patients taking levodopa for parkinsonism, contends that "the available literature data do not endorse the supposition that levodopa intake has an effect on malignant transformation of melanocytes." His conclusion seems somewhat curious but one gathers the question is still open.—Robert D. Currier, M.D.

High Dose Anticholinergic Therapy in Adult Dystonia
Anthony E. Lang (Toronto Western Hosp.)
Can. J. Neurol. Sci. 13:42–46, February 1986   9–7

High-dose anticholinergic therapy was attempted in 44 adult patients with various forms of dystonia (table). All patients were older than 18 years of age at the beginning of therapy, with the exception of 1 patient, aged 16 years, with idiopathic generalized dystonia.

Thirteen (37%) of the 35 patients with idiopathic dystonia had a mod-

PATIENT DETAILS

Type of Dystonia	Number	Sex M/F	Age of Onset Mean (range)	Duration of Dystonia Mean (range)	No. of Patients with Tremor	Family History Tremor	Family History Dystonia
Idiopathic Dystonia							
Generalized	5	1/4	19.2 (9-39)	9.4 (4-20)	1	1	1
Segmental	9	5/4	27.4 (7-55)	8.8 (2-18)	5	3	2
Cranial Dystonia	6	1/5	57.8 (42-80)	3.4 (1-14)	3	0	0
Spasmodic Torticollis	12	6/6	38.6 (25-55)	3.0 (0.3-8)	3	2	0
Focal Arm	3*	1/2	33.6 (28-43)	1.3 (1-2)	2	0	1
Sub-total	35	14/21	35.8 (7-80)	5.3 (0.3-20)	14	6	4
Symptomatic Dystonia							
Tardive: Segmental	3	2/1	25 (20-29)	4 (1-9)	—	—	—
Cranial	2	1/1	49 (45-53)	2.5 (1-4)	—	—	—
Hemidystonia	3*	2/1	43.3 (6-64)	7.8 (0.5-14)	—	—	—
Metachromatic Leukodystrophy	1	0/1	8	34	—	—	—
Sub-total	9	5/4	34.5 (6-64)	8.2 (0.5-34)	—	—	—
Total:	44	19/25	35.6 (6-80)	8.9 (0.3-34)			

*One patient had dystonia on many actions and two had simple writer's cramp.
†One patient had hemidystonia after trauma and two after stroke.
Courtesy of Lang, A.E.: Can. J. Neurol. Sci. 13:42–46, February 1986.)

erate-to-marked improvement with an average dosage of 21.5 mg. of trihexyphenidyl. Younger patients with a shorter duration of dystonia and those who tolerated higher doses tended to benefit most. However, there were exceptions to all of these factors. None of the 9 patients with symptomatic dystonias improved more than mildly and most had no benefit, despite the use of dosages similar to those resulting in improvement in patients with idiopathic dystonia. Side effects were common and often forced drug withdrawal at lower doses than those that might have resulted in improvement.

The potential benefit that might be obtained from high-dose anticholinergic therapy as shown in this and previous studies indicates that this should be the first line of therapy in patients with disabling dystonia.

▶ The administration of high-dose anticholinergic therapy in dystonia was first described by Fahn in 1979 (Fahn, S.: *Neurology* 29:605, April 1979). Since then, many studies have confirmed his results in both children and adults and in both idiopathic and symptomatic dystonia.—Russell N. DeJong, M.D.

The Heterogeneity of Parkinson's Disease: Clinical and Prognostic Implications

Walter J. Zetusky, Joseph Jankovic, and Francis J. Pirozzolo (Baylor College of Medicine)
Neurology 35:522–526, April 1985

9–8

The varying clinical features of Parkinson's disease (PD) suggest that subgroups of PD may exist, with the classification possibly related to different pathologic and biochemical mechanisms. Of 600 consecutive parkinsonian patients, 334 patients with idiopathic PD remained after those with a history of stereotaxic surgery, exposure to neuroleptic drugs or toxins, infectious or postinfectious parkinsonism, and other features were excluded. Patients with on-off clinical oscillations were also excluded. The mean age at onset of disease was 57.7 years, and the mean duration was 7.4 years. Mental status impairment was present in three fourths of the cases. More than one fifth of patients had a history of parkinsonism in first- or second-degree relatives.

Deterioration in mental status paralleled the severity of bradykinesia, postural instability, and gait difficulty in this patient sample. Tremor, however, was relatively independent of the other cardinal features, and was seen with relatively well-preserved mental status. Tremor was seen with an earlier age at onset of PD and was associated with a family history of parkinsonism, with a more favorable prognosis. Tremor did not contribute to functional disability.

There appear to be at least two subgroups of patients with idiopathic PD, one with postural instability and gait difficulty, and the other with tremor as the predominant feature. Tremor is relatively independent of other motor signs, except rigidity. It often is associated with slower progression of disease. Postural instability implies a poor outlook. Distinctions between subgroups of PD may have therapeutic implications.

Association Between Essential Tremor and Parkinson's Disease
John J. Geraghty, Joseph Jankovic, and Walter J. Zetusky (Baylor College of Medicine)
Ann. Neurol. 17:329–333, April 1985   9–9

A possible relation between essential tremor (ET) and Parkinson disease (PD) was explored in 211 consecutive patients with a primary or secondary diagnosis of ET. Patients with a combination of ET and PD (ETPD) were compared with a matched sample of patients with typical idiopathic PD. Criteria for ET were met by 130 of the patients, who had at least two of three specified features—a typical flexion-extension postural hand tremor or head tremor that preceded the onset of PD, improvement with alcohol or propranolol, and a family history of ET—and at least three of the four cardinal signs of PD: tremor at rest, bradykinesia, rigidity, and postural instability. Seventy-five patients had a family history of ET and 11 one of PD. Essential tremor alone was present in 105 patients.

Twenty-nine patients had focal dystonia besides ET, and 1 had both ET and Charcot-Marie-Tooth disease. Twenty-five patients had ETPD. The mean duration of ET was 16.6 years and that of PD 3.5 years. Nineteen of these 25 patients had a family history of ET, as did 2 with PD. Ten of 12 patients with ETPD responded to alcohol ingestion. All but 1 of 14 patients responded to propranolol. Bradykinesia and gait problems were less marked than in age-matched patients with idiopathic PD. Postural instability was also less severe in the patients with ET.

Several reports have suggested an increased prevalence of parkinsonism in patients with preexisting ET. The risk of PD in older patients with ET is much greater than that in the general population of similar age. A response to alcohol or propranolol is diagnostically helpful, as in patients with ET alone, but the mechanism of action of these agents is unknown. Neurophysiologic studies could provide understanding of the mechanisms of tremor in ET and PD and their possible association.

▶ I tend to agree with the authors that parkinsonism is not all one disease. The tendency for those with essential or familial tremor to develop parkinsonism may be greater in some cases, blurring the distinction between the two entities. It seems a bad idea to use Reserpine for ET, since it sometimes produces a permanent Parkinson's state. The question of the nature of depression in PD is still open. A recent thoughtful contribution is by Taylor et al. (Brain 109:279–292, April 1986), who found that "regardless of depression severity Parkinson's patients performed as well as control subjects on short term memory testing and did significantly better than those of the endogenously depressed patients."—Robert D. Currier, M.D.

A Comparison of Primidone, Propranolol, and Placebo in Essential Tremor, Using Quantitative Analysis
W. P. Gorman, R. Cooper, P. Pocock, and M. J. Campbell (Frenchay Hosp. and Burden Neurological Inst., Bristol, England)
J. Neurol. Neurosurg. Psychiatry 49:64–68, January 1986   9–10

Serious disability and embarrassment can result from benign essential tremor. The use of propranolol and primidone was evaluated quantitatively in 15 men and 4 women (mean age, 58 years) with a clinical diagnosis of benign essential tremor (mean tremor duration, 16 years). Nine patients had a positive family history, and 11 reported having improved with alcohol. A double-blind, randomized, cross-over study was performed, with an accelerometer and subsequent spectral analysis used to measure tremor. Primidone therapy was started in a dosage of 62.5 mg and raised to a maximum of 250 mg, three times daily. Propranolol therapy was begun at 20 mg and was raised to a maximum of 40 mg, three times daily. After 10 days at the maximum dosage treatment was withdrawn over a 5-day period.

Nine of 14 evaluable patients preferred primidone, and 5 propranolol. No patient preferred placebo to both active drugs. Accelerometer studies showed that both drugs significantly reduced tremor compared with placebo. The mean reduction was 60% with propranolol and 76% with primidone. The placebo response was small. Patients who responded to both drugs tended to have a higher mean dominant tremor frequency than the others.

Propranolol remains the drug of choice for the treatment of benign essential tremor, but patients with contraindications to β-blockers and those who fail to respond well may benefit from primidone. A useful additive effect of these drugs has been reported but requires confirmation in controlled trials.

▶ Years ago phenobarbital was used for the treatment of essential tremor, so it is not too surprising that primidone would also be useful. It certainly seems to have more side effects, at least in my experience, than propranolol.

Abila et al. (*J. Neurol. Neurosurg. Psychiatry* 48:1031–1036, October 1985) have pointed out that central adrenergic mechanisms are involved in the pathophysiology of essential tremor and suggested that α-adrenoceptor blockers may be useful therapy. This seems reasonable. They tried an α-adrenoceptor blocking drug, thymoxamine, and found that it did reduce essential tremor. So maybe the ideal drug would be a combined α- and β-blocker?—Robert D. Currier, M.D.

General Comments

The explosion of conjecture following the MPTP production of parkinsonism is continuing. A nice review on the mechanism of the neurotoxicity of MPTP is that by Snyder and D'Amato (*Neurology* 36:250–258, 1986). Barbeau et al. (*The Lancet* :1213–1215, Nov. 30, 1985) have found defective detoxification of debrisoquine in patients with parkinsonism. Alemany has suggested (*The Lancet* :737, March 29, 1986) that the calcium antagonists currently used for angina pectoris, hypertension, and migraine are structurally similar to MPTP and may increase the risk of parkinsonism; he recommended that a prospective study of the use of these drugs be done.—Robert D. Currier, M.D.

10 Headache and Migraine

Treatment of Intractable Cluster
Seymour Diamond, Frederick G. Freitag, Jordan Prager, and Sunil Gandhi
(Diamond Headache Clinic, Chicago, and Chicago Med. School, North Chicago, Ill.)
Headache 26:42–46, January 1986   10–1

Cluster headache appears to result from dilation of extracranial vessels, with some contribution from the internal carotid system, but the cause and the mechanisms involved are unclear. Data on 64 consecutive patients with intractable chronic cluster headache, 61 of them men, were reviewed. All had had headaches for 6 months or longer, despite treatment with steroids and erither methysergide or ergotamine tartrate. No patient had been free of pain for longer than 2 weeks in the previous 6 months. Histamine desensitization was carried out at an individualized histamine phosphate infusion rate, and oral prophylaxis with hydroxyzine and ci-metidine was instituted. Eleven patients received other prophylactic agents such as lithium carbonate or verapamil.

Twenty-five (40%) of the 64 patients had an excellent response (75%–100% reduction in headache frequency), 19% a good response (50%–74% reduction), and 16% a fair response (10%–49% reduction); the remaining 9 patients were considered refractive, with less than a 10% reduction in headaches. A number of patients benefited from prophylactic measures other than H_1 and H_2 blockers. Seven of 9 patients having cocainization of the sphenopalatine ganglion had an excellent or good response. A longer history of cluster headache was associated with poor response to treatment. Responses to histamine desensitization did not diminish over time.

Histamine desensitization is a useful approach to intractable cluster headaches. Lithium carbonate is a useful adjunctive measure. Cocainiza-tion of the sphenopalatine ganglion may be helpful in some cases, partic-ularly when surgery is under consideration.

▶ The histamine desensitization treatment of cluster headache appears to have been reborn. It's easy to see why when the difficulties of treating intractable cluster are considered.

Recently, herpes simplex virus was found to be associated with one patient with cluster headache, which is not too surprising (*Br. Med. J. [Clin Res]* 290:1625–1626, June 1, 1985). Other treatments are being evaluated. Fogan (*Arch. Neurol.* 42:362–363, April 1985) compared oxygen with air in the treat-ment of cluster headache and found a clear benefit to oxygen inhalation. Kit-trelle et al. found another old treatment, the use of local anesthetics in the area of the sphenopalatine fossa, to be useful, especially early in the course of the headache (*Arch. Neurol.* 42:496–498, May 1985). Solomon and Apfelbaum (Arch Neurol 43:479–437, May 1986), believing that the nervus intermedius may be responsible for the headache, surgically decompressed the root exit-entry zone of the facial nerve and found that it worked well in two of the five patients. Cluster headaches are a nice little mystery begging for a solution.—Robert D. Currier, M.D.

Cluster Headache: Local Anesthetic Abortive Agents
Jeffrey P. Kittrelle, David S. Grouse, and Marjorie E. Seybold (VA Med. Ctr. and Univ. of California at San Diego)
Arch. Neurol. 42:496–498, May 1985   10–2

It has recently been reported that dilute cocaine solution could abort cluster headache episodes, but it is unknown whether local anesthetics lacking the unique sympathomimetic properties of cocaine would be as effective. A trial of lidocaine hydrochloride was carried out in 5 patients with active cluster headache, 4 men and 1 woman aged 24–70 years. Three patients had a history of episodic unilateral attacks with extended periods of remission. Four patients had many autonomic accompaniments with each attack. Most supervised trials were performed after cluster headache was induced with 0.4 mg of nitroglycerin taken sublingually. The patient was placed supine 5–10 minutes after the onset of headache, and 1 ml of 4% lidocaine solution was slowly dropped into the ipsilateral nostril. Phenylephrine drops were used when necessary to relieve nasal congestion.

Ten headaches resembling spontaneous attacks were induced by nitroglycerin. Four patients had a 75% or greater reduction in headache intensity within 3 minutes of lidocaine application to the sphenopalatine fossa. Autonomic accompaniments were also relieved. Rhinorrhea stopped after 5–7 minutes. One patient failed to respond to either lidocaine or 5% cocaine solution. Three others reported excellent relief from spontaneous headaches with self-application of lidocaine.

Lidocaine, applied to the sphenopalatine fossa region, rapidly aborts cluster headaches; a local anesthetic action appears to be responsible. Lidocaine is potentially more useful than cocaine because it lacks abuse and habituation potential. Treatment is best given early in the course of headache, and concomitant use of a nasal decongestant may be necessary. A 1-ml dose of 4% lidocaine may be repeated once or twice within 15 minutes without significant risk.

▶ These results indicate that the anesthetic itself rather than the sympathomimetic effects are responsible for the cocaine-medicated abortion of acute cluster headaches.—Russell N. DeJong, M.D.

Do Certain Headache Syndromes Occur in "Pain-Prone" Patients?
Dewey K. Ziegler, Altan Kodanaz, and Ruth S. Hassanein (Univ. of Kansas)
Headache 25:90–94, March 1985   10–3

The clinical findings for 177 unselected patients with severe intermittent headaches were reviewed. The 130 female and 47 male patients had respective mean ages of 36 and 38 years (range, 13–75 years). Male patients had more frequent headaches and tended to report less energy. Pain at other sites was associated with an increased frequency of headache. Longer-lasting headaches occurred in female patients.

A history of fainting correlated both with inability to work during headache and patient perception of emotional stress as a precipitant of headache. Patients with arm or leg weakness before headache were more likely to report an increased frequency of fainting. Neither vomiting during headache nor unilateral pain was associated with other variables. High depression scores were associated with high anxiety scores and low energy levels. Younger patients with pain elsewhere tended to awaken with headache. Headache in the afternoon or evening was associated with advanced age, male sex, and a high energy level. No headache variables were associated with back pain.

A subgroup of persons with severe intermittent headaches appears to have emotional stress as a precipitant of headache. The "tension headache-neurosis" concept is of dubious value, however. Autonomic instability, as reflected in fainting, appears to be important in some headache syndromes. No specific headache characteristic has been associated with back pain, another common symptom.

▶ Garvey (*Headache* 25:101–103, March 1985) found that the frequency of headaches in patients given the diagnosis of anxiety disorder was no greater than that in nonanxious controls. Baier (*Neuropediatrics* 16:84–91, 1985), who studied the genetics of migraine, pointed out the largely maternal inheritance of the disorder. He also found that the prevalance of epileptic seizures was no greater in those with migraine.—Robert D. Currier, M.D.

Successful Migraine Prophylaxis With Naproxen Sodium
K. M. A. Welch, D. J. Ellis, and P. A. Keenan
Neurology 35:1304–1310, September 1985   10–4

Evidence of a role for prostaglandins in migraine led to a trial of the potent prostaglandin inhibitor naproxen sodium in patients with common or classic migraine who had had symptoms for at least 1 year and had had at least two attacks a month in 3 months. A double-blind, crossover trial was carried out with two 8-week treatment periods. Naproxen was taken in a dosage of 550 mg twice daily. Of the 35 patients who completed the study, 31 were evaluated.

Significant superiority of naproxen over placebo was evident (Fig 10–1). Fifty-two percent of patients were free from severe headache while taking naproxen and 19% while taking placebo. Patient records of attacks, nausea-vomiting, activity reduction, and use of other medications indicated substantially better results with naproxen than with placebo. The efficacy of naproxen did not correlate with the degree of platelet inhibition. Three

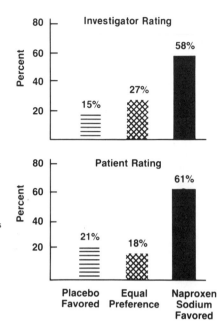

Fig 10–1.—The comparative rating of prophylactic efficacy for each treatment period is shown in terms of the percentage number of patients who preferred naproxen sodium over placebo on the basis of patient and investigator ratings. (Courtesy of Welch, K.M.A., et al.: Neurology 35:1304–1310, September 1985.)

patients had gastrointestinal disorder, including hematemesis, associated with naproxen use.

The efficacy of naproxen sodium in the treatment of migraine is not understood. Platelet inhibition was not significantly related to the clinical effect of the drug in this study. Changes in cranial blood flow or changes in control of the cerebral circulation could be involved. Naproxen can be recommended as the drug of first choice for the prevention of migraine.

▶ These observers state that naproxen sodium, a potent inhibitor of prostaglandin synthesis and platelet aggregation, can be recommended as "the drug of first choice for migraine prevention" in spite of uncertainty regarding its manner of action. This is a sweeping statement and further studies are necessary before this can be accepted.—Russell N. DeJong, M.D.

Naproxen in Prophylaxis of Migraine
Dewey K. Ziegler and David J. Ellis (Kansas Univ. and Syntex USA, Inc., Palo Alto, Calif.)
Arch. Neurol. 42:582–584, June 1985   10–5

Platelets from some patients with migraine aggregate more readily than normal and may release vasoactive products such as prostaglandins. The platelet-aggregating and prostaglandin synthesis inhibitor naproxen sodium was evaluated in a double-blind, placebo-controlled, cross-over study that involved 28 female patients and 6 male patients (mean age, 39.6 years). Naproxen was given in a dosage of 550 mg twice daily. The patients had had common or classic migraine headaches at a rate of at least two per month for a year or longer.

Patient ratings indicated that naproxen was preferred by far. Investigator ratings were similarly distributed. Patient diaries suggested that naproxen substantially reduced the severity and duration of headache, interference with activities, and use of medication. Substantially more patients had greater than 50% improvement during naproxen than with placebo. Nearly all side effects were mild, and their frequency was similar for the naproxen and placebo administration periods. One naproxen-treated patient withdrew because of stomach pain. No consistent drug-related laboratory abnormalities were seen.

A definite effect of naproxen is found in patients with classic or common migraine. The frequency and duration of episodes are reduced by naproxen. Whether the antiplatelet property of the drug, its antiprostaglandin activity, or both, is responsible remains to be established. Studies are needed to compare the efficacy of naproxen with that of the many other drugs used to prevent migraine.

▶ Naproxen sodium is a potent inhibitor of platelet aggregation and prostaglandin synthesis. It is also a significant anti-inflammatory and analgesic agent. This study demonstrates that it also shows promise in the prophylaxis of migraine. Further verification of the results is needed.—Russell N. DeJong, M.D.

Migraine Coma: Meningitic Migraine With Cerebral Oedema Associated With a New Form of Autosomal Dominant Cerebellar Ataxia

Robin B. Fitzsimons and W. H. Wolfenden (Sydney Hosp., Australia)
Brain 108:555–577, September 1985   10–6

Migraine is an infrequent cause of coma. However, data are presented on a family that for more than 40 years has had hemiplegic migraine associated with recurrent coma. Affected members of the family (Fig 10–2) also have cerebellar ataxia that is precipitated by migraine attacks, and ultimately they develop clinical features of autosomal dominant cerebellar ataxia.

Man, 30 years old (subject III.12), did not walk until age 2–3 years and apparently is mildly mentally retarded. Migrainous headaches have occurred since childhood, typically after trivial head injury. Tingling of the tongue, hemianopia, and numbness and weakness over the right extremities precede the onset of headache. Cerebellar signs were noted at age 11. Evaluation at age 23 and again at age 26 showed clear signs of a cerebellar abnormality and generalized hyperreflexia. Angiographic findings previously had been normal. An interepisode EEG showed dysrhythmia, with bursts of 4–6–Hz theta waves and of 3–4–Hz delta activity on hyperventilation. Computed tomography showed only cerebellar atrophy.

These cases are characterized by coma or profound stupor and are often precipitated by trivial head injury. Increased cellularity of the cerebrospinal fluid and fever were typical features. Hemispheric edema regularly developed in the week after onset of an attack, and massive hemispheric swelling could occur and prove life-threatening. The computed tomography findings

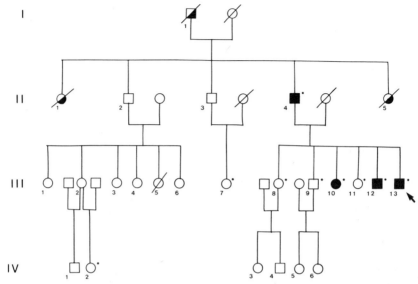

Fig 10–2.—Family pedigree. Cases examined and affected by the syndrome described are indicated by full-black shading. Cases affected by history are indicated by diagonal half-black shading. Subject III.7 (born in 1941), a British nursing lecturer, suffered from abdominal migraine in childhood and later from uncomplicated classic migraine. She has no signs of cerebellar abnormality. Subject IV.2 (born in 1977) had late motor and verbal milestones, but there is no present evidence of migraine, mental retardation, or cerebellar abnormality, and the EEG is normal. *Arrow* denotes the propositus. Cases examined by either author or another neurologist are indicated by *asterisk*. (Courtesy of Fitzsimons, R.B., and Wolfenden, W.H.: Brain 108:555–577, September 1985.)

for two family members are shown in Figure 10–3. Several patients have been intellectually slow or mentally retarded.

Possible causes of the cerebellar ataxia include damage from recurrent hyperthermia, phenytoin-induced degeneration, recurrent vascular insufficiency from vertebrobasilar ischemia, and a metabolic defect.

▶ Certainly, a very, very strange disorder. However, recalling my disbelief when I first heard of ataxia telangiectasia, there is little doubt that this peculiar collection of signs and symptoms also exists and is indeed hereditary. The authors note that members of this family tolerate cerebral angiography poorly and that the hemiplegia in these patients was probably associated with cerebral edema, as was the coma. How the ataxia fits in is uncertain. Blau and Solomon (*The Lancet* 2:718, Sept. 28, 1985) report a patient with migraine whose brain could be seen to swell through a craniotomy defect as the headache increased; the swelling was not delayed but was immediate. Meyer et al. (*The Lancet* 2:1308–1309, Dec. 7, 1985) took Blau to task.—Robert D. Currier, M.D.

Propranolol in the Prophylaxis of Migraine
J. W. Nadelmann, J. Stevens, and J. R. Saper (Ayerst Labs., New York, and Michigan Headache and Neurological Inst., Ann Arbor)
Headache 26:175–182, April 1986   10–7

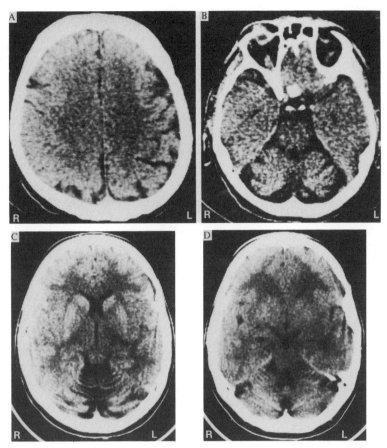

Fig 10–3.—A and B, noncontrast computed tomography scans of the father of propositus. A shows marked atrophy of the asymmetric cerebral hemisphere; B shows gross cerebellar atrophy, with enlargement of great horizontal fissure, cerebellar sulci, cerebellopontine angle cisterns, fourth ventricle, and pontine cisterns. C and D, noncontrast computed tomography scans of a sister of the propositus show marked atrophy in superior cerebellum, with involvement of lobuli simplices, quadrangular lobules, and semilunar lobules. (Courtesy of Fitzsimons, R.B., and Wolfenden, W.H.: Brain 108:555–577, September 1985.)

Several clinical trials have shown propranolol to be an effective means of preventing migraine. The present trial is the first with an upper dose range extending beyond 240 mg daily. Daily doses of 60–320 mg of propranolol were used in a 34-week, placebo-controlled, cross-over study conducted in a double-blind manner. The starting dosage of propranolol was 20 mg four times daily, with dose-finding at about 2-week intervals (Fig 10–4).

The 62 patients who completed the dose-finding phase exhibited fewer and/or less marked headaches after propranolol administration. Prophylaxis appeared to be effective in both severe and less marked cases of migraine (Fig 10–5). In 41 patients who completed the cross-over phase of the study, propranolol administration reduced migraine to a significant

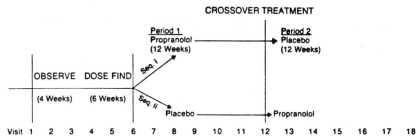

Fig 10–4.—Design of study. (Courtesy of Nadelmann, J.W., et al.: Headache 26:175–182, April 1986.)

degree with respect to both the headache itself and the therapeutic medication needed. Prophylaxis was effective against all types of migraine. Patients' weight increased with active prophylaxis. Both heart rate and blood pressure decreased. The changes were well tolerated and did not lead to withdrawals from the study. No significant chest radiograph or ECG changes were noted.

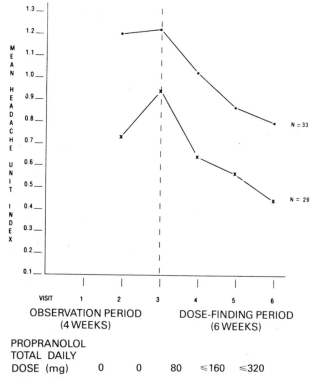

Fig 10–5.—Mean headache unit index by visit and final propranolol dosage for patients who completed the dose-finding period. (Courtesy of Nadelmann, J.W., et al.: Headache 26:175–182, April 1986.)

More than half of the patients in this trial received the maximum dose of propranolol—320 mg per day. Use of such a dose could lower the need for multiple ancillary medications in the treatment of acute migraine attacks. Propranolol prophylaxis was well tolerated. The lack of serious side effects and propranolol's usefulness in treating angina and hypertension make it a useful drug.

▶ This is a very carefully carried out, placebo-controlled, single cross-over, double-blinded study. It not only confirms what is now quite well accepted, that propranolol is an efficacious agent in the prophylaxis of common and classic migraine headache, but it also shows that propranolol in dosages larger than those usually prescribed for patient with migraine is well tolerated in outpatients, and that such dosages may reduce the need for multiple ancillary medications in the treatment of severe attacks of migraine. The value of the drug, not only in the control of migraine but also in the treatment of hypertension, angina, and thyrotoxicosis, makes it a valuable agent in the physician's armamentarium.—Russell N. DeJong, M.D.

General Comments

On the question of who gets a computed tomography (CT) scan in a migraine clinic Joseph et al. (*Practitioner* 229:447–481, May 1985) report on 1,900 consecutive patients seen in a headache clinic. Of 48 who were thought to have focal intracranial pathology, 6 were shown by CT scans to have mass lesions. Of the six, two had papilledema, one had a visual field defect, and the other three had recent changes in their neurologic state or in their headaches. So about one in 300 patients in a headache clinic really must have a CT scan, and the requirement for the CT scan can be determined by the history and examination.—Robert D. Currier, M.D.

11 Infections of the Nervous System

Meningitis Due to _Staphylococcus aureus_
James J. Gordon, Donald H. Harter, and John P. Phar (Northwestern Univ.)
Am. J. Med. 78:965–970, June 1985   11–1

Meningitis due to _S. aureus_ is an occasional complication of neurosurgery but is less frequent in the community setting. Information was reviewed on 10 adult patients treated for _S. aureus_ meningitis that was acquired in the community between 1976 and 1984. Of the seven men and three women (mean age, 57 years), four were diabetic, two had cancer, and two had a history of hypothyroidism. One patient each had a history of alcohol abuse and intravenous drug abuse, and 1 had recently had a myocardial infarction. All patients had a focus of infection outside the CNS. Acute bacterial endocarditis was present in 4. _Staphylococcus aureus_ was cultured from all peripheral sites of infection.

The presenting features included a mean oral temperature of 104.1 F, nuchal rigidity, headache, and deteriorating mental state. Half of the patients had myalgias, arthralgias, and weakness. The mean white blood cell count at admission was 19,400/cu mm. Hyponatremia was a constant feature; the 3 patients who later died were the most hyponatremic at presentation. The cerebrospinal fluid consistently showed marked pleocytosis with a predominance of polymorphonuclear cells. The average cerebrospinal fluid glucose concentration was 46 mg/dl. Six patients received nafcillin or oxacillin from the outset and did well, with no neurologic sequelae. Defervescence was especially rapid in patients given oxacillin or nafcillin plus rifampin. Three patients died with persistent or recurrent bacteremia and purulent bronchopneumonia, abscess formation, and cardiovascular collapse.

Combined treatment with rifampin and another antistaphylococcal antibiotic appears to be the most effective regimen for _S. aureus_ meningitis, but prospective randomized trials are needed. The high morbidity and mortality from community-acquired _S. aureus_ meningitis in adults warrant aggressive treatment.

▶ These investigators found that the administration of rifampin together with another antistaphylococcal antibiotic was the most effective regimen for the treatment of meningitis due to _S. aureus_. This should be proved by other investigators.—Russell N. DeJong, M.D.

Bacterial Antigen Detection in Cerebrospinal Fluid of Patients With Meningitis

D. J. Hoban, E. Witwicki, and G. W. Hammond (Univ. of Manitoba and the Cadham Provincial Lab., Winnipeg)

Diagn. Microbiol. Infect. Dis. 3:373–379, September 1985   11–2

The efficacy of four test systems in the detection of *Haemophilus influenzae* type b, *Streptococcus pneumoniae*, *Neisseria meningitidis*, and gram-negative organisms in the cerebrospinal fluid was assessed. The results obtained over an 18-month period with the Phadebact coagglutination (CoA) test, the Directigen latex agglutination (LA) test, counterimmunoelectrophoresis (CIE), and the Limulus amebocyte lysate (LAL) test were compared with the culture findings in patients with suspected meningitis or CNS shunt infection and more than 10 white blood cells in the cerebrospinal fluid (CSF). Ninety-nine specimens that were culture-positive for bacteria and 56 negative specimens from aseptic meningitis were studied.

Sensitivity for the detection of *H. influenzae* type b ranged from 67% for CIE to 78% for both the CoA and LA tests. The specificity of the tests was similar. The LA and CoA tests were most sensitive in detection of *S. pneumoniae* in the CSF, and all tests were quite specific. The LAL test was 77% sensitive in the detection of gram-negative organisms, but 8 false positive results were obtained, 2 in cases where no organism was present. The CoA test was most cost-effective for routine diagnostic use. The CIE test took considerably longer than either the CoA or LA tests.

Commerical agglutination tests are highly specific in the detection of bacterial antigen in CSF in patients with meningitis and are more sensitive than the CIE test. Detection of *N. meningitidis* is difficult with all test systems. It may be best to use both a rapid agglutination test and a method of detection of bacterial endotoxin. Rapid slide tests, such as the LA or CoA and LAL, are easier to use than is the CIE test and offer increased sensitivity.

▶ Rapid identification of the bacteria responsible for septic meningitis is necessary for specific antimicrobial therapy. Existing tests include the examination of fluid for bacteria by using various stains and detection of antigens. Microscopic examination has obvious limitations, particularly in pretreated meningitis. These authors present their experience with commercially available antigen detection tests and compare them to the more sophisticated method CIE. The commercial tests were more sensitive than CIE and were highly specific. Such tests should become a routine for evaluation of CSF in patients with suspected bacterial meningitis.—Owen. B. Evans, M.D.

▶ Once meningitis is diagnosed, the question is, what to use in the treatment? A recent survey (Schlech, W. F., III, et al.: *JAMA* 253:1749–1754, March 22/29, 1985) of 18,642 cases of meningitis in the United States that were reported to the Centers for Disease Control for a 3-year period from 1978 through 1981 showed that *H. influenzae* was the most frequent cause of bacterial meningitis, causing nearly half of the reported cases, followed by *N.*

meningitidis (20%) and *S. pneumoniae* (13%). Two recent reports of the third-generation cephalosporins ceftriaxone (Barson, W. J., et al.: *Pediatr. Infect. Dis.* 4:362–368, July/August 1985) and cefotaxime (Jacobs, R. F., et al.: *J. Pediatr.* 107:129–133, July 1985) show them to be as good as conventional therapy. But a lot more expensive. Chloramphenicol, after all these years, still appears to be a good drug.—Robert D. Currier, M.D.

Vidarabine Versus Acyclovir Therapy in Herpes Simplex Encephalitis
Richard J. Whitley, Charles A. Alford, Martin S. Hirsch, Robert T. Schooley, James P. Luby, Fred Y. Aoki, Daniel Hanley, Andre J. Nahmias, Seng-Jaw Soong, and the NIAID Collaborative Antiviral Study Group (Univ. of Alabama; Massachusetts Gen. Hosp., Boston; Univ. of Texas at Dallas-Southwestern; Univ. of Manitoba; Johns Hopkins Univ.; and Emory Univ.)
N. Engl. J. Med. 314:144–149, Jan. 16, 1986   11–3

In 1977, the National Institute of Allergy and Infectious Diseases Collaborative Antiviral Study Group demonstrated that mortality from biopsy-proved herpes simplex encephalitis decreased significantly 6 months after treatment with vidarabine (adenine arabinoside)—from 70% in placebo recipients to 44% in drug recipients. The introduction into pharmacokinetic studies and clinical trials of acyclovir, a selective inhibitor of herpes simplex virus replication, provided the opportunity to examine the activity of a more soluble and potent antiviral drug in the treatment of this disease.

A total of 208 randomly assigned patients who underwent diagnostic brain biopsy for presumptive herpes simplex encephalitis received either vidarabine (15 mg/kg per day) or acyclovir (30 mg/kg per day) for 10

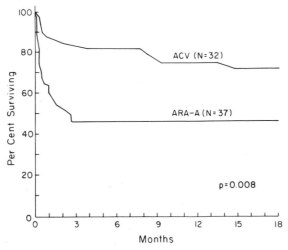

Fig 11–1.—Comparison of survival in patients with biopsy-proved herpes simplex encephalitis treated with vidarabine (ARA-A) or acyclovir (ACV); P = .008. (Courtesy of Whitley, R.J., et al.: N. Engl. J. Med. 314:144–149, Jan. 16, 1986. Reprinted by permission of The New England Journal of Medicine.)

days. Figure 11–1 contrasts the survival data for the 69 patients (33%) with biopsy-proved disease.

The mortality in the vidarabine recipients was 54%, compared with 28% in the acyclovir recipients ($P = .008$). The six-month mortality varied according to the Glasgow coma score at the onset of therapy. For scores of >10, 7–10, and <6, the mortality was 42%, 46%, and 67%, respectively, in the patients treated with vidarabine, compared with 0, 25, and 25%, respectively, in those treated with acyclovir. A 6-month morbidity assessment with the use of an adapted scoring system revealed that 5 (14%) of 37 patients receiving vidarabine compared with 12 (38%) of 32 receiving acyclovir were functioning normally ($P = .021$). Eight (22%) vidarabine-treated patients and 3 (9%) acyclovir-treated patients had moderate debility. Patients younger than 30 years of age and with a Glasgow coma score above 10 had the best results with acyclovir treatment.

Acyclovir is the treatment of choice for biopsy-proved herpes simplex encephalitis, particularly in the absence of serious toxicity. Although vidarabine was not as effective, it does have a role in treatment for this disease. The beneficial effects of early acyclovir therapy for herpes simplex encephalitis should advance the development of early noninvasive diagnostic procedures for deployment before irreversible brain damage occurs.

▶ Clearly, acyclovir is the treatment of choice for herpes simplex encephalitis. It seems a rather benign drug, and early treatment is so important that overusage is predictable and probably correct when herpes simplex encephalitis is suspected.—Robert D. Currier, M.D.

Antibodies to Human T-Lymphotrophic Virus Type I in Patients With Tropical Spastic Paraparesis

A. Gessain, F. Barin, J. C. Vernant, O. Gout, L. Maurs, A. Calender, and G. de Thé (Faculté de Medicine Alexis Carrel, Lyon, and Université F. Rabelais, Tours, France, and Centre Hospitalier Régional de Fort de France, Martinique)
Lancet 2:407–410, Aug. 24, 1985   11–4

Tropical spastic paraparesis (TSP) is a slowly progressive myelopathy involving mainly the pyramidal tracts. The finding of human T cell lymphotropic virus type I (HTLV-I) antibodies in two patients with TSP in Martinique led to a study of 17 patients in whom TSP was diagnosed between 1973 and 1981. The patients had spastic paraparesis or paraplegia with pyramidal signs, and some also had a mild distal sensory deficit or sphincter impairment. The onset was gradual and the progress slow. The 13 female and 4 male patients had a mean age of 52 years (range, 12–66 years) at the onset of disease. Controls included 24 neurologic patients without cord involvement, 27 healthy nurses or laboratory workers, and 252 blood donors.

All 5 patients with TSP and systemic symptoms and more than half of all those with TSP were positive for HTLV-I antibodies by enzyme-linked immunosorbent assay, compared with fewer than 5% of controls. All samples from patients with TSP positive for HTLV-I antibodies reacted in the Western blot test. No serum samples from patients with TSP were positive for HTLV-III antibody, although serum from one of 108 blood donors was positive.

These findings suggest either that HTLV-I is a neurotropic virus or that the virus or a related one contributes to the pathogenesis of TSP. Nearly 60% of the patients with TSP in this study and all those with systemic symptoms had antibodies to HTLV-I. There is evidence that HTLV-III is neurotropic. The association between HTLV-I and non-Hodgkin's lymphoma in the Caribbean islands has prompted a study of possible clustering of these disorders in HTLV-I-positive families.

Acute Syphilitic Meningitis: Its Occurrence After Clinical and Serologic Cure of Secondary Syphilis With Penicillin G
Lydia L. Bayne, James W. Schmidley, and Douglas S. Goodin (Univ. of California at San Francisco)
Arch. Neurol. 43:137–138, February 1986   11–5

A patient was encountered who developed acute syphilitic meningitis despite apparent clinical and serologic cure of secondary syphilis.

Man, a 36-year-old homosexual, developed lesions on the palms and soles with a reactive serum VDRL test. He received 2.4 million units of intramuscular penicillin G benzathine and promptly recovered. A bioccipital headache developed 3 months after presentation and recurred with fevers, mild neck stiffness, nausea, and vomiting. An episode of left ear tinnitus and hearing loss also occurred, and the right eye was blind for several seconds on standing.

The right optic disc margin was blurred, and the neck was stiff. The ankle jerks were absent bilaterally. The serum VDRL and fluorescent treponeural antibody absorption tests were positive. An EEG showed bursts of high-voltage slow waves in the right frontal region. The opening cerebrospinal fluid pressure was 180 mm H_2O. The fluid contained 140 leukocytes/cu mm with 95% mononuclear cells and a protein of 165 mg/dl. The VDRL was trace positive, and oligoclonal bands were present. Symptoms resolved with intravenous penicillin therapy over 10 days, and a cerebrospinal response was documented. The fundi were normal 5 months later, and hearing had improved. The patient was clinically unchanged 2 years later.

Five of seven patients seen in the past 3 years with meningeal or meningovascular syphilis had been treated with penicillin. Reinfection was convincingly ruled out only in the present case, but two other patients had a similar clinical picture. Failure of penicillin therapy may be seen more often as primary and secondary syphilis continue to increase. A history of treatment does not exclude a syphilitic cause of lymphocytic meningitis. It might be best to document treatment adequacy by lumbar puncture after 6 months.

▶ It is important to know that acute syphilitic meningitis may develop in a patient despite apparent clinical and serologic cure of primary and secondary syphilis when intramuscular penicillin therapy is used as recommended by the current Centers for Disease Control Guidelines. In this reported case, there was prompt clinical and serologic response to intravenous penicillin therapy. There have been several other case histories of this type reported in the recent literature (Moskovitz, B. L., et al.: *Arch. Intern. Med. 142:139–140, 1982;* Bayne, L. L., et al.: *Neurology* 34[Suppl. 1]:137, 1984). Syphilitic meningitis remains a difficult disease to treat.—Russell N. DeJong, M.D.

Inappropriate Use of the Cerebrospinal Fluid Venereal Disease Research Laboratory (VDRL) Test to Exclude Neurosyphilis

Peter E. Dans, Lee Cafferty, Sharon E. Otter, and Robert J. Johnson (Johns Hopkins Univ.)

Ann. Intern. Med. 104:86–89, January 1986   11–6

From 1977 to 1980, 24 (0.26%) of 9,200 cerebrospinal fluid (CSF) VDRL tests were positive. Because the rate of positivity for 1980 (0.12%) did not differ significantly from that for the other 3 years ($P = 0.015$), the authors concentrated their analyses on that year's data.

Of 1,598 serum fluorescent treponemal antibody absorption tests read as positive or borderline in 1980, only 226 (9%) were in patients who also had a CSF-VDRL test (table). Only 3 of 2,536 CSF-VDRL tests ordered in 1980 were positive. Records, which were available for 156 (69%) of the 226 patients, including all 3 with positive CSF-VDRL tests, were reviewed and showed that the diagnosis of neurosyphilis had been considered only in 44 (28%). One third of the records lacked notations of

RELATIONSHIP OF FINDINGS OF THE CEREBROSPINAL
FLUID-VDRL (CSF-VDRL) TEST AND THE SERUM
FLUORESCENT TREPONEMAL ANTIBODY ABSORPTION
(FTA-ABS) TEST

Serum FTA-ABS	CSF-VDRL			
	Positive	Negative	Not Done	Total
		n		
Positive or borderline	3*	223†	1372	1598
Negative	0	‡	N/A	392
Not done	0	‡	N/A	. . .
Total	3	2533	. . .	. . .

*All serum FTA-ABS tests were positive; serum VDRL titers were 2, 64, and 128 dilutions.

†Nine serum FTA-ABS tests were borderline.

‡Distribution of the remaining 2,310 results (those in patients in whom the serum FTA-ABS test was ordered and was negative and those for whom it was not ordered) is unknown because the records of negative tests were unavailable. Beginning in 1980, the laboratory had a policy of not doing the serum FTA-ABS test unless the rapid plasma reagin test was positive or, if negative, a specific request was made because of clinical suspicion. Thus, the number of instances in which the FTA–ABS test was ordered and was negative cannot exceed 392, which is the number of negative tests in 1980 from all the Johns Hopkins Hospital sources; the likely number is probably a tiny fraction of this number.

(Courtesy of Dans, P.E., et al.: Ann. Intern Med. 104:86–89, January 1986.)

historical and physical findings characteristic of neurosyphilis. Forty seropositive patients who had lumbar puncture to rule out asymptomatic neurosyphilis had negative CSF-VDRL tests; in none was a diagnosis of neurosyphilis made. Physicians documented the stage of syphilis in only 49 (31%) of the 156 patients; the predominant stages were late latent syphilis and adequately treated serofast syphilis. Two patients suspected of having neurosyphilis had positive CSF-VDRL tests and were diagnosed and treated accordingly. Two others in whom neurosyphilis was suspected had completely normal CSF results. Their discharge diagnoses were cardiovascular syphilis and "history of adequately treated neurosyphilis," respectively. Most patients (55%) had no neuropsychiatric diagnosis at discharge, but of those who did, the most common were cerebrovascular accident, dementia, seizures, syncope, and organic brain syndrome. The CSF findings appeared to lack specificity, because 14 (16%) of 86 patients with no neuropsychiatric diagnosis had abnormal findings. In contrast, of 70 patients with neuropsychiatric diagnoses, 51 (73%) had virtually normal CSF findings.

The CSF-VDRL test is better at "ruling in" than ruling out neurosyphilis. To prove this point, it may be assumed that the test has a sensitivity of 50% and a specificity of 99.95% and that the pretest probability of the disease is similar to that for the present overall study population, 60/10,000. A positive test raises the probability of neurosyphilis over 100-fold, to 30/35, whereas a negative test only lowers it two-fold to 30/9,965. The same holds if the test is used under the most favorable conditions, for example, in a seropositive patient with clinical findings suggestive of meningovascular syphilis. In this case, a pretest probability of 90%, a test sensitivity of 90%, and a test specificity of 99.95% are assumed. A positive CSF-VDRL test is virtually diagnostic, whereas the likelihood of neurosyphilis given a negative test is still 47%. As long as the CSF-VDRL test remains the test of choice for the diagnosis of neurosyphilis, it is best used either in seropositive patients with neuropsychiatric signs or in seronegative patients with neuropsychiatric signs suggestive of syphilis.

▶ The authors clearly point out that ordering a CSF-VDRL test without considering whether it is necessary is useless and wasteful. As a young man I ordered this test for years, not realizing that with a negative serum and an otherwise normal CSF and no reason to suspect syphilis the chance of finding anything with this test was nil.—Robert D. Currier, M.D.

Types of Progressive Paralysis: Not a Theme of the Past
A. Risse, A. Rohde, and A. Marneros (Univ. of Cologne, Federal Republic of Germany)
Dtsch. Med. Wochenschr. 110:1202–1205, 1985   11–7

Neurosyphilis is not a conquered disease. To the contrary, the number of registered new cases in the Federal Republic of Germany has shown a small but continuing increase in the past 10 years. In fact, since the end of the 1960s, the incidence has tripled. In this study, the following questions were considered: (1) What are the syndromatic forms of progressive paralysis? (2) What are the most common symptoms? (3) With which other pathologic conditions can the apparent symptoms of progressive paralysis be confused?

Investigations carried out between 1950 and 1979 on 293 patients with progressive paralysis showed that there is no classic form of this disease. Megalomania was found in only 13% of the patients and a manic state in fewer than 50%. Disturbances in affectivity, drive, and intellectual functions among patients with progressive paralysis were, in general, uncharacteristic of the disease and could appear in any psychotic syndrome.

Only about one third of the patients were found to be productively psychotic. Twenty-five percent of the 293 patients showed delusions, 17% hallucinations, and 1% identity disturbances. Symptoms of schizophrenia

MOST FREQUENT TYPES OF NEUROLOGIC DISTURBANCES IN PROGRESSIVE
PARALYSIS (n = 293)

Total neurologic disturbances	97%
Neurologically inconspicuous	3%
Dysarthria	64%
Pupil disturbances	64%
Argyll-Robertson-Pupil	34%
Anisocoria	30%
Absolute pupil rigidity	14%
Lazy light reaction	11%
Others	2%
Reflex anomalies	33%
Mimic quivering	14%
Gangataxia	14%
Pathological reflexes	12%
Convulsive attacks	12%
Dysdiadochokinesia	11%
Other coordination disturbances	9%
Hypoislands or analgesic islands	5%
Lancinating pain	4%
Slight tremor	4%
Aphasia	8%

(Courtesy of Risse, A., et al.: Dtsch. Med. Wochenschr. 110:1202–1205, 1985.)

were found in only 1% of the patients and optic and acoustic hallucinations in 9%. Depressive syndromes were relatively rare (6%) and syndromes that include a change between manic- and depressive-type symptoms were even rarer (2%). The largest group of nonproductive psychologic symptoms were the affectivity disturbances (79%). Ninety-seven percent of the patients had neurologic symptoms, the most frequent of which were pupil disturbances and dysarthria. However, it is suprising that one third of the patients did not show these typical neurologic symptoms of progressive paralysis (table).

In order to avoid misdiagnosis, a thorough neurologic examination is essential. Neurologic symptoms taken as characteristic for progressive paralysis such as the Argyll-Robertson phenomenon or mimic quivering are more the exception than the rule. Diagnosis with the serum and cerebrospinal fluid examination (TPHA test) is simple and effective. The possibility of progressive paralysis should be considered in patients with unclassifiable psychopathologic neurologic syndromes.

▶ I haven't seen a case of dementia paralytica of syphilis for I don't know how long. This is a timely reminder of the fact that it's still around and may not be classic in its presentation. However, Talbot and Morton (*Genitourin. Med.* 61:95–98, 1985) believe that neurosyphilis still looks like neurosyphilis ("the most common things are most common") and attribute the apparently uncommon presentation to many factors, including earlier presentation and partial treatment.—Robert D. Currier, M.D.

Late Effects of Poliomyelitis. Part I: Report of Five Cases
David O. Wiechers and Lauro S. Halstead (Ohio State University and Baylor College of Medicine)
South. Med. J. 78:1277–1280, November 1985   11–8

Five representative case reports concerning the development of muscle weakness, atrophy, and fasciculations many years after recovery from poliomyelitis were presented.

Male, age 47 years, contracted poliomyelitis at age 18. All extremities were involved, and a respirator was required. The muscles of both legs were of normal strength upon maximal functional and neurologic recovery 3 years later. The patient was extremely active physically in the following years. Sixteen years after the initial illness, muscle weakness and paresthesias developed. There were no metabolic abnormalities, and a computed tomography scan and lumbosacral spine radiographs were normal. The condition progressed, with generalized weakness, fatigue, and fasciculations. Electromyographic analysis showed extensive (90%) reinnervation of the motor units of the left tibialis anterior, with unstable and repetitive discharge on voluntary activation. The remaining case histories are summarized in the table.

Generally, muscle weakness is of gradual onset, increases with time, and is frequently associated with muscle pain. However, other coexistent medical problems must be ruled out. The cause of this delayed muscle weakness

CHARACTERISTICS OF FIVE PATIENTS WITH HISTORY OF ACUTE
PARALYTIC POLIOMYELITIS

Case	Age (Years)	Sex	Age at Onset	Year of Onset	Interval From Polio to New Symptoms (Years)	Clinical History and Diagnosis
1	47	M	18 yr	1954	28	Progressive weakness, muscle pain, and fatigue; cause unknown
2	49	F	2 yr	1936	30	Progressive weakness and fatigue; cause unknown
3	27	F	9 mo	1956	25	Diffuse muscle pain due to fibrositis syndrome
4	48	M	12 yr	1947	34	Back pain due to scoliosis, muscle imbalance, and obesity
5	42	F	6 yr	1948	36	Sudden onset of left arm weakness due to radiculopathy

(Courtesy of Wiechers, D.O., and Halstead, L.S.: South. Med. J. 78:1277–1280, November 1985. Reprinted by permission from the Southern Medical Journal.)

is not known, but recent evidence suggests the contribution of immuno-pathologic mechanisms in some patients. Abnormalities in the transmission of impulses to muscle fibers, as well as subsequent innervation of additional muscle fibers by the same motor neuron, may be pertinent factors. Motor neurons are also lost with age, a process that can further compromise muscle strength in these patients. The term *postpolio syndrome* should be reserved for only those patients with a definite progression of neuromuscular abnormalities in the absence of other medical problems.

Part II: Results of a Survey of 201 Polio Survivors
Lauro S. Halstead, David O. Wiechers, and C. Donald Rossi (Baylor College of Medicine and Inst. for Rehabilitation and Research, Houston, and Ohio State Univ.)
South. Med. J. 78:1281–1287, November 1985   11–9

A questionnaire concerning the late effects of poliomyelitis was sent to about 500 survivors of the disease in 1983, and 221 replies were received. Half of the 201 assessable respondents had acquired polio in 1949 or later; the peak year was 1952 (range, 1909–1963).

Sixty-three percent of subjects married after the onset of polio, and all but 5% have worked at least part-time. The age at onset and ventilator use at the onset also both increased over the years. Most subjects reported some neurologic and functional recovery regardless of the initial severity of involvement, with maximum recovery attained a median of 6 years after the onset. Peak recovery was sustained for a median of 26 years, before many patients developed significant new health problems and functional changes, especially wheelchair and ventilator use. New difficulty in walking, bladder problems, difficulties in dressing and in sexual function, sensory changes, and the need for more sleep also were described. Late effects were most frequent in those who at onset required hospitalization, were older than age 10 years, required ventilatory assistance, or had weakness or paralysis of all extremities.

Persons with a history of polio should use caution in undertaking exercise programs and strenuous activities but should remain as active as possible within the limits of comfort. Extended activities should be interrupted periodically by rest.

▶ The authors (Digests 11–8, 11–9) have done a service by clarifying the situation with this syndrome. It amounts to a rather benign worsening and affects those who were more severely paralyzed at onset.

Dalakas et al. (N. Engl. J. Med. 314:959–963, April 10, 1986), who studied the syndrome in 26 patients, found just about the same thing. The new difficulty began 25 to 30 years after the polio and was very slowly progressive. They feel that it is a "dysfunction of the surviving motor neurons that causes a slow disintegration of the terminals of the individual nerve axons".—Robert D. Currier, M.D.

Diagnosis of Creutzfeldt-Jakob Disease by Western Blot Identification of Marker Protein in Human Brain Tissue
Paul Brown, Millicent Coker-Vann, Kitty Pomeroy, Maryellen Franko, David M. Asher, Clarence J. Gibbs, Jr., and D. Carleton Gajdusek (Natl. Insts. of Health, Bethesda, Md.)
N. Engl. J. Med. 314:547–551, Feb. 27, 1986   11–10

A fibrillary structure containing a group of protease-resistant proteins having relative molecular weights of 27–30 kilodaltons has been found in brain tissue preparations from humans with Creutzfeldt-Jakob disease (CJD) and animals with scrapie. Immunologic study was made of brain tissue from 39 patients with CJD, kuru, or Gerstmann-Sträussler-Scheinker syndrome, and from 32 patients with other chronic neurologic disorders without spongiform degeneration. Western blots against antiserum to purified fraction of scrapie-infected hamster brain were used.

Western blot tests were positive in brain specimens from 81% of 31 patients with CJD, 3 of 4 with kuru, and 3 of 4 with Gerstmann-Sträussler-Scheinker syndrome. No positive tests were obtained in the neurologic control group. Sporadic and familial cases of CJD had similar findings, but specimens from patients who were ill for longer than 2 years were more often positive. Electron microscopy showed fibrils in all eight immunoblot-positive CJD specimens examined, but neither in two immunoblot-negative CJD cases nor in control cases. Specimens from both immunoblot-positive Gerstmann-Sträussler-Scheinker preparations examined contained fibrils.

Antiserum against purified scrapie-infected hamster brain reliably detects an antigen present in brain tissue from most patients with transmissible spongiform encephalopathies, but not in specimens from patients with other chronic neurologic disorders. Immunologic methods may provide a useful, rapid adjunct to neuropathologic study and animal transmission experiments in the diagnosis of spongiform encephalopathies.

▶ It appears that we are on the way to having a laboratory test in addition to neuropathologic examinations and animal transmission study for the diagnosis of these diseases. A piece of brain is still necessary, however. May we hope that a cerebrospinal fluid test will come along?—Robert D. Currier, M.D.

Sporadic Postinfectious Neuromyasthenia

Irving E. Salit (Toronto Gen. Hosp.)
Can. Med. Assoc. J. 133:659–663, October 1, 1985   11–11

Neuromyasthenia is characterized by fatigue, depression, myalgia, muscular weakness, headaches, and paresthesias. The illness occurs primarily in young and middle-aged women and may persist for years with frequent relapses. Fifty cases were reviewed, with an attempt at identification of the precipitating infectious agent, as well as clinical presentation and follow-up.

The cause of the initial infection was known in 28 of 50 patients; Epstein-Barr virus was identified in 16 of the 28 cases. Table 1 lists all identified infectious agents. The most common symptoms were "flu-like" (Table 2): upper respiratory tract infection, sore throat, and cervical lymphadenopathy. The chronic phase of the illness was characterized by incapacitating exhaustion, especially after exertion. This interfered considerably with the patient's work and activity. Physical examination and laboratory results were generally normal.

TABLE 1.—Infectious Agents Identified

Agent	No. of patients*
Epstein–Barr virus (EBV)	16
Coxsackievirus B	4
Giardia lamblia	2
Mycoplasma pneumoniae	2
Toxoplasma gondii	2
Hepatitis A virus	1
Herpes zoster virus	1
Cytomegalovirus	1
Unknown	22

*One patient and evidence of infection with both EBV and coxsackievirus.
(Courtesy of Salit, I.E.: Can. Med. Assoc. J. 133:659–663, October 1, 1985. Originally published in the Canadian Medical Association Journal.)

TABLE 2.—COMMON SYMPTOMS
OF NEUROMYASTHENIA

Symptom	No. of patients
Exhaustion	47
Malaise	40
Postexertional exacerbation of fatigue	38
Weakness	37
Headache	30
Fever	30
Subjective	26
Objective	4
Inability to concentrate	28
Frequent upper respiratory tract infections	27
Myalgia	25
Dizziness, lightheadedness	23
Allergies	21
Lymphadenopathy	21
Sleepiness	16

(Courtesy of Salit, I.E.: Can. Med. Assoc. J. 133:659–663, October 1, 1985. Originally published in the Canadian Medical Association Journal.)

Epidemic neuromyasthenia may be more a collection of symptoms than a disease and may have a marked psychologic component. However, data exist implicating chronic infection and subtle physiologic alterations in the etiology of this condition. Patients require continuing support, both emotional and, if possible, therapeutic. Specific therapy is unavailable, but symptomatic treatment can result in considerable improvement.

▶ This diagnosis sometimes is the only one that will fit certain situations and I am glad to hear that it has not been put in the psychogenic disease trash bin. It is interesting that the Epstein-Barr virus seems to be the commonest known cause in this series. Not so long ago we had no idea what the virus was.—Robert D. Currier, M.D.

12 Intoxications Affecting the Nervous System

Subacute Sequelae of Carbon Monoxide Poisoning
Roy A. M. Myers, Susan K. Snyder, and Timothy A. Emhoff (Maryland Inst. for Emergency Med. Services Systems, Baltimore)
Ann. Emerg. Med. 14:1163–1167, December 1985   12–1

A wide range of neuropsychiatric abnormalities, including Korsakoff's syndrome, cortical blindness, a syndrome resembling multiple sclerosis, peripheral neuritis, dementia, psychosis, parkinsonian syndromes, Wernicke's aphasia, manic-depressive psychosis, and almost every known neurologic syndrome, can occur following carbon monoxide (CO) poisoing.

From January 1980 to August 1983, 213 patients with CO poisoning were seen at the Hyperbaric Medicine Department, which has the only civilian hyperbaric chamber in Maryland. The 213 patients were divided into two groups as the result of the correlation of carboxyhemoglobin (HbCO) levels with clinical presentation and psychometric testing. The first group (131 patients) either had initial HbCO levels of more than 30% or presented with neurologic impairment. This group received hyperbaric oxygen therapy and had no sequelae. The second group (82 patients) had either initial HbCO levels of less than 30%, normal responses on psychometric testing, or low HbCO levels (< 30%), but showed borderline responses to the psychometric testing. These patients were treated with normobaric oxygen; 10 (12.1%) returned with clinically significant sequelae including headaches, irritability, personality changes, confusion, and memory loss. This recurrent symptomatology developed within 1–21 days (mean, 5.7 days) after the initial exposure, although no reexposure occurred. These recurring symptoms resolved rapidly with hyperbaric oxygen therapy.

The addition of the psychometric testing helped to define the group of patients requiring aggressive therapy (hyperbaric oxygen) and improved the ability to diagnose CO CNS involvement.

The resolution of symptomatology and return to the conscious level is far more rapid and possibly more complete with hyperbaric oxygen treatment than with normobaric or surface oxygen treatments. Hyperbaric oxygen therapy should be used whenever CO poisoning symptoms recur.

▶ The conclusion of this article is clear enough, namely, that any patient with a suspicion of carbon monoxide intoxication should receive hyperbaric oxygen therapy.—Robert D. Currier, M.D.

147

Association of High Cyanide and Low Sulfur Intake in Cassava-Induced Spastic Paraparesis

Julie Cliff, Per Lundqvist, Johannes Mårtensson, Hans Rosling, and Bo Sörbo (Ministry of Health, Lourenço Marques, Mozambique; and Linköping Univ. and Uppsala Univ., Sweden)

Lancet 2:1211–1212, Nov. 30, 1985   12–2

Nutritional neuropathies occur in several malnourished populations in tropical regions, and exposure to cyanide from the eating of cassava has been implicated in some of these areas in Africa. Cassava root contains cyanogenic glycosides that are ingested when it is eaten without processing, as with food shortage during a drought. A deficiency of sulfur-containing amino acids can impede cyanide detoxification. Acute spastic paraparesis has been described in a drought-affected area of Mozambique when toxic cassava types with a very high cyanide content were the only food available and the roots were eaten without being sun-dried.

The study was done in Nampula Province in northern Mozambique during the 1982 and 1983 harvests (after the epidemic of spastic paraparesis), when similar but less severe dietary circumstances prevailed. Urine was collected from 30 (1982) or 31 (1983) apparently healthy children in the school in a village located in the center of the epidemic. The children studied had increased thiocyanate and decreased inorganic sulfate excretion, a finding that suggests a high cyanide intake and a low intake of sulfur-containing amino acids. Children from a nearby area that did not have any cases of apastic paraparesis had lower thiocyanate and higher inorganic sulfate excretion. No differences in excretion of ester sulfate were noted.

Epidemic spastic paraparesis in Mozambique appears to be due to the combination of a high intake of cyanide and a low intake of sulfur amino acids. Cyanide itself may cause nervous system damage, or preferential use of sulfur-limited amino acids necessary to detoxify cyanide may lead to impaired synthesis of sulfur compounds needed for normal neural function. The disorder can be prevented by ensuring proper processing of cassava and by providing foods rich in sulfur amino acids, such as beans and fish.

► This is a very nice piece of work. Cassava may be the only edible crop that grows in these areas in times of severe drought. The provision of foods with sulfur-containing amino acids would evidently prevent this disease.—Robert D. Currier, M.D.

13 Multiple Sclerosis

General Comments

Geographic clusters of adult T cell leukemia/non-Hodgkin's lymphoma (ATLL) occur in southwest Japan, the Caribbean, and subSaharan Africa. Human T lymphotropic virus type-I (HTLV-I) has been implicated as the causative agent of ATLL. Osame et al. (*Lancet* 1:1031–1032, 1986) described their experience in Japan with a chronic myelopathy that closely resembles tropical spastic paraparesis and that occurred in patients with positive HTLV-I antibodies in serum and spinal fluid but without ATLL. Vernant et al. (Digest 11–4) reported positive serum HTLV-I antibodies in 80% of tropical spastic paraparesis patients from Martinique. Similar observations from Jamaica and Colombia (Rodgers-Johnson, P., et al.: *Lancet* 2:1247–1248, 1985) and from the Seychelles (Roman, G. C., et al., *N. Engl. J. Med.*, in press) support a possible neurotropic role for HTLV-I. Although tropical *ataxic* neuropathy has been linked with cyanide intake in Nigeria, Tanzania, and Mozambique, Carton et al. (*J. Neurol. Neurosurg. Psychiatry* 49:620–627, 1986) suggest that the cause of the epidemic spastic paraparesis of Zaïre could also be infectious. The role of HTLV-I in this and other clusters of tropical myeloneuropathies deserves further study.—Gustavo C. Román, M.D., F.A.C.P.

The Initial Diagnosis of Multiple Sclerosis: Clinical Impact of Magnetic Resonance Imaging

Stephen S. Gebarski, Trygve O. Gabrielsen, Sid Gilman, James E. Knake, Joseph T. Latack, and Alex M. Aisen (Univ. of Michigan)
Ann. Neurol. 17:469–474, May 1985

13–1

The diagnostic efficacy of magnetic resonance imaging (MRI) in multiple sclerosis (MS) was examined in 33 patients with an initial clinical diagnosis of MS. Thirty patients were evaluated by spin-echo sequencing in the axial and coronal planes. The average scan time was about 30 minutes. Eleven patients also underwent high-resolution computed tomographic (CT) scanning.

The spin-spin relaxation times (T_2) were prolonged in all lesions suggestive of MS in which such times could be calculated. Calculated spin-lattice relaxation times (T_1) were also prolonged. All but 4 patients had abnormal MR images, with at least one discrete high-signal focal lesion in the periependymal white matter of the cerebral hemispheres. All plaques were demonstrated on T_2-weighted images. Twelve patients also had more superficial lesions at the junction of gray and white matter. Seven patients had discrete high-signal lesions deep in the cerebellar hemispheres. Two patients had mesencephalic and 5 had pontine lesions. Most CT studies demonstrated only the largest lesions.

Plaques were demonstrated in most patients, all of whom had a recent onset of neurologic symptoms attributable to MS. The sensitivity of MRI for MS lesions was best in the cerebral white matter. Plaque detection was best in T_2-weighted images. A pattern of focal periependymal high-signal lesions may be specific for MS when definite clinical criteria are met. Similar findings, however, may be obtained in cases of progressive multifocal leukoencephalopathy, diffuse necrotizing leukoencephalopathy, and diffuse leukoencephalopathy.

▶ Magnetic resonance imaging is a good tool for finding MS lesions. Whether or not such lesions should be found is argued by Elian and Dean (*Lancet* 2:27–28, July 6, 1985), who conducted a survey of whether patients knew about their disease. A physician with multiple MS who wrote on the problem (Burnfield, *J. Med. Ethics* 1:21–26, 1984) stated, not unexpectedly, that although patients should be told about their disease, they should be told by someone with sufficient knowledge to discuss the disease at length and in a meaningful way. With the MRI scan showing lesions sometimes even before the patient or the doctor knows they are there, it is not unlikely that the diagnosis will come out of the closet even more than it has.—Robert D. Currier, M.D.

Magnetic Resonance Imaging and Other Techniques in Diagnosis of Multiple Sclerosis
Howard S. Kirshner, Stella I. Tsai, Val M. Runge, and Ann C. Price (Vanderbilt Univ.)
Arch. Neurol. 42:859–863, September 1985   13–2

The magnetic resonance (MR) imaging findings in 35 patients with multiple sclerosis (MS) were compared with the computed tomographic (CT) findings, studies of evoked potentials, and cerebrospinal fluid protein electrophoresis. The MR and CT studies were done within 1 month of each other. Twenty-seven patients had definite, 3 probable, and 5 possible or suspected MS. The 24 women and 11 men 25–68 years of age had been ill for 6 months to 40 years. Visual, brain stem auditory, and somatosensory evoked responses were recorded. Two spin-volume MR techniques and an inversion spin-echo recovery sequence were utilized.

The MR images showed multiple lesions in the periventricular white matter in all cases. Brain stem lesions were present in 15 cases but were not seen on CT scans. The MR findings did not correlate with duration of disease, functional state of the patient, positive oligoclonal banding, or evoked potential findings referable to the brain stem. The severity of the MR changes did correlate with the likelihood of an abnormal CT scan.

Magnetic resonance imaging appears to be a sensitive means of detecting lesions of MS. If, however, lesions are not apparent clinically, the detection of "silent" disease by MR imaging does not necessarily confirm the diagnosis of MS. Longitudinal studies may help relate the clinical and MR findings in MS. A recent patient with clinically definite MS had normal MR findings.

▶ Magnetic resonance imaging appears to be a sensitive indicator of the presence of lesions in MS and to give more diagnostic information than CT scanning, evoked potential testing, or cerebrospinal fluid analysis. In all cases, however, clinical assessment will continue to be crucial to diagnosis and evaluation of the patient.—Russell N. DeJong, M.D.

Use of Interferon in Multiple Sclerosis
Dale E. McFarlin (Natl. Insts. of Health, Bethesda, Md.)
Ann. Neurol. 18:432–433, October 1985   13–3

Recent findings in a double-blind trial of natural α-interferon in active multiple sclerosis (MS) are encouraging but inconclusive. The most improvement was found when the administration of interferon followed the use of a placebo. The systemic side effects that were associated with interferon suggested a learning effect. Increased synthesis of immunoglobulin G (IgG) in the cerebrospinal fluid has been demonstrated, with some antibody apparently directed at a non-interferon component of the preparation that was administered, possibly a Sendai viral protein. The α-interferon that was used in these studies was generated by incubating human lymphocytes with Sendai virus. Highly purified preparations of interferon that are made by using monoclonal antibody and recombinant DNA techniques are now available. Both β- and γ-interferon as well as α-interferon can be tried. At least 20 α-interferon genes have been identified, but it is not clear whether all are correlated with proteins.

Unexpected results and serious side effects can occur whenever a disease that is not understood is being treated. Careful design of trials, close monitoring, and critical evaluation of the findings are essential. Neither interferon nor any other treatment presently can be recommended for use by nonprotocol patients who simply wish to be treated. Patients who are interested in becoming research subjects should be referred to centers where such studies are conducted.

▶ This editorial, by a member of the Immunology Branch of the National Institute of Neurological and Communicative Disorders and Stroke, accompanies other articles dealing with immunologic studies on the use of interferon in the treatment of MS. The interferon system has been shown to be highly complex. Physicians will continue to face the difficult tasks of advising patients about entering new and experimental treatment regimens for MS. The present report certainly emphasizes that experimental trials should be approached as such and not as treatments and should not be recommended for sporadic patients with the disease.—Russell N. DeJong, M.D.

Intrathecal Interferon in the Treatment of Multiple Sclerosis: Patient Follow-up
Lawrence Jacobs, Judith A. O'Malley, Arnold Freeman, Roslyn Ekes, and Peter A. Reese (Dent Neurologic Inst., Roswell Park Mem. Inst., and State Univ. at Buffalo)
Arch. Neurol. 42:841–847, September 1985   13–4

A study of human fibroblast interferon (β-interferon) in multiple sclerosis (MS) had showed a significant reduction in exacerbation rates over about 1½ years. Data for 4½ years of follow-up are now available. Control patients have been followed for a mean of 2 years since cross-over to β-interferon. Fifteen women and five men with definite MS who participated in the study were randomly assigned to a recipient and a control group (mean duration of disease, about 8 years). Control patients received corticosteroids for exacerbations after the first year of the study. Interferon was first given semiweekly by lumbar puncture for 4 weeks and then once a month for 5 months. Each dose was 1×10^6 interferon reference units per sq m.

Exacerbations initially decreased from 1.8 to 0.2 per year in recipients during the study, with no significant change in rates for controls. The current mean number of exacerbations in recipients is 0.16 per year. Controls have had a reduction in exacerbations to 0.3 per year since cross-over. Unacceptable side effects have not occurred.

A sustained effect of intrathecal β-interferon therapy in reducing exacerbations of MS is evident in a small number of patients followed for more than 4 years. An effect is seen in control patients who were crossed over to active treatment. The severity of side effects may be much reduced by the administration of small doses of indomethacin. Further follow-up of these patients will be of great interest.

▶ One must always use caution in interpreting claims of success in the treatment of MS. This is especially true if intrathecal administration is used in therapy. The current study, however, appears to be a careful one, carried out accurately and reliably. The important question is, What is the experience of other investigators in the use of intrathecal interferon in the treatment of MS?—Russell N. DeJong, M.D.

Declining Incidence of Multiple Sclerosis in the Orkney Islands
Stuart D. Cook, James I. Cromarty, Walter Tapp, David Poskanzer, J. D. Walker, and Peter C. Dowling (VA Med. Ctr., East Orange; Univ. of Medicine and Dentistry of New Jersey, Newark; Natl. Insts. of Health, Bethesda, Md.; and Orkney Health Board, Kirkwall, Scotland)
Neurology 35:545–551, April 1985   13–5

A relation between multiple sclerosis (MS) and canine distemper virus (CDV) has been proposed. Persons with inadequate measles immunity might be most susceptible. An outbreak of MS in the Faroe Islands between 1943 and 1960 was preceded by a severe epizootic of CDV in the native dog population. The nearby Orkney Islands have had the highest rate of MS in the world for nearly a century. Epidemics of CDV appear to have been frequent and severe up to 1959 and less frequent since.

Review of the incidence of MS from 1941 through 1983 indicates a significant decline since 1965 (Fig 13–1). Changes in age-specific prevalence, the mean duration of illness, and the mean age of MS patients are consistent with the decline in the incidence of MS in recent years.

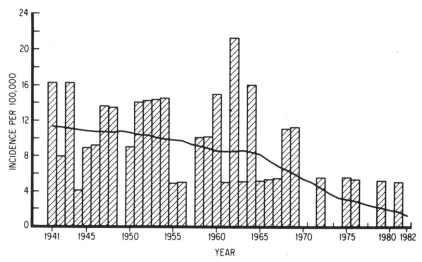

Fig 13–1.—Annual incidence of MS, probable cases per 100,000 per year. The *line* superimposed on the histogram represents the smooth trend in incidence as estimated by locally weighted robust regression. The change in slope at 1964–1965 can be noted. (Courtesy of Cook, S.D., et al.: Neurology 35:545–551, April 1985.)

The decreasing incidence of MS in the Orkney Islands is consistent with the hypothesis that MS may be caused by CDV. There is accumulating epidemiologic evidence of such an association. If it is confirmed, aggressive CDV vaccination programs for dogs could result in a decrease in the incidence of MS. Alternatively, measles boosters or CDV vaccination of humans might effectively prevent MS.

▶ This is an interesting finding and the first I'm aware of that shows a decrease in the incidence of MS. To this observer it seems unlikely that MS is a specific reaction to one virus, but of course it is possible. In a recent update on the situation in the Faroe Islands, Kurtzke and Hyllested (Digest 13–6) attribute the MS outbreak to the presence of British troops rather than dogs.

Compston et al. (*Brain* 109:325–344, 1986) recently confirmed the general increase in measles, mumps, and rubella antibody titers in patients with MS. The whole field of CNS-myelin-vascular-immunity in this disorder is in great ferment, and although I am greatly interested in it, I must say my understanding is limited. Koprowski et al. (*Nature* 318:154–160, Nov. 14, 1985) are finding in patients with MS increased antibody titers to human T cell lymphotropic virus type I, (HTLV-1) the same organism that is producing antibodies in tropical spastic paraparesis (Digest 11–4).—Robert D. Crowell, M.D.

Multiple Sclerosis in the Faroe Islands: II. Clinical Update, Transmission, and the Nature of MS
John F. Kurtske and Kay Hyllested
Neurology 36:307–328, March 1986   13–6

Multiple sclerosis (MS) remains an enigma. Epidemiologically, this seems a place-related disorder—an acquired, exogenous, environmental disease to which whites are especially prone. In this century, the case histories of 41 Faroese with MS were ascertained. The case reports of definite MS among native-born Faroese were divided into the 25 patients who had not been off the islands before clinical onset (group A), the 7 who had lived overseas for a total of less than 2 years (group B), and the 9 overseas for 3 or more years before onset (group C). In the Faroe Islands, MS occurred as three separate and decreasing epidemics beginning in 1943 and ending in 1973.

In 1940 and earlier, there were no cases of MS in the Faroes; at prevalence day in 1950, there were 15. The average calendar year of clinical onset had advanced from 1946 for the 1950 prevalence series to only 1953 for the 1980 series. Inclusion of 3 patients of postwar birth gave 1956 as onset for all 1980 prevalent cases. For patients born by 1940, the cumulative (43-year) risk of MS was 11.1/10,000 population, about that expected for a disease-free cohort of a high-risk populace. Risk for those younger than 20 years was 17/10,000, 12/10,000 for those aged 10–39 years, and 4/10,000 for those aged 40–49; no cases were found in persons older than 49 years (actually 44 years) in 1940. By either village or parish, there was a significant correlation between *residences* of prepubertal versus postpubertal patients. British troops had occupied the Faroes for 5 years, beginning early in 1940; through 1941, there were some 1,500 men. Residences of all MS patients during World War II, or at onset for postwar births, showed a striking concordance for both the pre- and postpubertal MS series cases when superimposed on the locations of the troops. Four postpubertal MS patients lived where no troops had been stationed.

Not one patient was found among native-born resident Faroese with onset of MS before 1943. Between 1943 and 1949, 16 cases appeared in this populace of less than 30,000. There were 32 patients with onset between 1943 and 1973, 25 of whom had never been off the islands, and 7 were off for less than 2 years before onset. Their cases of MS, then, were acquired in the Faroes. Furthermore, since one half of these patients had their onsets abruptly in the first 7 years of this 31-year interval, the introduction of the disease also had to be both abrupt and within a short period before 1943. Also, since early patients resided in widely scattered regions of the islands, this introduction had to be widespread. The Faroese are genetically Scandinavian with some Celtic admixture and are thus highly susceptible to MS.

It is believed that asymptomatic British troops brought MS to the Faroes during 1941 to 1942 and that affected Faroese later transmitted the illness to other Faroese. Multiple sclerosis is a widespread, systemic, specific infectious disease only rarely causing neurologic symptoms and transmissible at most from ages 13 to 26 years. The British must have communicated an infectious agent with unique properties, and the Faroese continued the chain of transmission.

▶ John Kurtzke and Kay Hyllested, who described the clinical epidemiologic features of MS in the Faroe Islands in 1977, now, in their detailed and meticulous fashion, update their material and present their inferences on the nature of the disease among the Faroese. They state that they believe that the disease was introduced into the Faroe Islands by asymptomatic British troops in 1941 and 1942 and that three separate and decreasing epidemics have occurred between 1943 and 1973. On the basis of these studies, they conclude that MS is a widespread, systemic, infectious disease, only rarely causing neurologic symptoms. They believe that it is not a primary neurologic disease.—Russell N. DeJong, M.D.

Clinical Viral Infections and Multiple Sclerosis
William A. Sibley, Colin R. Bamford, and Katherine Clark (Univ. of Arizona)
Lancet 1:1313–1315, June 8, 1985   13–7

Possible environmental factors in multiple sclerosis (MS) were evaluated over an 8-year period in 170 patients and 134 healthy control subjects matched with the patients for age. The average observation period was 5.3 years for patients with MS and 4.6 years for control subjects. The frequency of common viral infections was compared in the two groups.

Viral-like infections were significantly less frequent in patients than in control subjects, and the difference was most marked for patients with severe disability. Living sheltered lives may only partly explain this finding, since viral infections also were less frequent in patients with trivial disability. Differences were most evident for herpes simplex-like infections. Rates of exacerbation in at-risk periods, from 2 weeks before the onset of infectious symptoms to 5 weeks afterwards, were nearly three times higher than in other periods. The effect was seen for patients with all levels of disability. The exacerbation rate during at-risk periods in mildly disabled patients with frequent infections was five times greater than in similarly disabled patients with infrequent infections.

These findings suggest that patients with MS may have superior immune defenses against common viruses, but the effect of sheltering is difficult to assess. The observation of much more rapid progression in mildly affected patients with infrequent clinical infection suggests that overactive immune mechanisms determine not only a greater frequency of inapparent infection, but also more rapid progress of disease.

▶ This article reenforces the common opinion that MS is more likely to worsen after an infection. A recent study in England (Gay, D., et al.: *Lancet*:815–819, April 12, 1986) showing an association between sinusitis and MS attacks also found that sinusitis was more frequent in patients with MS than in controls, in contrast to the decreased frequency of viral infections found by Sibley et al.— Robert D. Currier, M.D.

Prevalence of Multiple Sclerosis in British Columbia
Vincent P. Sweeney, Adele D. Sadovnick and Vilma Brandejs (Univ. of British Columbia)
Can. J. Neurol. Sci. 13:47–51, February 1986   13–8

Epidemiologic studies of multiple sclerosis (MS) have made major contributions to the current understanding of this unique disease. Populations living in high-risk geographic areas are most susceptible. Migration studies and the demonstration of clusters suggest that an environmental factor, probably infectious, is involved in the etiology of MS. Genetic predisposition to MS is probably also a factor. Canada is considered a high-risk geographic zone, as are the northern states of the United States.

A provincewide prevalence study on MS was conducted in British Columbia (B.C.); the prevalence date was July 1, 1982. Most of this study was a review of all the files of neurologists practicing in B.C., since this was judged to be the most accurate source for identifying MS patients. A total of 239,412 neurologists' files were hand searched by one researcher using modified Schumacher criteria for classification. Other sources used during the study for the identification of patients with MS were the MS Clinic (University of B.C.), general practitioners, ophthalmologists, urologists, specialized facilities such as long-term care facilities and rehabilitation centers, and patient self-referrals.

A total of 4,620 nonduplicated cases were identified and classified, of which 4,112 (89%) were classified according to information contained in neurologists' records. The prevalence estimate for definite/probable MS in B.C. was 93.3/100,000 population. This increased to 130.5/100,000 population if possible MS and optic neuritis were also included. These rates are among the highest reported in Canada or elsewhere.

The prevalence of MS varies throughout the world, but areas of high prevalence include the British Isles and northern Europe. Multiple sclerosis is rare among persons of Asian, African, and Native Indian ancestry. Two factors may contribute to the high prevalence of MS in B.C.: (1) genetic predisposition, since the population of the province is largely made up of persons with British and northern European ancestry, and (2) geographic location, since the prevalence of MS has been observed to be higher in northern, as compared with southern, latitudes.

The high proportion of neurologist-confirmed cases of MS makes B.C. a suitable location to pursue further epidemiologic studies of MS.

▶ The geographic distribution of patients suffering from MS has intrigued and puzzled neurologic investigators, who have never completely understood the significance of its varying prevalence (Kurtzke, J. F.: *Neurology* 30:61–79, 1980; McDonald, W. I.: *Acta Neurol. Scand.* 68:65–76, 1983). Epidemiologic and migration studies, as well as the demonstration of clusters of the disease, suggest that an environmental factor, probably infectious in origin, is involved in the etiology of multiple sclerosis, although genetic predisposition is probably also a factor. The prevalence estimates herein reported are among the highest that have been described in Canada or elsewhere. The cooperation of the neurologists in British Columbia made this study unique in scope and in the accuracy of diagnosis.—Russell N. DeJong, M.D.

Primary Sjögren's Syndrome With Central Nervous System Disease Mimicking Multiple Sclerosis

Elaine L. Alexander, Kenneth Malinow, Jane E. Lejewski, Myles S. Jerdan, Thomas T. Provost, and Garrett E. Alexander (Johns Hopkins Med. Insts.)

Ann. Intern. Med. 104:323–330, March 1986   13–9

Sjögren's syndrome has been estimated to be the second most common connective tissue disorder, next to rheumatoid arthritis, which affects between 2% and 5% of the adult population over age 55 years. Central nervous system involvement has occurred in approximately 20% of patients with primary Sjögren's syndrome evaluated at The Johns Hopkins Medical Institutes. Characteristically, the neurologic dysfunction is multifocal, involving both the brain and spinal cord, and is recurrent over time.

For 20 patients (18 women) aged 26–61 years with primary Sjögren's syndrome, the clinical course and neurodiagnostic studies, including cerebrospinal fluid (CSF) and evoked potential testing, were indistinguishable from those of patients with multiple sclerosis (MS). All patients had symptoms of sicca complex with xerophthalmia, xerostomia, or recurrent salivary gland enlargement. Biopsy sample of the minor salivary gland was abnormal in all 18 tested. Agarose gel electrophoresis of CSF samples was done by standard techniques.

The mean age at the onset of CNS disease was 38 years, whereas the mean age at diagnosis of Sjögren's syndrome was 42 years. In 13 patients, Sjögren's syndrome was recognized only after the onset of neurologic complications, but sicca symptoms had been present for many years. In 3 patients, sicca symptoms and neurologic dysfunction emerged simultaneously. In only 4 had the diagnosis of Sjögren's syndrome been established before the development of neurologic abnormalities. All patients had multifocal CNS events that occurred over time. All patients met criteria for definite MS. All also had brain involvement. Sensory changes (hypesthesias) were the most common signs, occurring in 14 patients. Spasticity, hyperreflexia, or both were present in 12 patients. Seven patients had transient monocular visual loss. Cranial neuropathies were noted in 9. Seventeen had involvement of the spinal cord. In 13, psychiatric abnormalities were evident. Evoked potential testing showed abnormalities in 15 of 18 patients. Prolonged latencies were the most common abnormality (11 patients), with positive peaks in 4 and decreased amplitude and absent waves in 1. The electroencephalogram was abnormal in 5 patients, 4 of whom had focal abnormalities. Three of 18 patients tested had abnormal computed tomographic scans of the head (2 with cortical atrophy and 1 with two lucencies in gray matter). In no instances were attenuation defects or enhancing lesions noted in a periventricular location, as are often seen in patients with MS. Seventeen patients had myelograms, and all were normal. The CSF/serum glucose ratio was decreased in 11 patients. The following protein and immunoglobulin values were elevated: total protein (7 patients), IgG (5), IgG/total protein ratio (5), and IgG index (10). Sixteen of 18 patients tested had one or more oligoclonal bands: one in 11, two in 3, four in 1, and five in 1. In 1 patient who was found initially to have five oligoclonal bands, the number and intensity of bands decreased se-

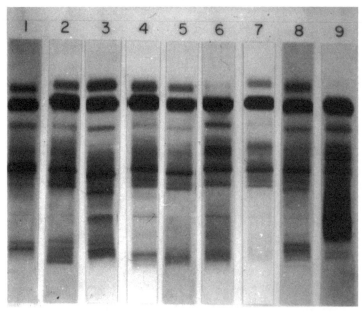

Fig 13–2.—Agarose gel electrophoresis of CSF samples from patients with Sjögren's syndrome with CNS disease mimicking MS. *Lane 1* shows a patient with two bands, and *lane 2* shows a patient with five bands. With corticosteroid therapy, the number of bands decreased to four (two discrete and two faint in *lane 3*); to three *(lane 4)*; to two *(lane 5)*; and then to one discrete and one faint *(lane 6)*. Control samples included CSF from a normal person *(lane 7)* and from a patient with MS *(lane 8)*, and serum from a patient with multiple myeloma *(lane 9)*. (Courtesy of Alexander, E.L., et al.: Ann. Intern. Med. 104:323–330, March 1986.)

quentially with corticosteroid therapy (Fig 13–2). Fourteen patients were treated with moderated daily doses of corticosteroids (40–60 mg of prednisone), all but one of whom showed an improvement or stabilization of neurologic function. All of the 6 patients not treated had deterioration in neurologic status ($P = .00036$).

Because of the similarity in the clinical presentations and laboratory findings in patients with MS and Sjögren's syndrome, Sjögren's syndrome should be added to the differential diagnosis of patients presenting with a syndrome that resembles MS.

▶ It is amazing how similar to MS this disease appears to be. I wonder how many cases I have missed.

Pachner and Steere (*Neurology* 36[suppl. 1]:286, April 1986) report a similar look-alike situation with Lyme disease, which can also manifest with intermittent and disseminated symptoms. It, however, is responsive to penicillin rather than steroids.—Robert D. Currier, M.D.

General Comments

Several interesting comments on multiple sclerosis (MS) come from the recent meeting of the American Academy of Neurology. Coyle, Sibony, and Johnson report finding oligoclonal banding in tears of MS patients.

Now this I don't understand. If the bands truly originate in the CNS, how do they get in our tears? (*Neurology* 36[suppl. 1]:315, April 1986). Paty et al. (*Neurology* 36[suppl. 1]:177, April 1986) report on the magnetic resonance imaging (MRI) changes of MS lesions over a period of time. They point out that the lesions come and go on the MRI scan without necessarily causing symptoms. Zimmerman et al. (*AJNR* 146:443–450, March 1986) helpfully clarify the situation regarding the periventricular abnormalities seen in MRI scanning. This is well worth reading for everyone like myself who really doesn't know what he or she is doing when looking at an MRI scan. Not everything that is white and periventricular is MS is the message, but there are ways of differentiating the other causes.

Ormerod et al. (*J. Neurol. Neurosurg. Psychiatry* 49:124–127, 1986) report that 61% of patients with optic neuritis are shown by MRI to have other lesions. It looks as though the MRI scan is going to give us more help in putting together the clinical picture of MS than anything that has come along so far.

Another double-blind hyperbaric oxygen MS treatment trial is reported from London by Wiles et al. (*Br. Med. J.* [*Clin. Res.*] 292:367–371, Feb. 8, 1986): they conclude that it does not work. On the other hand, Durelli et al. (*Neurology* 36:238–243, 1986) report success in the acute episode with high-dose intravenous methylprednisolone, but it does not prevent future bouts.

14 Myasthenia Gravis

Myasthenia Gravis Without Acetylcholine-Receptor Antibody: A Distinct Disease Entity
S. Mossman, A. Vincent, and J. Newsom-Davis (Royal Free Hosp. School of Medicine and Queen Square, London)
Lancet 1:116–119, Jan. 18, 1986   14–1

Weakness in myasthenia gravis is due to loss of functional acetylcholine receptors (AChR) at the postsynaptic membrane of the neuromuscular junction. Serum antibody against AChR can be found in 85%–90% of patients with generalized myasthenia gravis and about 70% of those with symptoms restricted to ocular muscles. It is bound to endplate receptor and is implicated in receptor loss. Some patients with myasthenia gravis whose serum is persistently "negative" for AChR antibody respond to plasma exchange or to immunosuppressive drug treatment; it has therefore been assumed that AChR antibody cannot be detected because critical determinants on the receptor are lost during solubilization required for the radioimmunoassay or because all measurable antibody is already bound to AChR.

Plasma was obtained at plasma exchange from eight patients with symptoms and signs typical of myasthenia gravis but for whom serum AChR antibody had been persistently undetectable by radioimmunoassay or by inhibition of ^{125}I-labeled α-bungarotoxin binding, with human AChR as antigen. Tendon reflexes were normal or brisk in all cases. One patient had autonomic disturbance (dry mouth). All patients had positive responses to treatment with intravenous edrophonium. Increased jitter on single-fiber electromyography was present in the seven patients tested, and three had abnormal decrement. Electromyographic features of the Lambert-Eaton myasthenic syndrome were absent. All six patients for whom plasma exchange was used therapeutically responded. In the other two patients, it was used to test whether a pathogenetic humoral factor (i.e., antibody) was present, with a view to introducing immunosuppressive drug treatment if necessary. One of these last 2 patients improved and was subsequently treated with prednisolone; the other patient did not respond, and no immunosuppressive treatment was given. Two of the patients had undergone a thymectomy 6 weeks before the exchange. No patient had received immunosuppressive drugs at the time of plasma exchange. Immunoglobulin preparations from the eight patients were injected intraperitoneally into mice. Neuromuscular transmission was significantly impaired compared with that of mice receiving control human immunoglobulin. No antibody bound to the mouse AChR was detected, but there was a small loss (9.4%) of AChR in the mouse diaphragms.

The results suggest that a pathogenetic immunoglobulin antibody interferes with neuromuscular transmission in these AChR-antibody-negative patients by binding to non-AChR determinants at the neuromuscular junction.

Several lines of evidence indicate that the antibody binds to determinants other than those on the AChR: (1) AChR antibody was not detected with the radioimmunoassay using an AChR mixture that is particularly effective in detecting low-titer AChR antibodies; (2) there was confirmation of the absence of antibodies to the α-bungarotoxin binding sites on the AChR by testing for inhibition of α-bungarotoxin binding; and (3) no antibody bound to mouse AChR could be demonstrated in mice treated with IgG from the eight AChR-antibody-negative patients, whereas it was in mice receiving AChR-antibody-positive immunoglobulin or injected with hybridoma cells secreting monoclonal anti-human-AChR antibody. Thus, the present patients appear to have a myasthenic disorder that is caused by antibodies to determinants at the neuromuscular junction other than the AChR and is thus immunologically and physiologically distinct from myasthenia gravis caused by AChR antibody. The typical myasthenic feature of thymic hyperplasia was absent in the two patients who underwent thymectomy before immunosuppressive drug treatment was started and in a further patient who had received treatment for only 5 days. This raises the question of whether thymectomy is appropriate management for this group of patients, in view of evidence that the response to thymectomy is positively correlated with the degree of thymic hyperplasia.

Further studies will be needed to define the precise site of action at the neuromuscular junction of these patients' antibodies and to evaluate methods of treating this form of myasthenia.

▶ These authors are to be congratulated on suggesting a solution to the problem of the myasthenic patient with a negative antibody test. Such patients are then either early myasthenics, with the test not yet positive, or members of the group reported here, who have antibodies to something other than the acetylcholine receptor. The clinical importance of this finding is, of course, that the patients do have myasthenia, but may require other treatment considerations. Perhaps they are not proper subjects for thymectomy, since the thymus is not found to be hyperplastic at operation.—Robert D. Currier, M.D.

Antiacetylcholine Receptor Antibodies in Myasthenia Gravis: Part 3. Effect of Thymectomy

H. J. G. H. Oosterhuis, P. C. Limburg, E. Hummel-Tappel, W. Van den Burg, and T. H. The (Univ. Hosp., Groningen, The Netherlands)
J. Neurol. Sci. 69:335–343, July 1985 14–2

Immune and immunoregulatory abnormalities may help explain why thymectomy is generally effective in younger patients with myasthenia but less effective in older patients with thymoma. The clinical and immunologic response to thymectomy was evaluated in 30 patients with generalized myasthenia gravis for whom antibody to acetylcholine receptor (AChR) was detected preoperatively. Thymectomy was performed in the first year of disease in 11 of the patients, and in the 2nd, 3rd, or 4th years in the remaining patients (mean age at operation, 26 years).

Severe hyperplasia was found in 11 patients and atrophy in 1 patient. Titers of AChR antibody before thymectomy were related to both the clinical severity of myasthenia and the degree of hyperplasia. Both disability scores and antibody titers generally fell significantly after thymectomy, and correlation between these measures was more apparent over time after operation. Four prednisone-treated patients improved after thymectomy while their antibody titers declined steeply. Changes in AChR antibody titers were not attributable to concomitant changes in total immunoglobulin G levels in most cases.

AChR antibody titers vary widely in patients with myasthenia gravis. In most patients a clear change in clinical state after thymectomy is associated with a definite change in AChR antibody titer. Improvement presumably is related to an increase in functioning receptors, but myasthenia may improve after thymectomy in the absence of detectable levels in serum of AChR antibody.

▶ It is nice to know that reasonable things are reasonable and that the antibody titer does fall in the three years after thymectomy. A nearly identical study from Japan (Kagotani, K., et al.: *J. Thorac. Cardiovasc. Surg.* 90:7–12, 1985) in which patients were followed up for the same length of time resulted in the same improvement in the myasthenia gravis and decrease in the antibody titer.—Robert D. Currier, M.D.

Thymectomy in Myasthenia With Pure Ocular Symptoms
F. Schumm, H. Wiethölter, A. Fateh-Moghadam, and J. Dichgans (Univ. of Tübingen and Univ. of Munich, Federal Republic of Germany)
J. Neurol. Neurosurg. Psychiatry 48:332–337, April 1985   14–3

The indications for thymectomy in purely ocular myasthenia are uncertain, but it generally is not recommended. Eighteen of 42 patients seen since 1978 with ocular myasthenia underwent thymectomy, after favorable experience in two cases incorrectly thought to be thymoma on the basis of the mediastinal computed tomographic scan. All of the patients, 13 men and 5 women with respective mean ages of 39 and 32 years, had purely ocular symptoms and a positive edrophonium test. The mean follow-up after operation was 27 months.

There was no surgical morbidity. Acetylcholine antibody titers declined postoperatively in 8 of 9 patients, in 6 by more than 40%. Ocular symptom scores decreased in all patients but 1. Half the patients still had slight ocular symptoms at the last follow-up. Improvement nearly always occurred in the first 6 months after operation. Thymic hyperplasia was the usual finding, but 1 patient had a lymphocytic thymoma.

The lack of operative morbidity in this series suggests that thymectomy be considered for patients with purely ocular myasthenia if there is no satisfactory response to treatment with cholinesterase inhibitors and no spontaneous remission within a 6-month period. Early surgery probably inhibits generalization of the disorder, which otherwise can be expected to occur in about 50% of patients within 2 years. Surgery can often avoid the risks of long-term prednisone and azathioprine therapy.

▶ So, ocular myasthenia responds in the same way as general myasthenia. None of the 18 patients developed generalized myasthenia in an average follow-up of two years. Perhaps the operation should be considered for ocular myasthenia in adults.—Robert D. Currier, M.D.

15 Myopathy

Mitochondrial Myopathies
Salvatore DiMauro, Eduardo Bonilla, Massimo Zeviani, Masanori Nakagawa, and Darryl C. De Vivo (Columbia Univ.)
Ann. Neurol. 17:521–538, June 1985   15–1

The mitochondrial myopathies are a clinically heterogeneous group of disorders affecting systems other than skeletal muscle. Morphologically distinct syndromes include Kearns-Sayre syndrome with ophthalmoplegia and pigmentary retinal degeneration, myoclonus epilepsy with ragged-red fibers, and mitochondrial myopathy with encephalopathy, lactic acidosis, and strokelike episodes.

Electron microscopic examination shows large aggregates of mitochondria, usually under the sarcolemma but also between myofibrils. The mitochondria may appear normal in size but often are enlarged up to 5 μ in diameter. Cristae may be increased in number or irregularly oriented, or few cristae may be present. Various abnormal inclusions such as "paracrystalline" inclusions may be seen. Excessive accumulation of glycogen particles and triglyceride droplets is characteristic. The morphologic abnormalities do not differentiate among the various mitochondrial myopathies.

Mitochondrial myopathies can be classified biochemically as defects of substrate utilization, oxidation-phosphorylation coupling, and the respiratory chain. Deficiencies of carnitine or carnitine palmitoyl transferase, necessary for transfer of long-chain fatty acids across the inner mitochondrial membrane to be oxidized, have been described. Carnitine deficiency may be a systemic disorder. Several clinical syndromes have been associated with cytochrome c oxidase deficiency in muscle or in multiple tissues, including benign infantile mitochondrial myopathy, subacute necrotizing encephalomyelopathy, and trichopoliodystrophy (Menkes' disease). Much remains to be done in the biochemical definition of the mitochondrial myopathies.

Mitochondria have their own DNA and their own translating and transcribing mechanism. Mitochondrial myopathies therefore can be due to defects of either a nuclear or a mitochondrial genome and can be transmitted by mendelian or maternal inheritance.

▶ Mitochondrial myopathies are morphologic abnormalities of muscle mitochondria. Biochemical investigations have led to the identification of several specific errors of mitochondrial metabolism. Modern techniques in molecular genetics hold great promise for the study of these diseases.—Russell N. DeJong, M.D.

Cramps, Spasms and Muscle Stiffness
Lewis P. Rowland (Columbia-Presbyterian Med. Center)
Rev. Neurol. (Paris) 141:261–273, 1985   15–2

Involuntary painful shortening of muscle in phosphorylase deficiency was the first momentary condition in humans to be called *contracture*. In a true cramp, there is a sudden, involuntary, and painful shortening of muscle that is relieved by stretching or massage. The prominence of cramps in motor neuron disease and their absence in any known metabolic myopathy suggests a neurogenic origin. The Denny-Brown and Foley syndrome (1948) consists of benign fasciculation and cramping. Tetany, a state of increased sensitivity to emotional or sensory stimuli, can be induced by hyperventilation and respiratory alkalosis. Painful tonic seizures are seen in multiple sclerosis. Isaacs' syndrome is characterized by myokymia, or continuous muscular twitching, as well as by pseudomyotonia and abnormal posturing of the hands and feet. Central disorders that include cramping, spasms, and muscle stiffness are stiff-man syndrome and writer's cramp, or occupational cramps.

The term *severe cramps* may be applied to isolated cramping not associated with other neurologic abnormalities. Benign fasciculation is not accompanied by wasting, weakness, or reflex changes. Isaacs' syndrome is diagnosed if widespread fasciculation or myokymia is present, along with abnormal posturing or difficulty relaxing after a forceful movement. Hyperventilation tetany should be considered in any case where Isaacs' syndrome is proposed. The stiff-man syndrome is characterized by leg and trunk stiffness without abnormal corticospinal signs or basal ganglia disease. The term *continuous motor activity* must be more precisely defined. Specific syndromes include the spasticity of amyotrophic lateral sclerosis, the stiffness of "rigid spine syndrome," Emery-Dreifuss muscular dystrophy, tetanus, and dystonic reactions to phenothiazines and other drugs.

▶ Dr. Rowland has long been interested in muscle abnormalities characterized by cramps, spasms, and muscle stiffness. This study, from a lecture given at the Fifth International Congress on Neuromuscular Diseases in Marseilles, France in 1982, is a scholarly discussion of these phenomena.—Russell N. DeJong, M.D.

General Comments

The review by Mastaglia and Ojeda of Inflammatory Myopathies (*Ann. Neurol.* 17:215–227, March 1985; 17:317–323, April 1985) appears up to date and complete. In Israel Benbassat et al. (*Arthritis Rheum.* 28:249–255, March 1985) have recently analyzed data for their patients with myositis; the average survival after diagnosis was five years. Unfavorable prognostic signs were failure to induce remission, leukocytosis, fever, older age, a shorter disease history, and dysphagia. A comprehensive review of myopathies due to enzyme deficiencies is that of Cornelio and DiDonato from Italy (*J. Neurol.* 232:329–340, 1985). The localization of myotonic dystrophy on chromosome 19 is proved with the recent work of Yamaoka et al. (*J. Neurogenetics* 2:403–412, 1985), and Bakker et al. (*Lancet* 1:655–658, March 23, 1985) have gotten close enough to the gene for Duchenne's dystrophy, so that their markers have been used in prenatal diagnosis. The Japanese are using coenzyme Q_{10} to treat patients with the Kearns-Sayre syndrome (Ogasahara, S., et al.: *Neurology* 36:45–53, January 1986).—Robert D. Currier, M.D.

16 Neuro-Ophthalmology

Reversible Optic Neuropathy Due to Carotid-Cavernous Fistula
Thomas R. Hedges, III, Gerard Debrun, and Samuel Sokol (Tufts Univ., Massachusetts Gen. Hosp., and Harvard Univ., Boston)
J. Clin. Neuro Ophthalmol. 5:37–40, March 1985   16–1

Visual loss complicating carotid-cavernous fistula may result from ocular ischemia or several different forms of optic neuropathy. A patient had deteriorating vision weeks after trauma that resulted in a carotid-cavernous fistula, and for whom vision was completely restored by occluding the fistula with an intra-arterial balloon.

Man, 21 years old, incurred a mandibular fracture when thrown from a motor bicycle and striking a pole. The right eye protruded, with limitation of all extraocular movements, especially abduction. Vision was normal 4 weeks later, but at 7 weeks it was reduced on the right, and orbital congestion had worsened. Proptosis was more marked on the right, and a loud bruit was audible over most of the skull. Minimal retinal venous dilatation was seen. Visual evoked potential amplitudes were markedly reduced on the right. Angiography showed a high-flow carotid-cavernous fistula with swelling of the cavernous sinus and distention of the ophthalmic artery. A detachable balloon was placed in the right cavernous sinus via the internal carotid artery, with immediate improvement. The bruit recurred and more balloons were placed to close the cavernous carotid artery. Vision was 20/15 on the right 6 days later, and visual evoked potential amplitudes were normal.

This type of visual impairment may be more frequent in patients with large carotid-cavernous fistulas requiring treatment before ophthalmologic investigation is possible. The patient's visual loss resolved completely after intra-arterial balloon placement. Delayed optic neuropathy is a strong indication for intervention in a patient with carotid-cavernous fistula.

▶ By carefully monitoring visual function in patients with traumatic carotid-cavernous fistulas, delayed optic neuropathy can be recognized early in its development and can thus be treated successfully.—Russell N. DeJong, M.D.

17 Neuropathies

Guillain-Barré Syndrome: Clinicoepidemiologic Features and Effect of Influenza Vaccine
Ettore Beghi, Leonard T. Kurland, Donald W. Mulder and Wigbert C. Wiederholt (Mayo Clinic and Found. and Univ. of California at San Diego)
Arch. Neurol. 42:1053–1057, November 1985   17–1

Analysis of the centralized diagnostic index at the Mayo Clinic yielded 48 cases of Guillain-Barré syndrome (GBS) in Olmsted County, Minnesota, in 1935–1980. The age- and sex-adjusted incidence was 1.8 per 100,000 person-years. The diagnosis was based on progressive motor weakness in the upper and/or lower extremities and a loss or marked reduction of muscle stretch reflexes. Supportive findings included a rapid development of signs and symptoms peaking within 1 month, relatively symmetric weakness, and a high level of recovery.

The rate of GBS per 100,000 person-years increased over time, from 1.2 in 1935–1956 to 2.4 in 1970–1980. Male and female persons had respective age-adjusted rates of 2.3 and 1.2 per 100,000 person-years. The rate of GBS increased with advancing age, from 0.8 before age 18 years to 3.2 for persons aged 60 years and older. Influenza-like infectious disease in the 4 weeks preceding the onset of neurologic symptoms was reported in 31 (65%) of the 48 cases. Only six patients (12%) had respiratory insufficiency; three of the required tracheostomy and mechanical ventilation.

Negative findings such as the lack of variation in numbers of cases in relation to swine flu vaccine use and the lack of an increase with earlier influenza vaccination programs call the presumed association of GBS with vaccination into question. Any increased risk in the vaccinated population is probably limited to the first 5–6 weeks after immunization.

▶ The reported increase in the incidence of GBS following the national swine influenza vaccination program in 1976–1977 has been questioned by many authorities. This study by epidemiologists at the Mayo Clinic in Rochester, Minnesota, questions the validity of the diagnosis in these cases. In 20% of the patients, there was no confirmation of the diagnosis by a neurologist, and in 80% there was no indication of recovery.

In another article in this same issue of the *Archives of Neurology,* two of the authors of this article and three associates recommend that a panel of neurologists with expertise in the diagnosis of GBS review the medical records of each of these patients and classify them on the basis of reasonable diagnostic criteria; the Director of the Centers for Disease Control reportedly favors such a reappraisal (Kurland, L. T., et al.: *Arch. Neurol.* 42:1089–1090, 1985). In the same issue, C. M. Poser (Harvard Univ.) makes similar recommendations

(*Arch. Neurol.* 42:1090–1092, 1985) and V. Hachinski (Univ. of Western Ontario) states that such review can only enhance the likelihood, not of an ultimate answer, but of a workable approximation to the truth (*Arch. Neurol.* 42:1092, 1985).—Russell N. DeJong, M.D.

Guillain-Barré Syndrome: Current Methods of Diagnosis and Treatment
Robert G. Miller (Univ. of California at San Francisco)
Postgrad. Med. 57:57–64, May 15, 1985   17–2

Guillain-Barré syndrome (GBS), the most common cause of acute weakness in persons younger than age 40 years, is an acute, symmetric limb weakness that sometimes follows viral or *mycoplasma* infection, surgery, or immunization. Cranial nerve involvement and dysautonomia may be present. Spontaneous improvement is characteristic. Radicular deficits, sensory disturbance, areflexia, and absence of fever may aid diagnosis of GBS. Weakness tends to begin in the legs and spread to the upper limbs and respiratory muscles. The cerebrospinal fluid protein concentration is usually elevated after the first week of neuropathic symptoms. Most patients have electrophysiologic findings of acquired demyelinating neuropathy. Fibrillation and postitive-wave activity on electromyography are proportional to the amount of axonal degeneration. There is increasing evidence for a role of humoral mechanisms in the pathogenesis of GBS.

The prognosis is excellent for most patients with GBS, but up to 20% have significant residual weakness, and mortalities range from 1.5% to 8%. About one fifth of patients require ventilatory assistance for respiratory failure. Low-dosage heparin has been used to prevent pulmonary embolism in extremely weak patients. Nutritional support, usually by nasogastric tube feeding, is essential. Hypotension is more of a problem than hypertension. Most patients require physical therapy and intensive psychologic support. High-dosage corticosteroid therapy is no longer considered to be beneficial to patients with GBS. Plasma exchange has appeared to be helpful but is risky in patients with autonomic dysfunction.

► This is a rather elementary, but helpful, discussion of GBS. Its reference to plasmapheresis is not as positive as that of the report of the Guillain-Barré Syndrome Study Group, which calls it the first treatment shown to benefit patients with the acute syndrome (Digest 17–3).—Russell N. DeJong, M.D.

Plasmapheresis and Acute Guillain-Barré Syndrome
Guillain-Barré Syndrome Study Group
Neurology 35:1096–1104, August 1985   17–3

A randomized comparison of plasmapheresis with traditional measures was carried out in 245 patients with severe, acute Guillain-Barré syndrome (GBS) at 21 centers. From 200 to 250 cc of plasma/kg was exchanged in

7 to 14 days; Plasmanate or 5% salt-poor albumin was used for replacement, or pooled plasma in a few cases. Among conventionally treated patients receiving corticosteroids, the dosage was lowered to 5 mg daily or the patient was excluded.

Complications did not differ significantly in the two groups. The overall mortality was 3%. Patients undergoing plasmapheresis did better than controls in terms of clinical improvement at 4 weeks, time to improve one clinical grade, time to independent walking, and status at 6 months. Plasmapheresis was especially effective in patients treated within a week of the onset of GBS and those requiring mechanical ventilation after entry into the study. Plasmapheresis remained significantly effective when patients not completing the protocol were included in the evaluation.

Plasmapheresis is the first treatment shown to benefit patients with acute GBS. Lessening of the time to independent walking and the time for patients receiving mechanical ventilation to improve has substantial economic implications. Plasmapheresis should be used early in the course of acute GBS. Complications have not been significantly increased, but it may be necessary to use this treatment in an intensive care setting with experienced staff at hand.

▶ Since the marked decline in the incidence of poliomyelitis in the United States, GBS has become the major cause of rapid-onset flaccid paralysis in healthy persons. This paper reports the first mode of therapy shown to benefit patients with the acute syndrome. The paper stresses, however, that to be effective plasmapheresis must be started early in the course of the disease.— Russell N. DeJong, M.D.

Plasma Exchange in Chronic Inflammatory Demyelinating Polyradiculoneuropathy

Peter James Dyck, Jasper Daube, Peter O'Brien, Alvaro Pineda, Phillip A. Low, Anthony J. Windebank, and Carol Swanson (Mayo Clinic and Found.)

N. Engl. J. Med. 314:461–465, Feb. 20, 1986   17–4

Chronic inflammatory demyelinating polyradiculoneuropathy (CIDP) is a chronic neuropathy thought to be mediated by the immune system. Characteristically, its onset is insidious, developing over weeks, months, or years. The cause of the disease is unknown. There is a need to improve therapy, because CIDP may cause prolonged periods of disability and even death. Plasma exchange has been reported to be efficacious in CIDP.

The present study was initiated to assess (1) whether plasma exchange ameliorates neurologic dysfunction, (2) which types of patient improve, (3) how long the improvement lasts, and (4) whether plasma exchange can be performed safely in patients with the disease. The study patients had to have a protein concentration in cerebrospinal fluid of 60 mg/dl or higher; be 18 years of age or older; agree to random assignment either to plasma exchange or sham exchange; have a neurologic-disability score of

50 points or higher; and have a neurologic status that was static or worsening. Immunotherapy or prednisone therapy was not to have been changed in the preceding 6 weeks.

A prospective double-blind trial was performed in which patients with static or worsening disease were randomly assigned to plasma exchange (n = 15) or to sham exchange (n = 14) for 3 weeks. Patients who had received sham exchange (controlled trial) were offered plasma exchange, administered twice weekly for the next 3 weeks (open trial). Neurologic assessment continued as in the controlled trial. In plasma exchange, after removal of plasma, cells were suspended in 5% normal serum albumin and 0.9% sodium chloride solution and reinfused into the patient. In sham exchange, after the cells were separated from the plasma, they were recombined and reinfused.

There was not a significant difference in subjective responses between

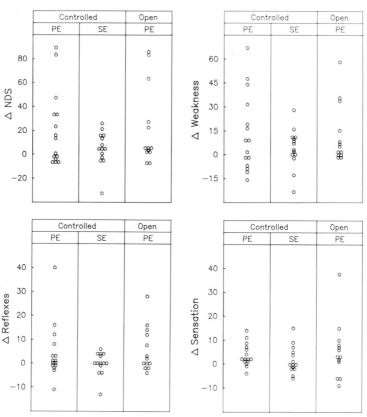

Fig 17–1.—Changes in the neurologic-disability score (NDS) and in the tendon-reflexes, weakness, and sensation subsets of the neurologic-disability score 3 weeks after plasma exchange (PE) or sham exchange (SE) in the controlled trial and after plasma exchange in the open trial. Each symbol represents the response of 1 patient. Positive values indicate improvement. (Courtesy of Dyck, P.J., et al.: N. Engl. J. Med. 314:461–465, Feb. 20, 1986. Reprinted by permission of The New England Journal of Medicine.)

the groups. Striking differences were found between the two treatment groups in the distribution of changes in the neurologic-disability score and its subsets (Fig 17–1). In the controlled study, 5 patients receiving plasma exchange had an improvement in their scores at 3 weeks, compared with base-line scores, that exceeded the largest improvement attained by any patient receiving sham exchange ($P = .025$). Four patients receiving plasma exchange had greater improvement in the weakness and reflexes subsets than did those receiving sham exchange ($P < .057$). In the open study, an approximately similar rate of improvement was observed. Changes in the neurologic-disability score were associated with improvement in nerve conduction ($P = .032$; Spearman's rank-sum correlation coefficient).

For some patients with CIDP, plasma exchange has an ameliorating effect on neurologic dysfunction and nerve conduction, but in others no improvement is noted. Because plasma was replaced with normal serum albumin, a humoral factor(s) may have a role in the neurologic deficit of this disorder.

▶ Chronic inflammatory demyelinating polyneuropathy has a longer disability duration and a higher mortality rate than the acute disorder (Dyck, P. J., et al.: *Mayo Clin. Proc.,* 1979). In the acute type it has been demonstrated that plasmaphoresis is definitely effective (Digest 17–3). In this therapeutic trial of the chronic disorder it was demonstrated that plasma exchange therapy appeared to have an ameliorating affect on neurologic dysfunction and nerve conduction in some patients, while no improvement was observed in others. Unfortunately, this study fails to provide helpful therapeutic suggestions for patients with chronic inflammatory demyelinating polyradiculoneuropathy.—Russell N. DeJong, M.D.

Transient Conduction Block Following Acute Peripheral Nerve Ischemia
Gareth J. Parry, David R. Cornblath, and Mark J. Brown (Univ. of Pennsylvania)
Muscle Nerve 8:409–412, June 1985   17–5

Nerve conduction abnormalities reflecting axonal loss are often found in human ischemic neuropathy, but the roles of metabolic and morphologic factors are uncertain. Femoral artery ligation was used to assess the physiologic and morphologic sequelae of transient focal nerve ischemia in adult rats. Percutaneous electrodes stimulated the sciatic and posterior tibial nerves, with subcutaneous recording electrodes over the intrinsic plantar muscles, and the femoral artery was ligated to produce proximal posterior tibial nerve ischemia. Electrophysiologic studies were repeated at intervals up to 24 hours after ligation.

Falling evoked muscle and nerve action potential amplitudes reflected focal and generalized impairment of impulse conduction within 10 minutes of femoral occlusion. Conduction failure was most marked at 45 to 60 minutes and resolved within 24 hours. The fastest motor and mixed nerve conduction velocities were reduced by less than 15% of baseline at the time of acute conduction block. Morphologic studies showed no evidence of segmental or paranodal demyelination or degeneration of myelinated or unmyelinated axons.

Transient nerve ischemia leads to a reversible conduction block without significant morphologic changes in the nerve. Slower-conducting myelinated fibers appear to be most sensitive to the effect of acute ischemia. The rapid reversibility of ischemic conduction failure suggests that metabolic, rather than morphologic, changes underlie the electrophysiologic abnormalities, although severe ischemia may lead to axonal infarction and segmental demyelination. An element of chronic entrapment neuropathies may have an ischemic basis. Compression-induced nerve ischemia could lead to transient conduction block, and relief from compression could explain the rapid improvement in pain and nerve conduction observed clinically.

▶ As stated in the article's own abstract, the fall in amplitude without significant conduction slowing implies that slower conducting myelinated fibers are relatively more sensitive to the effect of acute ischemia.—Russell N. DeJong, M.D.

Reactivity of Serums and Isolated Monoclonal IgM From Patients With Waldenström's Macroglobulinaemia With Peripheral Nerve Myelin
H. Harbs, M. Arfmann, E. Frick, Ch. Hörmann, U. Wurster, U. Patzold, E. Stark, and H. Deicher (Medizinische Hochschule Hannover and Univ. of Munich, Federal Republic of Germany)
J. Neurol. 232:43–48, March 1985   17–6

A peripheral polyneuropathy (PN) is found in 8% of cases of Waldenström's macroglobulinemia, and the actual incidence may be much higher. Peripheral polyneuropathy has been associated with benign monoclonal immunoglobulin M (IgM) paraproteinemia and benign monoclonal gammopathy. Twenty-three patients, aged 57 to 78 years, with biopsy-proved Waldenström's macroglobulinemia (range of duration of disease, less than 2 years to 12 years) were investigated. Nerve conduction velocity was measured in the median and peroneal nerves in the 12 patients who showed clinical evidence of PN.

Six patients had sensory and 6 had sensorimotor PN. Involvement of the CNS was not observed. Only 3 patients had received Vinca alkaloids. Nine of the 11 patients with disease for longer than 5 years had signs of PN. Indirect fluorescence studies gave similar results in patients with and in those without PN. Sera from patients with Waldenström's macroglobulinemia reacted mainly with structures at the border of the myelin sheath and occasionally with the axon itself. Fifteen of 23 serum samples were reactive in an antibody-dependent, lymphocyte-mediated cytotoxicity reaction (ADLC) with peripheral nerve myelin and to a lesser degree with myelin basic protein. Five of 6 monoclonal IgM preparations yielded ADLC reactions. Results of a complement fixation assay were normal.

These findings support an immunologic mechanism in the pathogenesis of PN in Waldenström's macroglobulinemia. Further work is needed to determine the number and identity of the nerve antigens involved, but there appears to be a restricted number of antigen specificities of the monoclonal IgM.

▶ These results provide additional evidence for an immunologic mechanism in the pathogenesis of the PN in Waldenström's macroglobulinemia.—Russell N. DeJong, M.D.

Tropical Myeloneuropathies: The Hidden Endemias
Gustavo C. Román, Peter S. Spencer, and Bruce S. Schoenberg (Texas Tech Univ., Albert Einstein College of Medicine, and Natl. Insts. of Health, Bethesda, Md.)
Neurology 35:1158–1170, August 1985   17–7

Myeloneuropathologic conditions of unknown origin have been described in geographic isolates throughout the tropics since the turn of the century. Reports went unnoticed in the United States and Europe until World War II, when neurologists became aware of the relationship between their occurrence and climatic, environmental, and nutritional factors. Tropical myelonephropathies pose a serious public health problem in certain affected countries because of the large number of disabled persons and the prevailing lack of preventive measures. Most of the disorders probably are multifactorial in origin, but malnutrition appears to be a common factor.

Tropical ataxic neuropathy (TAN) is an indolent myeloneuropathy usually affecting large populations in the tropics. It is characterized by severe loss of position and vibration sensation, touch, and pressure, particularly distally in the legs. Lower motor neuron signs may be present. Association with orogenital dermatitis and amblyopia led to the implication of malnutrition. The TAN and other neurologic syndromes were found in prisoners of war in tropical and subtropical regions. Deficiencies of the B-group vitamins have been implicated, as has tropical malabsorption. Painful neuropathy and ataxia are features of cassava neurotoxicosis, the result of a cassava-based diet that is prominent throughout the tropics. Yams, beans, and maize also contain cyanogenic alkaloids.

Tropical spastic paraparesis is less prevalent than TAN. The classic cause of epidemic outbreaks in the tropics is lathyrism. Malnutrition is a prominent factor, but cases not associated with malnutrition or vitamin deficiency have been reported in south India, South Africa, the Seychelles Islands, Jamaica, and Colombia. An unknown neurotoxic factor or, possibly, endemic treponemal infection, may be involved.

▶ The tropical myeloneuropathies constitute a serious, widespread health problem. They are multifactorial conditions that provide unsurpassed opportunities for international cooperation and neurologic research.—Russell N. DeJong, M.D.

Progressive, Predominantly Motor, Uraemic Neuropathy

R. J. S. McGonigle, M. Bewick, M. J. Weston, and V. Parsons (Dulwich Hosp., London)
Acta Neurol. Scand. 71:379–384, May 1985   17–8

A small proportion of uremic patients develop a severe, progressive neuropathy with chiefly motor involvement, producing muscle wasting and weakness. Four such cases were encountered among young men with end-stage renal failure, three of whom had accelerated hypertension. Symptoms began after the start of regular hemodialysis and in all cases were associated with septicemic illness.

Man, 19 years old, was seen, 3 years after the initial finding of proteinuria, with blurred vision and headaches. Blood pressure was 250/150 mm Hg, and he had grade IV retinopathy. The creatinine clearance was 9 ml per minute. The renal biopsy showed mesangial IgA nephropathy. Renal function continued to decline. The patient began to have painful feet and weak legs a few weeks after hemodialysis, after an episode of *Staphylococcus aureus* septicemia from an infected arteriovenous shunt. The neuropathy progressed rapidly, with gross wasting of the lower limbs and hands, dysarthria, and difficulty standing. Good dialysis control did not limit the neurologic disorder. Bilateral nephrectomy and cadaver kidney transplantation were performed after 7 months of hemodialysis. A perinephric abscess had to be drained, and several acute rejection episodes occurred, but renal function eventually returned to normal. Mobility improved gradually over the next 18 months, but clinical wasting persisted (Fig 17–2). Electrophysiologic study showed grossly impaired nerve conduction, with complete denervation of the distal hand and foot muscles. Sensory changes were less marked.

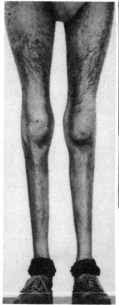
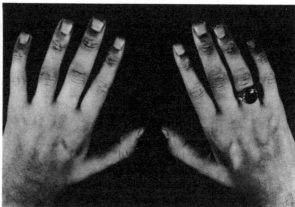

Fig 17–2.—Gross muscle wasting of the lower limbs and hands 15 months after successful renal transplantation is evident. (Courtesy of McGonigle, R.J.S., et al.: Acta Neurol. Scand. 71:379–384, May 1985.)

Renal transplantation led to considerable improvement in two of these patients, and the condition of a third stabilized after charcoal hemoperfusion was carried out. Nerve conduction, however, remained grossly impaired. Three of the four patients had severe, poorly controlled hypertension. Septicemia could exacerbate the neuropathy through endotoxin-mediated ischemia or through the accumulation of metabolites having a toxic effect on nerves compromised by ischemia. The neuropathy is partly irreversible.

▶ A severe progressive, predominantly motor, uremic neuropathy is described in four young men with end-stage renal failure. In three of the patients there was accelerated hypertension. Renal transplantation and charcoal hemoperfusion was followed by some clinical improvement in three patients, but there was no associated improvement in nerve conduction studies. A possible ischemic etiology related to accelerated hypertension and septicemia is suggested for this unusual, serious and partly irreversible variant of uremic neuropathy.—Russell N. DeJong, M.D.

Polyneuritis Cranialis Associated With *Borrelia Burgdorferi*
E. Schmutzhard, G. Stanek, and P. Pohl (Univ. Hosp. of Innsbruck and Univ. of Vienna, Austria)
J. Neurol. Neurosurg. Psychiatry 48:1182–1184, November 1985   17–9

Three cases of typical polyneuritis cranialis associated with the spirochete *Borrelia burgdorferi* without involvement of peripheral nerves, nerve roots, or the brain were encountered.

Woman, 39 years old, developed right facial paresis and, a few days later, left-sided facial paresis. Taste was impaired, but there were no other abnormal neurologic signs. Lymphocytic pleocytosis was found in the cerebrospinal fluid, as were markedly elevated immunoglobulin indices. Electroencephalograms and computed tomography scans were normal, and complement fixation studies were negative for neurotropic viruses. Antituberculosis treatment was instituted. Facial paresis began improving within a week and resolved totally after about 3 weeks, but the cerebrospinal fluid abnormalities persisted for more than 3½ months. Subsequently, antibodies against *B. burgdorferi* were found, and antituberculosis drugs were replaced by penicillin G, with positive serologic effects. The patient had not been bitten by ticks or tabanidae in the previous year.

The three patients had isolated polyneuritis cranialis; two had a history of tick bite, and one had erythema chronicum migrans. The neurologic manifestations of tick-transmitted Lyme disease are those of meningoradiculoneuritis. Infection by *B. burgdorferi* should be considered when osteomyelitis of the skull base, basal meningitis, diabetes, tumor, and granulomatous meningitides are excluded. Penicillin G therapy has been very effective.

▶ Perhaps some unexplained cranial nerve palsies are due to the Lyme-Bannwarth syndrome caused by *B. burgdorferi* in which case they may be treatable.—Robert D. Currier, M.D.

Idiopathic (Bell's) Facial Palsy: Natural History Defies Steroid Or Surgical Treatment

Mark May, Susan R. Klein, and Floyd H. Taylor (Univ. of Pittsburgh)
Laryngoscope 95:406–409, April 1985   17–10

Idiopathic (Bell's) facial palsy is a self-limiting condition that is spontaneously remitting and has a favorable natural history. The prognostic efficacy of evoked electromyography (EEMG) and the benefits of transmastoid facial nerve surgical decompression for relief of Bell's palsy were investigated.

Two hundred and seventy-three patients with unilateral paralysis were studied. Surgery was recommended for 38 patients on the basis of complete paralysis and a response to EEMG of 10% or less of normal; their results, including those for the 13 patients who did not have the operation are summarized in the table. Results were classified by use of a modification of the House system, a comprehensive, accurate, valid, and reproducible method of reporting recovery. There were no statistically significant differences between the results obtained with surgery and those occurring without surgery. Evaluation of all 273 patients by EEMG revealed that this procedure is the test of choice for predicting which patients are most likely to have spontaneous recovery of facial function. Of 204 patients with an EEMG response ≥25% of normal, 98% had a satisfactory recovery.

Although the number of patients who had surgery in this study was small, it appears from these results that surgery did not improve the outcome for these patients. The authors feel that surgery can no longer be justified for Bell's palsy.

▶ Well, this is a surprise to me. I thought that surgery probably was helpful in selected cases.—Robert D. Currier, M.D.

INFLUENCE OF TRANSMASTOID SURGERY ON RECOVERY FROM
BELL'S PALSY IN 38 PATIENTS WITH POOR PROGNOSES*

Treatment	No.	Results Satisfactory		Results Unsatisfactory	
		I	II	III	IV
				(% unsatisfactory)	
No surgery	13	1	2	9 (77%)	1
Surgery	25	0	5	11 (80%)	9

*Poor prognosis was based on results on EEMG of 0% to 10% of normal and complete palsy.

(Courtesy of May, M., et al.: Laryngoscope 95:406–409, April 1985.)

Hemifacial Spasm: Results of Electrophysiologic Recording During Microvascular Decompression Operations

Aage R. Møller and Peter J. Jannetta (Univ. of Pittsburgh)
Neurology 35:969–974, July 1985   17–11

Hemifacial spasm (HFS) is ascribed to facial nerve injury from cross-compression by blood vessels at the root entry zone in most cases, but it is unclear whether nerve injury in the facial motonucleus or the formation of artificial synapses is responsible. Neural conduction was measured in the antidromic and orthodromic parts of the facial nerve in 24 patients with classic HFS who underwent microvascular decompression of the nerve with general anesthesia. The marginal mandibular nerve and zygomatic branch of the facial nerve (Fig 17–3) were stimulated, and the supraorbital nerve was stimulated with a surface electrode.

The orbicularis oculi response to stimulation of the marginal mandibular nerve had a latency 2.2 msec longer than the sum of the conduction times of the parts of the facial nerve that would be involved were the response a result of ephaptic transmission at the root entry zone of the facial nerve. Similar results were obtained when the zygomatic branch of the facial nerve was stimulated. Several tests were done to insure that the response to stimulation of the peripheral part of the facial nerve was mediated by antidromic activity in the facial

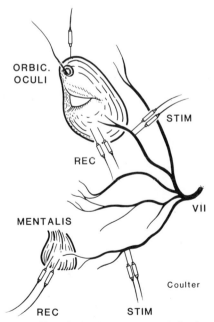

Fig 17–3.—Schematic illustration of how the facial nerve (VII) is stimulated (STIM) and the electromyographic response of the muslces (ORBIC. OCULI, MENTALIS) recorded (REC). (Courtesy of Møller, A.R., and Jannetta, P.J.: Neurology 35:969–974, July 1985.)

nerve and did not result from simultaneous stimulation of a trigeminal nerve branch.

The findings suggest that the facial motonucleus is involved in HFS, and that it is unlikely that ephaptic transmission in the facial nerve near its root entry zone is responsible for synkinesis and spasm. Activity generated at the lesion site propagates in both directions and, when impinging on the facial motor nucleus over a long time, may set up abnormal neural circuits that in turn give rise to abnormal facial muscle contractions.

▶ These results document the fact that the motor nucleus of the facial nerve is involved in hemifacial spasm.—Russell N. DeJong, M.D.

18 Miscellaneous Topics

The Neurologic Content of Family Practice: Implications for Neurologists
James Q. Miller (Univ. of Virginia School of Medicine)
Arch. Neurol. 43:286–288, March 1986   18–1

Recent publications by Murray and Kurtzke have provided information on the nature and prevalence of neurologic disorders in the United States. Other authors have discussed issues of neurologic manpower and the future oversupply or undersupply of neurologically competent physicians. To address the related question of what neurologic problems come to family and general practitioners—those members of the medical community most frequently contacted for initial diagnosis and subsequent management or referral—a survey was conducted in which 23 of 40 physicians identified by the Virginia State Board of Medicine as family or general practitioners participated. Neurologic questions were addressed in 9% of patient visits. A total of 9,500 patient visits provided approximately 11,500 health problems. Neurologic patient complaints were grouped into the following categories: pain; peripheral nerve problems; dizziness, vertigo, tinnitus; cerebrovascular disease; epilepsy; dementia; involuntary movements; head or spine trauma; weakness; and other such important neurologic conditions as amyotrophic lateral sclerosis, multiple sclerosis, meningitis, mental retardation with neurologic deficits, static encephalopathy, neoplasm, and syncope. The responses were compared with other surveys.

Pain was the most common complaint among patients with probable or possible neurologic disorders in this survey. Back pain and headache together made up about 50% of "neurologic" visits; low-back pain was the single most frequent entity. The frequency of this common complaint indicates that neurologists should increase their role in its management. Nonmigraine patient visits were more frequent that migraine ones. Dizziness, vertigo, or tinnitus, followed by cerebrovascular disorders, were frequent diagnostic and management challenges. Relatively few patients presented to the family physician with recognized evidence of problems related to multiple sclerosis, amyotrophic lateral sclerosis, static encephalopathies, neoplasia, infections, or weakness, a finding in significant contrast with the usual content of neurologic specialty practice.

Generalists see few patients with progressive diseases of nervous system or muscle but frequently encounter patients complaining of back pain, headache, peripheral nerve problems, or dizziness, and they experience more uncertainty in treating these patients than those with equivalent internal medical conditions. An in-depth knowledge and expert clinical application of neurologic pathophysiology should be the basis for answering neurologic-patient-care questions, and neurologists are the practitioners most able to diagnose and treat neurologic disease. Residency-training programs should train and evaluate graduates in the management of patients with cervical and lumbosacral back pain, headache, peripheral nerve disorders, and dizziness, since these patients will constitute the majority for whom their colleagues in general or family practice will seek consultation.

▶ After looking at our local medical school neurologic curriculum, it is clear that our teaching is not attending properly to the most frequent neurologic disorders complained of by patients. We do include a lecture each on peripheral neuropathy, disk disease, and headache, but nothing on dizziness and nothing on the treatment of low-back pain in general.—Robert D. Currier, M.D.

Neuropsychiatry . . . Again
Eric D. Caine and Robert J. Joynt (Univ. of Rochester, NY)
Arch. Neurol. 43:325–328, April 1986   18–2

There has recently been a renewed interest in neuropsychiatry. During the first half of the 20th century, many psychiatrists considered neuropsychiatry synonymous with general psychiatry. An enthusiasm for the clinical-neuropathologic correlation of cerebral disorder, which developed from the study of aphasia, was encouraged further by the recognition that general paresis of the insane was an acquired disease and later by the successful treatment of general paresis and pernicious anemia. However, other behavioral abnormalities proved more resistant to organic approaches; for example, neuropathologic studies failed to clarify the pathophysiology of schizophrenia or depression.

In 1952, Cobb attempted to blend the perspectives of psychiatrists and neurologists. Neuropharmacology has dominated psychiatric research during the past 20 years, with the neuronal synapse as the focus for study. The emergence of neuropsychiatry coincides with the appearance of "behavioral neurology," the growing prominence of "clinical neuropsychology," and the preeminence of "biologic psychiatry." The roots of neuropsychiatry are embedded in both neurology and psychiatry, whereas behavioral neurology draws its inspiration from the former. Clinical neuropsychology shares a common theme with neuropsychiatry in relating brain function to mental processes. Although neuropsychiatry is built on a neurobiologic scientific foundation, it does not stand in opposition to other modes of considering human behavior. Like neurology, neuropsychiatry deals with brain diseases. The brain is regarded as the site of interaction between what is inherited and what is learned or acquired. Treatment is planned according to the presentation of symptoms of disturbances in (1) arousal, attention, and concentration; (2) mood and affect; (3) perception (both internal and external, ideational, and physical); (4) intellectual function (e.g., language and memory); and (5) personality. Neuropsychiatry is an amalgam of psychiatry, neurology, and neuropsychology. Patients with cerebral infarctions, degenerative diseases, and persistent neurophysiologic abnormalities come to the attention of the neuropsychiatrist. Such involuntary movement disorders as drug-induced dyskinesia or Gilles de la Tourette's syndrome are focal points for neuropsychiatric research.

To overcome the traditional schism between psychiatry and neurology, new patterns of training are being developed. The American Board of Psychiatry and Neurology has recently changed its eligibility requirements for dual certification in Neurology and Psychiatry. As of January 1, 1987, a prior approved combined residency program must include, following internship, at least two years of psychiatry, two years of neurology, and one jointly supervised year.

▶ Robert J. Joynt, Chief Editor of the *Archives of Neurology,* makes a plea for the resurgence of the term *neuropsychiatry.* The movement to unify mental disorders and brain diseases begun by Greisinger in 1845 was gradually discarded between the two world wars by increasing regard for psychoanalysis and social psychiatry. Now, with growing interest in behavioral neurology, clinical neuropsychiatry, and biological psychiatry, neuropsychiatry is emerging again, and, after a century of separation, psychiatry and neurology are uniting. With such clinical activists as Robert Joynt and such investigators as the late Norman Geschwind, there will obviously be continued progress in our understanding of disorders of behavior.—Russell N. DeJong, M.D.

Neuroleptic Malignant Syndrome
Moonasar P. Rampertaap (Univ. of Missouri and Truman Med. Ctr., Kansas City)
South. Med. J. 79:331–336, March 1986   18–3

The neuroleptic malignant syndrome (NMS), first reported by Delay and Deniker in 1968, is a lethal complication of neuroleptic medication. This syndrome may be underdiagnosed because it is poorly understood and often unrecognized. It affects all age groups and has a 20% mortality, which is predominantly from respiratory failure. Men are affected five times as often as women. Presenting features include extrapyramidal symptoms, altered mental consciousness, autonomic dysfunction, and hyperthermia. Since neuroleptic drugs exert both therapeutic and adverse effects through dopamine-receptor blockade in the basal ganglia and hypothalamus, the best hypothesis for the cause of NMS is that, given the proper (though as yet unknown) neurobiochemical conditions, dopamine-receptor blockade can produce the clinical features of the syndrome. Three case histories are presented.

CASE 1.—Woman, 43 years old, during the first episode of psychosis was treated with 5 mg of intramuscular haloperidol, followed by the oral administration of 2 mg three times a day. Two days after the initiation of haloperidol therapy, altered responsiveness, rigidity, and a two-day history of incontinence were noted. The patient stared fixedly at the wall and was mute, with ptyalism. Forty-eight hours after admission, the patient became semistuporous with marked "lead-pipe" rigidity, claw-like hands, and mask-like face. Temperature was 99 F, respiration 12 per minute, and pulse 40 per minute, with fluctuating blood pressure. When NMS was diagnosed, the haloperidol therapy was immediately discontinued and oral bromocriptine therapy initiated at 5 mg three times daily. By the second day of bromocriptine therapy, the patient became responsive, autonomic functions were stable, and extrapyramidal symptoms had greatly decreased. The patient was able to walk on the fifth day of bromocriptine therapy, with normal extrapyramidal functions and biochemical parameters.

Neuroleptic malignant syndrome is a life-threatening illness that does not lend itself to study by controlled trials. Fluphenazine and haloperidol, the two neuroleptics most commonly associated with NMS, were given to the 3 patients in the present case reports. In case reports previously cited, patients treated with oral bromocriptine had regained stability of autonomic functions and consciousness and showed improvement of other extrapyramidal symptoms within 5–48 hours. Bromocriptine is the drug of choice because it has decreased overall mortality. Patients treated with this dopamine agonist have responded rapidly, usually within hours, which is noted by improvement in the clinical features of this lethal syndrome. Because bromocriptine's effect is exerted in small increments, it is less likely to produce additional adverse effects when used to treat NMS in patients who are already severely debilitated.

Bromocriptine has been proved efficacious and should be further evaluated in the treatment of NMS.

▶ The neuroleptic malignant syndrome, first reported in 1968 (Delay, J., Deniker, P.: *Handbook of Clinical Neurology* [Vol. 6], Vinken, P., and Bruyn, G. [eds.], Amsterdam: North Holland Publishing Co., 1968) is a rare but potentially fatal disorder associated with the administration of neuroleptic agents. These authors have found that bromocriptine, a dopamine agonist, is effective in the treatment of this syndrome and recommend that its use be further investigated.—Russell N. DeJong, M.D.

A Neuroleptic Malignant-Like Syndrome Due to Levodopa Therapy Withdrawal

Joseph H. Friedman, Stanford S. Feinberg, and Robert G. Feldman (Brown Univ., Boston Univ., and Boston VA Hosp.)
JAMA 254:2792–2795, Nov. 15, 1985   18–4

Three cases of a disorder resembling neuroleptic malignant syndrome (NMS) were encountered in three patients undergoing discontinuation of levodopa therapy for long-standing Parkinson's disease. None had been exposed to neuroleptics at any time. Three similar cases, one of them fatal, have previously been reported.

Man, 71 years old, was admitted to the hospital with fever, rigidity, and diaphoresis after 10 years of idiopathic Parkinson's disease. His mother had tremors only, and a brother had amyotrophic lateral sclerosis. The patient had responded to levodopa therapy for 10 years, but function had declined in the past 2 years while he was receiving constant carbidopa-levodopa therapy. Sudden freezing episodes developed, with increased stiffness and tremor. Marked rigidity was accompanied by tachycardia and a diffuse erythematous rash. Ethopropazine and diphenhydramine were given along with carbidopa-levodopa at the time the episode began. Carbidopa-levodopa and benztropine produced improvement. Over the next 6 days, carbidopa-levodopa treatment was tapered and benztropine therapy continued, and less severe episodes of increased rigidity and tremor occurred, apparently in relation to benztropine. A very severe episode occurred on the seventh day without carbidopa-levodopa, and the patient became comatose, hypotensive, and bradycardic. Renal failure occurred the next day, and the patient died a week later of aspiration pneumonia.

All three patients had a long history of Parkinson's disease and had received carbidopa-levodopa therapy. Two developed the syndrome when therapy was temporarily discontinued. There probably is dysfunction at more than one level of the neuroaxis in these cases. The neuroleptic malignant syndrome has been ascribed to dopamine receptor blockade. The syndrome should be considered in patients undergoing drug holiday. Determination of the creatine kinase level may be useful in febrile patients. Patients with evidence of NMS may be poor candidates for drug holidays.

▶ The neuroleptic malignant syndrome evidently can be associated with drugs that are antidopaminergic or withdrawal of drugs that are directly or indirectly dopaminergic. There are two good reviews, one by Guze and Baxter in *The New England Journal of Medicine* (313:163–166, July 18, 1985) and the other by Gibb and Lees in the *Quarterly Journal of Medicine* (56:421–429, August 1985). Treatment consists of discontinuing the administration of whatever drug caused it, the administration of dantrolene plus possibly other drugs including bromocriptine and amantadine, and cooling the patient. Since NMS may be precipitated by drug holidays, perhaps the appropriateness of such holidays should be carefully reconsidered.—Robert D. Currier, M.D.

Neurologic Complications of Gastric Partitioning
George W. Paulson, Edward W. Martin, Cathy Mojzisik, and Larey C. Carey (Ohio State Univ.)
Arch. Neurol. 42:675–677, July 1985   18–5

Six patients had severe, complex neurologic disturbances after gastric reduction for morbid obesity. All were profoundly weak or paraplegic, had encephalopathic features, and had prolonged and incomplete recovery. Encephalopathy was documented by neurologic examination and the EEG findings. Confusion, agitation, and inappropriate behavior led to an initial diagnosis of hysteria in all cases. No patient had overt liver failure or a significant ammonia elevation. The patients had normal vitamin B_{12} concentrations, and more than one patient had normal folate, magnesium, heavy metal, and cortisol values. Tests for mononucleosis and porphyria were negative, as were thyroid tests and viral or complement studies.

The symptoms in these patients resembled those of hyperemesis gravidarum. Sudden, massive weight loss might produce toxic effects. Patients who vomit or lose weight abruptly require attention to vitamin and protein status. Those seen after surgery should not initially be labeled as hysterical. Malnutrition is a possibility even in the presence of massive obesity. Preoperative and postoperative EEG and electromyographic recordings may be useful in this setting. The syndrome may have more than one cause, but vitamin deficiency is a useful postulate in terms of treatment and prevention. Extremely rapid metabolism of fat in the context of acute starvation may damage the nervous system.

▶ This contribution calls attention to the possibly dangerous and even potentially fatal complications of this elective relief for extreme morbid obesity.— Russell N. DeJong, M.D.

Reversible "Locked-in" Syndromes

G. Ebinger, L. Huyghens, L. Corne, and W. Aelbrecht (Vrije Universiteit Brussel, Brussels)

Intensive Care Med. 11:218–219, July 1985   18–6

"Locked-in" syndrome connotes a state of quadriplegia and paralysis of the lower cranial nerves with preservation of consciousness. Patients can communicate by blinking their eyes. The cerebro-medullospinal disconnection usually results from ventral pontine infarction after basilar artery occlusion. Patients rarely survive more than a few days or weeks, but significant recovery has been described.

Two young patients were encountered who made good recoveries from a locked-in syndrome presumed to be due to ventral pontine ischemia.

Woman, aged 19 years, developed seizures during cisplatinum therapy for metastatic ovarian cancer. Consciousness returned within 24 hours, although the patient was able to reply to questions only by closing her eyes or looking up or down. She was quadriplegic and had flaccid tone in all extremities, as well as jaw and facial muscle paralysis. She eventually recovered completely from quadriplegia and mutism, suggesting that a basilar artery spasm was responsible. Neurologic findings were normal 2 months after presentation.

Woman, aged 31 years, developed seizures following a respiratory arrest during nasal surgery (from which she had recovered except for slight dysarthria and mild spasticity). Leg movement returned 3 weeks after onset of the locked-in syndrome. After 2 years, the patient was totally independent. Pontine infarction was ascribed to a basilar artery spasm or occlusion that was related to nasal infiltration with local anesthetic containing adrenaline.

Patients can make a good recovery from a locked-in syndrome, a finding that warrants aggressive supportive measures in the first weeks or months. The syndrome often is overlooked or misdiagnosed as true coma.

▶ Since patients may recover nearly completely from a locked-in syndrome, aggressive supportive therapy seems justified during the initial weeks or months.—Russell N. DeJong, M.D.

Randomized Clinical Study of Thiopental Loading in Comatose Survivors of Cardiac Arrest

Brain Resuscitation Clinical Trial I Study Group (Univ. of Pittsburgh)
N. Engl. J. Med. 314:397–403, Feb. 13, 1986   18–7

To determine the efficacy of thiopental loading in the amelioration of brain damage after severe global ischemic insults to the brain and to identify the risks and complications of this experimental treatment, 12 hospitals in nine countries participated in a randomized clinical trial. After restoration of spontaneous circulation and adequate oxygenation, 262 comatose survivors of cardiac arrest were randomly assigned to receive standard brain-oriented intensive care or the same standard therapy plus a single intravenous loading dose of thiopental (30 mg/kg). Three fourths of the patients were male (mean age, 58 years; range, less than 1 to 88 years). After restoration of spontaneous circulation, patients were observed for 10 minutes to verify both eligibility and cardiovascular stability. The thiopental-loading group received a single-loading dose of up to 30 mg of intravenous thiopental/kg, given as soon as possible after the 10-minute observation period and as rapidly as the circulation would tolerate. For each patient, the cerebral and overall performances were evaluated 48–72 hours, 10 days, and 1, 3, 6, and 12 months after cardiac arrest. Determinations of prearrest status were accomplished through family member interviews.

Base-line characteristics were similar in the two groups. By the end of the 1-year follow-up, 77% of the patients in the thiopental group, compared with 80% of those in the standard-therapy group, had died. Most deaths occurred within the first month (Fig 18–1). The causes of death were similar: cerebral failure caused 37% of the deaths in the thiopental

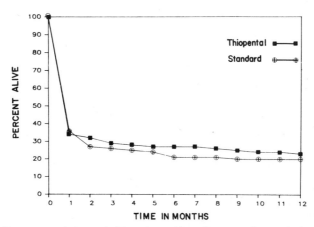

Fig 18–1.—One-year cumulative survival in patients with cardiac arrest who remained comatose after the restoration of spontaneous circulation. (Courtesy of Brain Resuscitation Clinical Trial I Study Group: N. Engl. J. Med. 314:397–403, Feb. 13, 1986. Reprinted by permission of The New England Journal of Medicine.)

group vs. 36% of those in the standard-therapy group. The mortality among 18 patients who received 20 mg or less/kg of thiopental was 78%, compared with 77% among those who received more than 20 mg/kg. After 1 year of follow-up, 18% of the patients in the thiopental group had recovered and were functioning at their prearrest level of cerebral function, compared with 15% of those in the standard-therapy group. Five percent of both groups were conscious but had some degree of permanent neurologic damage compared with their prearrest state. The incidence of postresuscitation complications, with the exception of hypotension, was similar. Hypotension developed during the first 8 hours after resuscitation in 60% of the thiopental group, compared with 29% of the standard-therapy group. Early arrhythmias and rearrests occurred with approximately equal frequency in both groups.

In skilled hands thiopental can be safely administered immediately after cardiac arrest for such purposes as sedation, anticonvulsant therapy, or reduction of intracranial pressure. However, the hypothesis that high-dose thiopental administered 10 minutes or more after restoration of spontaneous circulation ameliorates neurologic damage in comatose survivors of cardiac arrest was not supported.

▶ Recent evidence indicates that the resistance of neurons to ischemia exceeds the commonly accepted time limit of 4–6 minutes and that potentially treatable neuronal damage occurs during and after reperfusion (Ames, A., III, et al.: *Stroke* 14:219–226, 1983; Safar, P., et al.: *Arch. Neurol.* 33:91–95, 1976). In the present study, 262 comatose survivors of cardiac arrest, were randomly given, after restoration of spontaneous circulation and adequate oxygenation, either standard brain-oriented intensive care or the same standard therapy plus a single intravenous loading-dose of a barbiturate, thiopental (Brievik, H., et al.: *Anesthesiology* 49:390–398, 1978). At the end of a 1-year follow-up, there was no statistically significant difference between the two treatment groups. The results of this study do not support the use of barbiturates for brain resuscitation after cardiac arrest.—Russell N. DeJong, M.D.

Serum Creatine Kinase Level as a Screening Test for Susceptibility to Malignant Hyperthermia
Rein T. Paasuke and A. Keith W. Brownell (Univ. of Calgary)
JAMA 255:769–771, Feb. 14, 1986   18–8

Relatives of persons susceptible to malignant hyperthermia (MH) may also be susceptible, and the only definitive way of making a diagnosis is with an in vitro muscle contracture test, a cumbersome and invasive procedure, or a definite MH reaction under anesthesia. Many patients still are advised on the basis of serum creatine kinase (CK) levels or its isoenzymes, although this method can result in underidentification of susceptible individuals. Muscle biopsy and in vitro caffeine contracture studies were performed on more than 130 patients who either had a suspected MH reaction or were relatives of MH-susceptible persons. Muscle specimens were taken from the vastus lateralis muscle during anesthesia with a known safe agent or with procaine nerve block.

All 87 patients not susceptible to MH had normal prebiopsy serum CK levels, as did 34 MH-susceptible patients without other muscle disease. The mean CK level was slightly higher in the MH-susceptible group, but the test was nondiagnostic. Four of 10 patients with other muscle disease had normal CK values. All 10 of these patients had positive caffeine contracture test findings, and several had a clinical MH reaction under anesthesia.

The practice of diagnosing MH susceptibility by measuring the serum CK level should be abandoned because of the frequency of false positive and false negative findings. Myopathy may be present even if physical signs are absent, and skeletal muscle biopsy should be done, along with an in vitro muscle contracture test if feasible. If there is no evidence of myopathy despite an elevated CK level, no special precautions for MH need be taken.

▶ This news is unfortunate. The in vitro caffeine test sounds somewhat cumbersome and certainly must be more difficult and time-consuming than obtaining a serum creatine kinase level. Perhaps someone will eventually come up with a better test.

Pamphlett et al. (*Aust. N.Z. J. Med.* 15:199–202, April 1985) and Greig et al. (*Surg. Gynecol. & Obstet.* 160:466–468, May 1985) have recently commented on the vacuum or suction needle biopsy test for muscle disease. Both give it good marks. It certainly does sound easier and quicker and probably has fewer postbiopsy complications. Shri Mishra, our local muscle expert, continues to prefer the open biopsy since it gives better fiber orientation and allows the obtaining of a larger specimen. One would presume that both methods will survive.—Robert D. Currier, M.D.

Treatment of Pathologic Laughing and Weeping With Amitriptyline
Randolph B. Schiffer, Robert M. Herndon, and Richard A. Rudick (Strong Mem. Hosp., Rochester, N.Y.)
N. Engl. J. Med. 312:1480–1482, June 6, 1985   18–9

Disorders damaging subcortical forebrain structures can disinhibit the motor systems for emotional expression and result in pathologic laughing and weeping. The use of tricyclic drugs has been suggested in stroke patients. A double-blind, cross-over trial of amitriptyline was carried out in 12 patients with bilateral forebrain disease due to multiple sclerosis. Two patients had episodes of laughing, 8 of weeping, and 2 of both. Amitriptyline was given for 30 days, as was placebo. The mean daily dose of amitriptyline was 58 mg (maximum daily dose, 75 mg).

Eight patients were thought to improve with amitriptyline therapy, and 7 of them improved dramatically. The drug effect was significant when measured both by lability counts and clinical judgments. One patient improved with placebo. The responders and nonresponders could not be distinguished clinically or demographically or in degree of compliance with treatment. Because of side effects 4 responders required a dose reduction, as did 2 placebo patients. Symptoms of depression were not prominent at baseline and did not change significantly during the study, as measured by the Beck Inventory and the Hamilton Scale.

Low-dose amitriptyline is an effective treatment of patients with multiple sclerosis and pathologic laughing and weeping. Partial restoration of inhibitory transmission via subcortical relays may be responsible. The effective drugs potentiate transmission of the inhibitory neurotransmitter dopamine in the caudate nucleus. A trial of amitriptyline seems to be worthwhile in patients with forebrain disease causing pathologic laughing or weeping.

▶ This treatment is also recommended for the emotional lability of the bulbar paralysis of amyotrophic lateral sclerosis.—Robert D. Currier, M.D.

Chronic Idiopathic Anhidrosis
P. A. Low, R. D. Fealey, S. G. Sheps, W. P. D. Su, J. C. Trautmann, and N. L. Kuntz (Mayo Clinic and Found.)
Ann. Neurol. 18:344–348, September 1985   18–10

Generalized sudomotor failure occurs in various peripheral autonomic neuropathies, such as acute panautomatic, diabetic, and amyloid neuropathies, but relatively isolated thermoregulatory sudomotor failure is less well known. Eight affected patients (4 men) aged 23–62 years were encountered in a 2-year period. Symptoms had been present for 1 to 10 years. Symptoms of heat intolerance included subjective heat, dizziness, dyspnea, weakness, and flushing in the absence of sweating. The patients rapidly learned to avoid hyperthermia. The general medical history was unremarkable except for one patient with hypertension and one with breast cancer. Vasospastic symptoms were frequent.

Sural nerve biopsies performed on two of the patients showed a minor reduction in myelinated fibers density. Electromyography showed no marked abnormalities. No patient had orthostatic hypotension. Skin vasomotor reflexes were abnormal in three of the seven patients tested. The quantitative sudomotor axon reflex test responses in the forearm and foot were reduced or absent in four of the eight patients. Three patients had pupillary abnormalities.

The term *chronic idiopathic anhidrosis* is suggested for this disorder. Thermoregulatory impairment produced symptoms in all these patients, who had widespread anhidrosis or hypohidrosis. Whether the lesion is in the central or in the peripheral nervous system is unclear. The prognosis appears to be relatively good. None of the eight patients have developed widespread autonomic failure or symptomatic peripheral neuropathy during long-term observation. Other disorders associated with generalized anhidrosis carry a relatively poor prognosis.

▶ Here is lack of the ability to adjust to heat caused by a nervous system disorder. In reference to the last article one might ask which comes first, the loss of heat regulating neurons or the heat causing a loss of spinal cord and possibly other neurons?—Robert D. Currier, M.D.

Hypoglycemia: Causes, Neurological Manifestations, and Outcome
Renée Malouf and John C. M. Brust (Columbia Univ.)
Ann. Neurol. 17:421–430, May 1985   18–11

An attempt was made to define symptomatic categories for 125 patient visits to an emergency room in a 12-month, prospective study for symptomatic hypoglycemia. Only subjects aged 18 and older were included. The total number of patients was 116. Seventy-one visits led to admission.

The clinical presentation is outlined in Table 1. A cause of hypoglycemia was identified in all cases. Diabetes, alcoholism, or sepsis accounted for 90% of the cases. Fasting alone explained symptomatic hypoglycemia in five instances. No patient had an insulin-secreting tumor. There was no case of uncomplicated reactive hypoglycemia or surreptitious insulin administration. A wide range of blood glucose concentrations was apparent in most groups. The cause of hypoglycemia was not predictive of the symptoms, although most patients with bizarre behavior were diabetic and/or alcoholic. The blood glucose concentration also was not predictive of the symptoms. The degree of hypoglycemia did not predict hypothermia, nor did hypothermia itself predict symptoms.

Mortality was 11%, but only one death was attributable to hypoglycemia itself. Four patients had residual focal neurologic signs, but it was impossible to assess subtle changes in cognitive function or behavior.

Potentially hypoglycemic agents are listed in Table 2. Nearly half the patients in this study were alcohol abusers. Residual abnormalities were unexpectedly infrequent, but subtle mental impairment may have gone

TABLE 1.—CLINICAL PRESENTATION

Presenting Symptom	No. of Patient Visits
Depressed sensorium	
Coma	39
Stupor	16
Obtundation	10
Behavioral change	
Confusion	24
Bizarre behavior	14
Dizziness, tremor	10
Seizures	9
Sudden hemiparesis	3
Total	125

(Courtesy of Malouf, R., and Brust, J.C.M.: Ann. Neurol. 17:421–430, May 1985.)

TABLE 2.—POTENTIALLY HYPOGLYCEMIC AGENTS

Agents

Phenylbutazone	Pentamidine
Aspirin	Dextropropoxyphene
Halofenate	Orphenadrine
Dicumarol	Ethylenediaminetetra-acetate
Sulfa drugs	Manganese
Chloramphenicol	Amphetamine
Propranolol	Lithium
Acetaminophen	Disopyramide
Oxytetracycline	Hypoglycin (akee nut)
Monoamine oxidase inhibitors	Quinine
Phenothiazines	Kerola (herb)
Haloperidol	Onion extract

(Courtesy of Malouf, R., and Brust, J.C.M.: Ann. Neurol. 17:421–430, May 1985.)

unnoticed in alcoholic or elderly patients. Coma is less dangerous when caused by hypoglycemia than by anoxia-ischemia. Severely symptomatic hypoglycemia, however, is a medical emergency. Patients with unexplained behavioral change, seizures, or coma should receive glucose with thiamine. Most patients should be admitted, since relapse can occur some hours after apparently effective treatment.

▶ The causes of true hypoglycemia were diabetes, alcohol, and sepsis. The list of potentially hypoglycemic agents is an eye opener.

An editorial in *The Lancet* (2:759, October 5, 1985) discusses hypoglycemia and in particular the hemiparesis, which is quickly corrected with glucose, and concludes that there is no clear understanding of it. However, an article by Frier and Hilsted appearing the following month in *The Lancet* (2:1175–1177, November 23, 1985) lists several hemostatic variables that alter with hypoglycemia, including changes in platelet function, fibrinogen and thromboglobulin levels, and rises in hematocrit values, all of which I suppose could explain hypoglycemia.—Robert D. Currier, M.D.

Treatment by Progabide in One Case of Painful Legs and Moving Toes
Ph. Bovier, H. Hilleret, and R. Tissot (Institutions Universitaries de Psychiatrie, Geneva)
Rev. Neurol. (Paris) 141:422–424, 1985   18–12

First described in 1971, the painful legs and moving toes syndrome associates painful lower extremities with spontaneous movements of the toes of flexion-extension and adduction-abduction type. This "dance of the toes" may be stopped voluntarily but resumes as soon as attention is no longer focused on the foot. The physiopathology of this phenomenon remains unexplained, although one hypothesis suggests that stimuli arising from intervertebral disk lesions, the posterior radix or peripheral nerve, join the pathway implicated in the control of pain at the medullary level, whereas others stimulate the medullary motoneurons by way of the interneurons, giving rise to the toe movements. There being no currently recognized treatment for this syndrome, the authors report the effect of progabide, a gamma-aminobutyric acid (GABA)-agonist, in one patient.

Woman, aged 64 years, when hospitalized in March 1984 for involutional melancholia was found to have "painful legs and moving toes" syndrome. Historical data included coxalgias following her first delivery and subsequent repeated bouts of lumbar pain. At age 40 years, there was an onset of episodic pain in both legs, which was attributed to bilateral hallux valgus. At age 63 years, the spontaneous movements of the toes were noted in the left foot.

Clinical examination confirmed bilateral hallux valgus, hammer toes, collapsed plantar arch, and a luxation of the big toe. Aside from a hyperalgesic zone at the plantar base of the big toe, findings were normal. Radiologic investigation showed a sesamoid bone, general osteoporosis, and hemisacralization of the last lumbar vertebra.

Progabide therapy was started at 40 mg/kg (1,800 mg/24 hours), associated with active physiotherapy of the left foot. Within 2 weeks abnormal movements diminished in amplitude and frequency. At 5 weeks clomipramine was added to the patient's regimen to combat the depressive state, with resultant mood elevation and parallel diminution of pain. At 6 months, all abnormal movements had disappeared.

Further observations will have to confirm the effect of progabide in this type of affliction.

▶ This is a rare syndrome of unknown etiology. This report of the relief of one case by the administration of a GABA-agonist needs further confirmation.— Russell N. DeJong, M.D.

Somatosensory Evoked Potentials in Cervical Spondylosis: Correlation of Median, Ulnar and Posterior Tibial Nerve Responses With Clinical and Radiological Findings
Y. L. Yu and S. J. Jones (Natl. Hosp. for Nervous Diseases, London)
Brain 108:273–300, June 1985   18–13

The diagnosis of myelopathy associated with cervical spondylosis may be problematic, and there is little correlation between the degree of radiologic spondylosis and the presence or severity of myelopathy. Somatosensory evoked potentials (SEPs) after median, ulnar, and tibial nerve stimulation were recorded from shoulder, neck, and scalp sites in 34 patients with symptomatic cervical spondylosis, 20 men (mean age, 60 years) and 14 women (mean age, 58 years). Twenty controls were also evaluated. Fifteen study patients had myelopathy alone on clinical grounds, 6 had radiculopathy and myelopathy, 6 had radiculopathy alone, and 7 had neck pain without sensory and motor signs.

Abnormalities of SEPs correlated closely with clinical myelopathy but not with radiculopathy. Tibial nerve responses were most often abnormal, even with myelopathy above the C6 level. Tibial nerve SEP changes correlated with ipsilateral posterior column signs but not with anterolateral column sensory signs. In cases of myelopathy, SEP changes were a more sensitive indicator of sensory pathway involvement than were the findings on clinical sensory testing. The SEP findings generally did not correlate well with the radiologic findings. Follow-up SEP recordings reflected clinical improvement after surgical treatment. Abnormalities of SEPs were infrequent in patients with radiculopathy alone or neck pain.

Recording of SEPs with lower limb stimulation may be a useful adjunct to clinical and radiologic assessment in the differential diagnosis of cervical cord lesions and in the detection of subclinical posterior column involvement. The finding of SEP changes in cases of myelopathy unassociated with radiologic evidence of posterior cord compression suggests that direct compression may not be the only mechanism of cord damage in cervical spondylosis, but that local impairment of blood supply may be equally important.

▶ The detection of SEPs in patients with cervical spondylosis may show evidence of posterior column involvement and may assist in the differential diagnosis from disorders such as multiple sclerosis and amyotrophic laterial sclerosis.—Russell N. DeJong, M.D.

Changing Concepts in Treatment of Severe Symptomatic Hyponatremia: Rapid Correction and Possible Relation to Central Pontine Myelinolysis
J. Carlos Ayus, Rhada K. Krothapalli, and Allen I. Arieff (Ben Taub Gen. Hosp. and Baylor College of Medicine, Houston, and VA Med. Ctr. and Univ. of California at San Francisco)
Am. J. Med. 78:897–902, June 1985   18–14

Hyponatremia is frequent and usually mild, but severe, symptomatic hyponatremia with a serum sodium concentration of less than 120 mEq/L often leads to permanent neurologic damage or death. Aggressive and rapid correction of hyponatremia is not always necessary. Rapid correction with hypertonic saline should be considered in severe cases, after cardiopulmonary status is carefully assessed so that congestive failure and pulmonary edema will not occur. Diuresis should be established with intravenous furosemide in normovolemic or volume-overloaded patients before treatment. Patients with a serum sodium concentration of more than 120 mEq/L and no symptoms generally do well with water restriction only. Central pontine myelinolysis may complicate treatment of hyponatremia, but little clinical support has been obtained.

Mortality from severe hyponatremia is especially high in alcoholics and in severely malnourished patients. Rapid correction of symptomatic hyponatremia with hypertonic saline at the rate of 2 mEq/L per hour has led to good survival rates, but the data are not definitive. Prospective observations are needed to determine the best means of correcting severe symptomatic hyponatremia. Alcoholic patients have had high mortality when hyponatremia was corrected slowly, at a rate of less than 0.7 mEq/ L per hour, and nonalcoholic patients have done better in recent years with rapid correction. If the serum sodium concentration is less than 105 mEq/L, it may be safe to raise it by only 20 mEq/L. Acute correction to normonatremia or hypernatremia should be avoided.

▶ The treatment of mild and severe and of asymptomatic and symptomatic hyponatremia must be individualized for each patient. This is an important article for the clinician.—Russell N. DeJong, M.D.

Persisent Vegetative State: Review and Report of Electrodiagnostic Studies in Eight Cases
Phiroze L. Hansotia (Marshfield Clinic, Wis.)
Arch. Neurol. 42:1048–1052, November 1985   18–15

"Persistent vegetative state" (PVS) is the clinical term used when responsiveness limited to postural and reflex movements of the extremities and eyes and absence of cortical function last longer than 2 weeks. The condition raises several humanitarian and socioeconomic questions and will occur more often as mortality from severe brain damage declines. Review was made of eight patients of PVS seen among 81 comatose patients encountered in a 2-year period; four of the patients died.

Patients in PVS are awake without being aware. All 8 patients had findings of wakefulness without cognitive function. The EEGs showed a range of patterns—from diffuse polymorphic slow waves to alpha-theta coma and spindle coma—that were unchanged from the comatose through the vegetative state. Brain stem auditory evoked responses were normal, but median somatosensory evoked responses showed a prolonged central conduction time. The amplitude of the N20 (cerebral) response was diminished. The delay in central conduction time from N13 (spinal) to N20 may reflect selective synaptic delay, mainly in certain vulnerable regions such as the thalamus, as is observed during general anesthesia.

The PVS can be recognized electrodiagnostically, and its course can be followed by median somatosensory evoked potential recording. The EEG and brain stem auditory evoked response recordings provide little help once PVS is diagnosed. An increasing duration of central conduction time may indicate deteriorating brain function and, when accompanied by loss of the N20 response, approaching death.

▶ This investigator describes electrodiagnostic studies that may serve to identify and monitor patients with PVS and that may accurately predict outcome. A related article states that PVS is a feature of the terminal phase of several progressive neurologic disorders and that patients with it should be treated without excessive intervention (Walsh, T. M., and Leonard, C.: *Arch. Neurol.* 42:1045–1047, 1985).—Russell N. DeJong, M.D.

Spinal Cord Lesions in Heat Stroke

Gabriel Delgado, Teresa Tuñón, Jaime Gállego, and José A. Villanueva (Hospital de Navarra, Pamplona, Spain)
J. Neurol. Neurosurg. Psychiatry 43:1065–1067, October 1985   18–16

Signs and symptoms of neurologic involvement are characteristically present with heat stroke. The clinical and pathologic findings are described

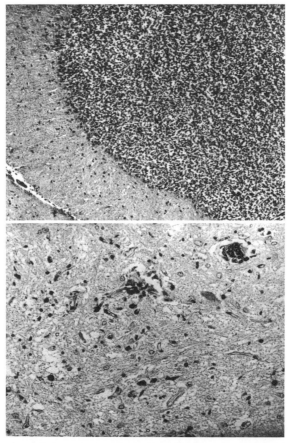

Fig 18–2 (top).—Cerebellar cortex shows marked loss of Purkinje cells without proliferation of Bergmann glia. Necrosis of cells of granular layer can be seen. Hematoxylin-eosin; bar = 25 μm.

Fig 18–3 (bottom).—Anterior horn of the lumbar spinal cord shows total loss of motor neurons, abundant macrophages loaded with lipofuscin, and fibrillar and hypertrophic gliosis. Periodic acid; Schiff; bar = 25 μm.

(Courtesy of Delgado, G., et al.: J. Neurol. Neurosurg. Psychiatry 43:1065–1067, October 1985.)

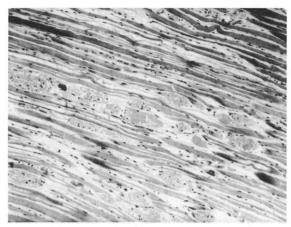

Fig 18–4.—Longitudinal section of quadriceps femoris. Numerous muscle fibers are necrotic, others show regeneration. Hematoxylin-eosin; bar = 25 μm. (Courtesy of Delgado, G., et al.: J. Neurol. Neurosurg. Psychiatry 43:1065–1067, October 1985.)

in a patient who was being treated institutionally for manic depressive psychosis after classic heat stroke.

Man, 66 years old and obese, was admitted to the hospital with somatomotor partial seizures with secondary generalization after a local heat wave. Seizures abated after he was given 2 mg of clonazepam. The rectal temperature was 42.5 C and the blood pressure was 120/70 mm Hg. Neurologic examination revealed drowsiness and confusion; the EEG was diffusely slowed. The computed tomography scan, cerebrospinal fluid, pH, electrolytes, and clotting time were normal. Endotracheal intubation was required 12 hours after admission because of acute respiratory insufficiency. Quadriplegia was observed at this time, with muscular hypotonia, retention of urine, fecal incontinence, and anhidrosis. The patient died 14 days later.

At autopsy, cerebral hemispheres and brain stem were found to be normal. Figure 18–2 shows neuronal loss without gliosis in the cerebellum and dentate nucleus. The anterior and intermediolateral horns revealed chromatolysis and neuronophagia (Fig 18–3). Skeletal muscle showed severe rhabdomyolysis with regeneration (Fig 18–4).

Unlike most cases of heat stroke, which involve serious electrolyte disturbances, disseminated intravascular coagulation, and circulatory collapse, this case had no demonstrable physiopathologic mechanism other than hyperthermia. The clinical picture was completely accounted for by the spinal cord lesions. Anhidrosis may be a consequence, rather than a mechanism, of hyperthermia. The spinal cord, as well as the cerebellum, is particularly sensitive to hyperthermia.

▶ This is an intriguing situation. It does appear the anterior horn cell loss was due to the heat. On the other hand, what about the antipsychotic drugs the patient was taking? If heat alone were responsible one would think this disorder would be present in the patients being treated with hyperthermia for cancer.—Robert D. Currier, M.D.

Human Histocompatibility Leukocyte Antigen (HLA) Haplotype Frequencies Estimated from the Data on HLA Class I, II, and III Antigens in 111 Japanese Narcoleptics

Kazumasa Matsuki, Takeo Juji, Katsushi Tokunaga, Tohru Naohara, Masahiro Satake, and Yutaka Honda (Tokyo Women's Med. College Hosp., Tokyo Univ. Hosp., Tokyo Univ., and Neuropsychiatric Research Found., Tokyo; and Tohoku Univ., Sendai, Japan)
J. Clin. Invest. 76:2078–2083, December 1985   18–17

Narcolepsy is a sleep disorder characterized by recurrent napping in the daytime that persists for years (napping habit), irresistible attacks of sleep (sleep attacks), and sudden loss of tone in the striated muscles, which typically occurs at moments of increased emotion (cataplexy). Other characteristics of narcolepsy are sleep paralysis, which is often accompanied by vivid and frightening hallucination, and a rapid eye movement period at the onset of sleep.

One-hundred eleven Japanese patients with narcolepsy and six multiple-case families were studied for HLA class I and class II antigens and for class III HLA-linked complement markers to determine the predominant haplotypes in Japanese narcoleptics.

In Japanese narcoleptics, the most frequent haplotypes were B35-DR2, B15-DR2, and B51-DR2, haplotypes that were rare in normal Japanese; among Caucasian narcoleptics, the haplotype found more frequently is A3-CW7-B7-DR2-DQw1. In contrast, the most frequent haplotype of HLA-DR2 in normal Japanese had a decreased frequency, as low as one third of that of the normal controls. Haplotype analysis on six families showed that B35-DR2 and other rare haplotypes in normal Japanese were associated with narcolepsy.

Four persons in three of the six families who had the disease susceptibility haplotype did not show any signs or symptoms of narcolepsy. In the six families studied, 19 subjects had disease susceptibility haplotypes. Among them, 8 subjects were suffering from narcolepsy, 3 from essential hypersomnia, 4 from excessive daytime sleepiness, and 4 had no symptoms of excessive daytime somnolence. These data show that there were subjects who did not develop narcolepsy, even if they had a disease susceptibility HLA haplotype. This incomplete penetrance of the disease and the multiform appearance of both narcolepsy and essential hypersomnia suggest that factors other than a HLA-DR2-linked disease susceptibility gene(s) are also required for the full manifestation of narcolepsy. This finding agrees with a previously proposed two-threshold multifactorial inheritance model. In some cases, environmental factors seem to play a precipitating role in the development of narcolepsy.

Haplotype analysis of the family members is useful for the early detection of the high-risk children to narcolepsy and also for the possible prevention of the development of narcolepsy by the avoidance of precipitating environmental factors that may contribute to the development of the disease.

▶ This is a comprehensive report of the association between narcolepsy and HLA-DR2. It is with great relief that we heard Neely et al. (*Neurology* 36 [Suppl. 1]:299, April 1986) report at the recent Academy meeting that of 11 Chicagoans with narcolepsy, 2 did not have DR2. This represents possibly the first reported negative association of narcolepsy and DR2. It is much easier for me to understand an imperfect association of some component of the immune system with narcolepsy. A perfect correlation would mean that the DR2 gene is directly responsible for narcolepsy or is associated with another gene elsewhere directly responsible for narcolepsy, which would be hard to swallow.—Robert D. Currier, M.D.

Prolactinomas in Men: Clinical Characteristics and the Effect of Bromocriptine Treatment
A.-L. Hulting, C. Muhr, P. O. Lundberg, and S. Werner (Karolinska Hosp., Stockholm, and Univ. Hosp., Uppsala, Sweden)
Acta Med. Scand. 217:101–109, 1985   18–18

A study was carried out in 37 men (mean age, 47 years; range, 25–73 years) with prolactin (PRL)-producing pituitary adenomas to determine if the patient's delay in seeking medical attention might cause the predominance of large tumors in men as compared with women, for whom microadenomas predominate.

The 37 patients were grouped according to radiographic findings. Group I had sellae of normal size with asymmetries indicating microadenomas (5 patients). Group II had enlarged sellae (13), and group III enlarged sellae with local bone erosions as signs of invasive tumor growth (6). Group IV consisted of 13 patients with enlarged sellae, bone erosions, and signs of parasellar tumor growth according to encephalography or computed tomography. Groups III and IV thus comprised invasively growing adenomas. Perimetry and visual acuity were examined in all patients. Pituitary surgery was performed in 11 patients, and external irradiation was given to 11, in 8 after previous surgery. All patients were treated with bromocriptine (1.25–10 mg per day). Follow-up varied between 6 months and 5 years in all but 1 patient, who died of pneumonia 3 months after commencement of treatment.

Tumor size, as reflected by the radiographic findings, correlated with PRL levels. Four patients in group I and 2 in group II had PRL levels ≤100 μg/L. These patients had no signs of suprasellar disorders or medical treatment that could have caused moderate increase in PRL levels. However, moderately elevated PRL levels in a pituitary adenoma do not per se prove the adenoma to be actually PRL-producing. No patient was asymptomatic at the time of diagnosis. The most common symptom was decreased libido and/or potency (29 patients). Headache (16) and eye symptoms (16) were also frequent. Increased weight (>4 kg) occurred during the first year (13) together with other subjective symptoms of the disease. Secondary hypothroidism (11) and secondary cortisol insufficiency (7) were noted. Galactorrhea was infrequent (2). Decreased libido and impotence were the first subjective symptoms in 18 patients, but only 5 patients consulted a physician for the condition. Usually, patients with visual symptoms or headache contacted a physician. Duration of symptoms varied from 5 months to 35 years. Fifty percent of the patients had a subjective history of disease for 4 years or less. There was no correlation between the size of the sella and the duration of symptoms. Of 13 men with symptoms for less than 1 year, 7 had enlarged sellae with bone erosions and parasellar tumor growth. In contrast, 4 of 6 patients with symptoms for more than 10 years presented with enlarged sellae without bone erosions. There was no correlation between PRL and testosterone levels.

The reason for the predominance of large PRL-producing tumors in men remains to be elucidated. However, this predominance depends not on a patient's or physician's delay, but rather on a high frequency of presumably rapidly growing PRL-producing tumors in men. Clinical symptoms improved and PRL levels were normalized during bromocriptine therapy in 34 of the 37 patients and tumor size in 8 of 10 patient was markedly diminished. Since bromocriptine-induced effects on PRL-producing adenomas are reversible, continuous treatment with dopamine agonists such as bromocriptine seems advisable in men with prolactinomas of benign as well as fulminant clinical course.

▶ Prolactinomas (PRL-producing pituitary tumors) are usually larger at the time the diagnosis is made in men than they are in women, and such focal signs as visual field defects and headaches are much more common than endocrine signs (decreased libido, impotence, and infertility). Surgery and irradiation are unsatisfactory in the treatment of tumors that are large at the time of diagnosis, but bromocriptine therapy is effective in patients with both focal and endocrine signs and brings about improvement in focal signs and in the normalization of prolactin levels. These studies also suggest that the predominance of large tumors in men does not depend on the delay in diagnosis on the part of either the patient or the doctor, but rather on the high frequency of rapidly growing prolactin-producing tumors in male patients.—Russell N. DeJong, M.D.

Public Health Service Study of Reye's Syndrome and Medications: Report of the Pilot Phase
Eugene S. Hurwitz, Michael J. Barrett, Dennis Bregman, Walter J. Gunn, Lawrence B. Schonberger, William R. Fairweather, Joseph S. Drage, John R. LaMontagne, Richard A. Kaslow, D. Bruce Burlington, Gerald V. Quinnan, Robert A. Parker, Kem Phillips, Paul Pinsky, Delbert Dayton, and Walter R. Dowdle (Public Health Service Reye's Syndrome Task Force)
N. Engl. J. Med. 313:849–857, Oct. 3, 1985   18–19

Case-control studies have shown a significant excess risk of Reye's syn-

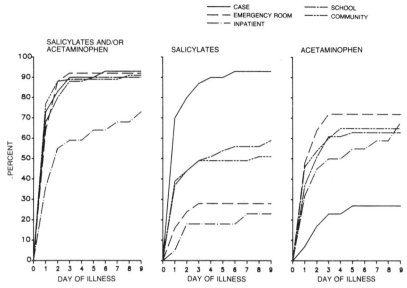

Fig 18–5.—Cumulative percentage of study subjects exposed to salicylates or acetaminophen or both, according to day of illness. (Courtesy of Hurwitz, E.S., et al.: *N. Engl. J. Med.* 313:849–857, Oct. 3, 1985. Reprinted by permission of The New England Journal of Medicine.)

drome in association with ingestion of salicylates during antecedent chicken pox and respiratory illnesses. A pilot study was carried out in early 1984 to assess methods for use in a larger study of this reported association. Thirty patients seen at 16 pediatric tertiary care centers in 11 states, whose diagnoses were confirmed by an expert panel, were matched with 145 control subjects for age, race, and antecedent illness. Controls came from the emergency room, hospital, school, and community.

Salicylates had been given to 93% of cases and 46% of controls during matched antecedent illnesses, for an odds ratio of 16.1 and a lower 95% confidence limit of 4.6. Exposure to salicylates or acetaminophen or both is shown in Figure 18–5. The prevalence and severity of signs, symptoms, and selected events during antecedent illness tended to be lower in cases than in controls, so that differences in the severity of antecedent illness could not explain the differences in medication exposure.

The results of this pilot study support an association between Reye's syndrome and the use of salicylates during antecedent illness. The association was strong and is consistent with the results of earlier studies. A large study involving more than 50 pediatric tertiary care centers throughout the United States is under way.

▶ This study, even though it is called a pilot study, solidifies the relationship between aspirin use and Reye's syndrome. Further confirmation is a study by Remington et al. (Am. J. Dis. Child. 139:870–872, 1985), who found that three children receiving long-term salicylate therapy for rheumatoid arthritis developed Reye's syndrome. The incidence in children receiving aspirin therapy regularly was substantially higher than that in the general population. The Food and Drug Administration finds an encouraging increase in the awareness of parents of the danger of giving children aspirin as treatment for flu or chicken pox—31% in 1981, but 88% in 1985 (FDA Drug Bull. 15:40–41, 1985)—the result of an education campaign that worked quickly and well.—Owen B. Evans, M.D., and Robert D. Currier, M.D.

Epilepsy After Penetrating Head Injury: I. Clinical Correlates: A Report of the Vietnam Head Injury Study
Andres M. Salazar, Bahman Jabbari, Stephen C. Vance, Jordan Grafman, Dina Amin, and J. D. Dillon (Walter Reed Army Med. Ctr. and George Washington Univ.)
Neurology 35:1406–1414, October 1985   18–20

An association between epilepsy and brain trauma has long been recognized, but the pathogenesis of posttraumatic epilepsy remains incompletely understood. Review was made of the data on 421 Vietnam veterans who incurred penetrating brain wounds 15 years earlier. The mean age at the time of injury was 21 years. Posttraumatic epilepsy developed in 53% of subjects, and half of these still had seizures 15 years after injury. The overall mean duration of epilepsy was 93 months.

Total brain volume loss (as evidenced on computed tomography), early evidence of hematoma, and retained metal fragments all correlated signifi-

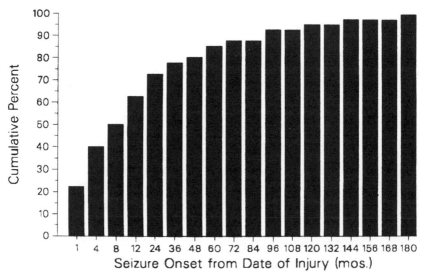

Fig 18–6.—Cumulative percentage of 197 patients with seizures, by time after injury. The time scale is expanded for the first year. Only patients in whom epilepsy developed by 180 months after injury are represented; new patients are expected to enter this group at a slow rate in the future. Although most epileptics have had their first seizure within 2 years of injury, more than 15% will not manifest epilepsy until 5 or more years later. (Courtesy of Salazar, A.M., et al.: *Neurology* 35:1406–1414, October 1985.)

cantly with seizures. Neurologic outcomes associated with posttraumatic epilepsy included hemiparesis, aphasia, organic mental disorder, visual field loss, and headache. Seizures began within a year of injury in 57% of cases, but more than 5 years after injury in over 18% (Fig 18–6). The time of onset within 5 years after injury was not related to seizure frequency, duration, or persistence. About 70% of patients had partial seizures or a partial onset, and 70% also had at least one generalized seizure. Seizure type tended to remain stable or to improve. Seizure frequency in the first year predicted the future severity of seizures. Persistent epilepsy was most frequent in patients with partial seizures.

Posttraumatic epilepsy persisted 15 years after injury in half of the affected veterans in this study. Phenytoin therapy early in the course of epilepsy did not prevent later seizures. The risk was increased in patients with focal neurologic signs or large lesions. Lesion site may be more important than lesion size.

▶ Epilepsy developed in 53% of Vietnam veterans with penetrating brain wounds. About half of the patients with seizures were still having seizures 15 years after injury. Prophylactic phenytoin was useless in preventing the development of seizures, and a family history of epilepsy had no effect on their occurrence or nonoccurrence.

This is a significant and very helpful study.—Robert D. Currier, M.D.

Prognosis After a First Untreated Tonic-Clonic Seizure
R. D. C. Elwes, P. Chesterman, and E. H. Reynolds (London)
Lancet 2:752–753, Oct. 5, 1985   18–21

Up to 5% of the population will have at least one afebrile seizure at some time, but little is known of the early prognosis for seizure recurrence.

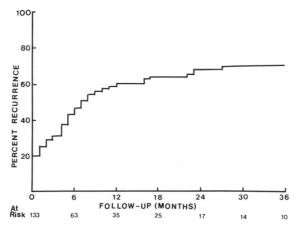

Fig 18–7.—Cumulative probability of seizure recurrence in 133 patients presenting with a single seizure. (Courtesy of Elwes, R.D.C., et al.: *Lancet* 2:752–753, Oct. 5, 1985.)

A total of 328 patients with previously untreated seizures were seen in 1978–1983. Of the 214 patients with tonic-clonic seizures, 133 presented after a single seizure, and 73 of these patients were seen in emergency rooms. No patient was treated after the initial seizure. The cumulative risk of seizure recurrence during a median follow-up of 15 months is shown in Figure 18–7. The risk was 62% by 1 year and 71% after 3 and 4 years.

The time between first and second seizures is likely to be less than a month in at least one third of cases of established epilepsy. It is unknown what proportion of patients who experience a single seizure are not referred to a hospital. Most neurologists do not treat a single seizure, but immediate treatment after a first seizure might reduce the recurrence rate and improve the prognosis. More than two thirds of the present patients eventually had recurrent seizures.

NEUROSURGERY

ROBERT M. CROWELL, M.D.

Introduction

Nineteen eighty-six continued the course of rapid change in neurosurgery. Several megatrends can be identified: (1) New technology plays a dramatic role in improving patient care. Magnetic resonance imaging, interstitial radiation therapy, and detachable balloon catheters are prominent examples. (2) Statistical analysis shapes clinical practice. As a powerful example, the negative results of the Extracranial-Intracranial Bypass Study have sharply curtailed performance of bypass grafts. (3) Extra medical forces profoundly affect neurosurgical activities. Highly visible examples are cost containment and liability. Neurosurgery must adapt to meet these challenging changes.

In DIAGNOSTICS, magnetic resonance imaging is revolutionizing the evaluation of many neurosurgical problems. For intracranial tumors, it is usually more helpful than computed tomography (Digests 19–1, 19–4), except for meningiomas, where calcification eludes detection (Digest 19–5). Surface-coil technology has produced excellent images of spinal pathology, including syrinx and herniated intervertebral discs (Kokmen et al.: *Neurosurgery* 17:267–270, 1985, Digest 19–14). Portable isotope angiography can provide a reliable, practical means of confirming brain death (Digest 19–11).

New TECHNIQUES have been described for adjunctive radiotherapy of brain tumors. Intracavitary instillation of P^{32} is helpful in treating cystic craniopharyngiomas and astrocytomas (Digest 20–3). Interstitial radiation therapy may be helpful for certain skull base tumors (Digest 20–4), and heavy particle therapy seems beneficial for intracranial chordoma (Digest 20–6). In preliminary studies, computed tomography-guided laser vaporization of deep-seated gliomas produces remarkable reduction in tumor bulk with low risk (Digest 20–8). Percutaneous transvascular occlusion of basilar aneurysms has been achieved in a few cases with detachable balloon catheters (Zeumer: *Acta Neurochir.* 78:136–142, 1985). Fibrin glue is a new material with promise for transvascular obliteration of carotid-cavernous fistulae (Digest 20–13).

In the TUMOR field, serum and cerebrospinal fluid levels of markers may be helpful in guiding therapy of germ cell tumors (Digest 21–1). Interleukin-2 and monoclonal antibodies hold promise in the treatment of gliomas (Digests 21–3, 21–5). Drug therapy for pituitary tumors was advanced; a somatostatin analogue can control acromegaly (Digest 21–12). Transventricular excision of colloid cysts of the third ventricle gives excellent results that are hard to beat by other methods (Digest 21–24).

In ISCHEMIA, the Extracranial-Intracranial Bypass Study (Digest 22–23) gave negative results, but some questions on methodology have been raised, and some indications for the procedure remain valid, e.g., giant aneurysms. Emergency endarterectomy is advocated for certain cases, with good salvage results (Digest 22–18). Medical therapy for ischemia (Digest 22–14) may salvage some of the 25% of stroke cases that worsen in the hospital (Digest 22–5). A new operation—"synangiosis"—produces new collateral circulation for moyamoya disease; the superficial temporal artery is simply laid over the cortex (Digest 22–27).

As for HEMORRHAGE, polyvinyl alcohol embolization seems an advance in the treatment of intracranial and spinal arteriovenous malformations (Digest 23–6). Drake and Peerless report good results in many posterior fossa arteriovenous malformations, but poor results in 14% of the cases and deaths in 15% remain formidable statistics (Digest 23–3). Delay of referral of aneurysm cases continues to cause additional morbidity (Digest 23–1).

In the area of TRAUMA, the expensive policy of admission for loss of consciousness has been questioned (Digest 24–7). General surgeons have claimed a role in the emergency management of head trauma in rural settings (Digest 24–3). Magnetic resonance can image pathology in head injury cases in which computed tomography scans are normal (Digest 24–4). Type III fractures of the dens often lead to instability (Digest 24–8). Acrylic can be used for simple cervical fusion after injury (Digest 24–9).

For SPINE, transoral removal of the dens is advocated for several conditions (Digest 25–1). Chemonucleolysis is more helpful than placebo, according to analysis of available randomized studies (Digest 25–7). Radical transthoracic decompression and fusion gives effective palliation for neoplastic cord compression (Digest 25–15). Radical excision of intramedullary cord tumors can give good results (Digest 25–20).

In PEDIATRICS, results of surgery for brain tumors in infants remain discouraging (Digest 26–7). Guidelines for management of fetal hydrocephalus have appeared, and ventriculoamnionic shunting remains of uncertain value (Digest 26–9). Separation of craniopagus twins is aided by tissue expanders to assist scalp coverage (Digest 26–7).

For NERVE surgery, a variety of sheaths offer promise in improving results of suture and grafting (Digest 28–8).

In FUNCTIONAL surgery, commissurotomy appears effective in the treatment of certain seizure disorders (Digest 29–2).

NEUROSCIENCE has demonstrated remarkable regeneration of CNS elements in vertebrates under certain conditions (Digest 30–2).

Among a variety of MISCELLANEOUS TOPICS, discussion of Diagnostic Related Groups (DGRs) gives an upbeat suggestion on adaptation for survival (Digest 31–1).

Robert M. Crowell, M.D.

19 Diagnostics

Introduction

Magnetic resonance (MR) imaging holds center stage. The paramagnetic contrast agent gadolinium-diethylenetriamine penta-acetic acid (Gd-DTPA) has been used for contrast enhancement of MR images. Two major studies have demonstrated utility for such enhancement in the depiction of brain tumors (Digests 19–1, 19–2). In two other studies, MR images clearly demonstrated brain stem tumors through increased T1 and T2 values and mass affect. The superior ability of MR to localize these tumors may enhance brain stem biopsy (Digests 19–3, 19–4). Magnetic resonance was less successful in the specific diagnosis of brain radiation lesions (Digest 19–5). MR depicts these lesions with great sensitivity but the findings are not specific and do not distinguish between necrosis and tumor. Nor is MR superior in the imaging of meningiomas (Digest 19–6). Sometimes lesions are not seen, calcification is not well shown, and angiography may still be needed for evaluation of venous occlusion. On the other hand, the contents of the cavernous sinus and its involvement by masses encroaching may be detected better by MR than by computed tomography (Digest 19–7).

Several other modalities showed special prominence for intracranial diagnosis: positron emission tomography (PET) has been used to study blood flow and metabolism in brain tumors (Digest 19–8). These studies demonstrate the effects of Dexamethasone upon tumor and peritumoral flow and metabolism. Positron emission tomography scanning, which has been shown to discriminate radiation necrosis from tumor, is now found to bear useful prognostic information in patients with high-grade gliomas (Digest 19–9). Posterior fossa tumors may be depicted well in direct coronal computed tomography (CT) to demonstrate the orientation for surgical dissection. In a landmark study, Goodman et al. (Digest 19–11) demonstrated in a series of 204 cases the efficacy of portable isotope angiography in confirmation of brain death. Preserved somatosensory evoked potentials in the face of apparent inability to move the lower extremities and denial of sensation of a stimulus provide objective evidence of hysteria (Digest 19–13).

Advances in spinal diagnosis have been reported. Surface coil for MR imaging of the lumbar spine can demonstrate disk herniation as well as can CT or myelography (Digest 19–14). In selected patients, CT myelography with low doses of metrizamide can achieve satisfactory studies with minimal side effects in outpatients (Digest 19–15). "Squeezing" of contrast under pressure has been suggested to provide demonstration of the superior end of a block, with contrast administered by lumbar puncture (Digest 19–16).

Robert M. Crowell, M.D.

Magnetic Resonance Imaging

Contrast-Enhanced MR Imaging of Malignant Brain Tumors

Moshe Graif, Graeme M. Bydder, Robert E. Steiner, Peter Neindorf, David G. T. Thomas, and Ian R. Young (Hammersmith and Maida Vale Hosps., London; Schering AG, Berlin; Picker Internatl., Wembley, England)
AJNR 6:855–862, Nov.–Dec. 1985   19–1

The paramagnetic contrast agent gadolinium-diethylenetriamine penta-acetic acid (Gd-DTPA) has been studied in animals and in pilot clinical studies. The enhancement obtained with various pulse sequences was assessed in 12 patients with primary cerebral tumors demonstrated histologically, and in another patient who refused biopsy. Two other patients had histologic evidence of secondary brain involvement. One inversion-recovery sequence and two spin-echo pulse sequences were utilized before and after injection of 0.1 mM/kg of Gd-DTPA.

Contrast enhancement was evident in 16 of 17 cerebral tumors, most often in a ring-shaped or diffuse pattern. A mean 22% reduction in T1 and a mean decrease of 21% in T2 were noted. Primary tumors of low-grade malignancy showed a mean decrease in T1 of 16%, compared with 29% for high-grade lesions. The mean T1 decrease in metastases was 33%. In terms of changes in signal intensity with pulse sequence, maximal enhancement was seen 20–40 minutes after injection for low-malignant lesions, and at 40–60 minutes in the other cases. The decrease in signal occurred earlier with spin-echo sequences than with inversion-recovery sequences in all groups. Some apparent areas of peritumoral edema showed a decrease in signal intensity after contrast injection. Separation of tumor from edema was as good as with CT or better in all cases. There were no serious side effects.

Injection of Gd-DTPA is an effective means of enhancing malignant brain tumors. Inversion-recovery sequencing is most sensitive to contrast enhancement. The findings compare favorably with those of CT. Toxicity has not been significant.

▶ Contrast enhancement with gadolinium-DTPA appears to be a common feature of cerebral tumors. It seems likely that this approach will be helpful in the differential diagnosis of demonstrated anatomic intracranial lesions. Data so far indicate that histologic verification will remain necessary.—Robert M. Crowell, M.D.

Brain Tumors: MR Imaging With Gadolinium-DTPA

Roland Felix, Wolfgang Schörner, Michael Laniado, Hans-Peter Neindorf, Claus Clausen, Wiland Fiegler, and Ulrich Speck (Free Univ. of Berlin and Schering A G)
Radiology 156:681–688, September 1985   19–2

It has proved difficult to consistently distinguish between tumor and

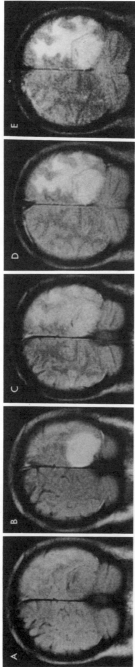

Fig 19–1.—Coronal MR images through a meningioma of the tentorium cerebelli (patient 29). **A**, precontrast, spin-echo (SE), 800/35. Tumor and brain tissue display nearly the same signal intensities. A thin rim of decreased signal partly delineates the meningioma from adjacent brain tissue. **B**, postcontrast, SE, 800/35 (Gd-DTPA, 0.1 mmol/kg body wt, intravenous). The homogeneous signal enhancement of the meningioma results in excellent tumor display. **C**, precontrast, SE, 1,600/35. Tumor and perifocal edema are displayed as slightly hyperintense areas. No separation between tumor and edema is seen in this sequence. **D**, pre-contrast, SE, 1,600/70. Meningioma and perifocal edema are hyperintense relative to normal brain tissue. The extension of the edema through the white matter is clearly displayed. A thin rim of reduced signal around the tumor provides for tumor delineation. **E**, precontrast, SE, 1,600/105. The edema is more intense than the meningioma. This difference in signal intensities, and the thin rim of low signal intensity between tumor and edema, slightly improve tumor delineation compared with **D**. (Courtesy of Felix, R., et al.: Radiology 156:681–688, September 1985. Reproduced with permission of the Radiological Society of North America.)

SUMMARY OF TUMOR DELINEATION

Before Gd-DTPA

	SE, 400/35	SE, 800/35	SE, 1,600/35	SE, 1,600/70	SE, 1,600/105 SE, 1,600/120	After Gd-DTPA SE, 800/35
No tumor delineation	25	38	22	21	6	4
Diagnostically sufficient tumor delineation	4	2	5	8	4	9
Excellent tumor delineation	0	0	0	2	2	28
Total studies	29	40	27	31	12	40

(Courtesy of Felix, R., et al.: Radiology 156:681–688, September 1985. Reproduced with permission of the Radiological Society of North America.)

chronic infarction or perifocal edema by magnetic resonance (MR) imaging. The value of gadolinium-diethylenetriamine penta-acetic acid (Gd-DTPA) enhancement was assessed in 40 patients with intracranial tumors, including 28 with primary tumors and 12 with cerebral metastases. Contrast-enhanced computed tomography also was done in all cases. The MR imaging was done using spin-echo pulse sequences before and after the intravenous injection of 0.1 mM Gd-DTPA/kg.

The results are given in the table. T2-weighted MR images showed anatomic effects of masses in many instances and consistently demonstrated a difference in signal intensity between the lesion and normal brain tissue (Fig 19–1). Increased signal intensity from the tumor was observed in all cases after Gd-DTPA injection. Tumor delineation was considerably improved in all but 4 cases. Glioblastomas and intracranial metastases were reliably demonstrated only after Gd-DTPA administration. No adverse effects resulted from Gd-DTPA injection.

Most meningiomas, neuromas, and adenomas can be demonstrated by routine MR imaging, but injection of Gd-DTPA is helpful in the delineation of glioblastomas and intracranial metastases. The appropriate imaging time following contrast injection remains to be determined. Technical parameters have to be optimized to assure effective administration of paramagnetic contrast agents in MR imaging.

▶ In another study of MRI-enhancement, gadolinium-DPTA demonstrated marked contrast enhancement in tumor tissue in all 14 patients with glioblastoma and 7 with intracranial metastases (Claussen, C., et al.: AJNR 6:669–674, 1985).—Robert M. Crowell, M.D.

Nuclear Magnetic Resonance Imaging (NMR), (MRI), of Brain Stem Tumors
S. B. Peterman, R. E. Steiner, G. M. Bydder, D. J. Thomas, J. S. Tobias, and I. R. Young (Hammersmith Hosp., Inst. of Neurology and Natl. Hosp. for Nervous Diseases, Univ. College Hosp., London, and Picker Internatl., Wembley, England)
Neuroradiology 27:202–207, 1985

19–3

It may be difficult to evaluate the brain stem thoroughly with computed tomography (CT), even with intrathecal contrast enhancement. Bone artifacts are avoided by magnetic resonance (MR) imaging, and direct sagittal and coronal views are readily obtained. Review was made of the MR scan findings in 26 patients who were clinically suspected of or known to have brain stem tumor. Twenty-one patients, including 11 children, had MR findings that were positive for tumor. Tumor was confirmed histologically in 9 cases, while clinical findings in the other patients were suggestive enough to warrant radiotherapy. Patients also had contrast-enhanced CT scans. The MR imaging employed saturation-recovery, inversion-recovery, and spin-echo pulse sequences. Two patients received the paramagnetic contrast agent gadolinium-diethylene triamine penta-acetic acid (Gd-DTPA).

All but one of the 21 patients with MR findings of tumor had an increased T1 and T2 in the region of the tumor. Cysts and areas of necrosis were evident in five cases, and hemorrhage was apparent in two. Mass

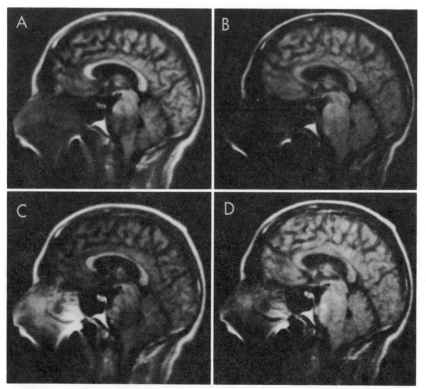

Fig 19–2.—Brain-stem tumor with gadolinium-diethylenetriamine penta-acetic acid (Gd-DTPA) enhancement: **A,** sagittal inversion-recovery (IR) 1500/500/44 precontrast; **B,** sagittal spin-echo (SE) 544/44 precontrast; **C,** sagittal IR 1500/500/44 postcontrast; and **D,** sagittal SE 544/44 postcontrast scans. A mass is seen within and anterior to the pons (**A** and **B**). Administration of intravenous Gd-DTPA shows ring enhancement of the lesion that is more obvious on **C.** The enhancement of nasal mucosa (**D**) can be noted. (Courtesy of Peterman, S.B., et al.: Neuroradiology 27:202–207, 1985: Berlin-Heidelberg-New York; Springer.)

effect was apparent in 20 cases. Hydrocephalus was seen in 3 of the 6 cases for which the ventricles were included in the images; an increased T2 was noted in the periventricular region. Tumor enhancement by Gd-DTPA is shown in Figure 19–2. It was difficult to distinguish between residual or recurrent tumor and postradiation changes. The MR images showed more extensive abnormalities than CT in nearly all cases. In 3 cases, cysts and focal necrosis were seen only on MR images.

Brain stem tumors show up well on MR images through their increased T1 and T2 values and mass effect. The superior ability of MR to localize these tumors in several planes may enhance brain stem biopsy analysis and aid in the delineation of radiotherapy fields. Calcification is better shown by CT.

▶ This report and the one that follows (Digest 19–4) indicate clearly that MRI is the diagnostic study of choice for brain stem tumors. To settle questions of calcification, CT scanning may be needed as well. Since direct biopsy via stereotactic means is now feasible (Digest 20–7), careful MRI evaluation of such cases is imperative in this day and age. One can imagine that the marriage of stereotaxic technique and MRI guidance may be of value in some lesions poorly discerned by the CT technique.—Robert M. Crowell, M.D.

MR Imaging of Brainstem Tumors
B. C. P. Lee, J. B. Kneeland, R. W. Walker, J. B. Posner, P. T. Cahill, and M. D. F. Deck (New York Hosp.-Cornell Univ. Med. Ctr., Memorial Sloan-Kettering Cancer Inst., Cornell Univ., and Polytechnic Inst., New York)
AJNR 6:159–163, Mar.–Apr. 1985   19–4

A distinction between intrinsic and extrinsic brain stem tumor is very important in patients with posterior fossa symptoms, since intrinsic tumors usually require radiotherapy, whereas extraaxial lesions can be removed surgically. Computed tomography (CT) is less accurate in older children and adults than in younger patients. Magnetic resonance (MR) imaging was performed in 18 patients (age range, 4–72 years) with intrinsic brain stem tumors, including 16 with primary gliomas and 2 with metastases. Three of the patients with gliomas had received radiotherapy. The CT scan was done with and without intravenous contrast, and with intrathecal metrizamide in 3 cases. The MR sagittal and axial images were obtained by use of spin-echo sequencing. Inversion-recovery sequences also were used in some cases.

The CT scan was equivocal in three cases of brain stem glioma and normal in three others. Sagittal MR images showed brain stem enlargement in all 16 cases. Four studies showed exophytic growth posteriorly into the fourth ventricle, and 3 showed growth anteriorly into the pontine cistern (Fig 19–3). A definite diagnosis of brain stem tumor was made by MR imaging in all cases. In one of the 2 cases metastases was not diagnosed by CT whereas both cases were diagnosed by MR imaging.

Thus, MR imaging is a sensitive means of detecting brain stem tumors

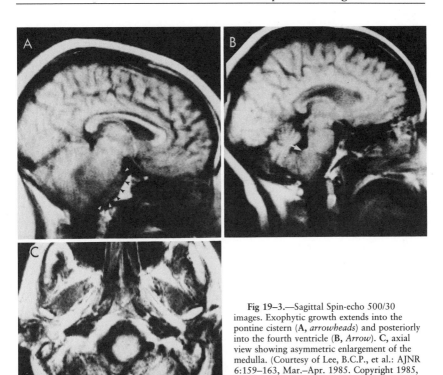

Fig 19–3.—Sagittal Spin-echo 500/30 images. Exophytic growth extends into the pontine cistern (**A,** *arrowheads*) and posteriorly into the fourth ventricle (**B,** *Arrow*). **C,** axial view showing asymmetric enlargement of the medulla. (Courtesy of Lee, B.C.P., et al.: AJNR 6:159–163, Mar.–Apr. 1985. Copyright 1985, by the American Roentgen Ray Society.)

and is superior to CT for this purpose. The precise location and extent of brain stem enlargement are consistently shown by MR imaging. The exact pathology of brain stem tumors is not predicted, and it is not clear whether MR imaging can distinguish between brain stem tumor and encephalitis.

▶ Magnetic resonance, particularly in sagittal images with surface coil technique, depicts the anatomic relations of the jugular foramen with good resolution (Daniels, D. L., *et al.: AJNR* 6:699–703, September/October 1985).— Robert M. Crowell, M.D.

Brain Radiation Lesions: MR Imaging
Georges C. Dooms, Stephen Hecht, Michael Brant-Zawadzki, Yves Berthiaume, David Norman, and T. Hans Newton (Université Catholique de Louvain, Belgium, and Univ. of California at San Francisco)
Radiology 158:149–155, January 1986   19–5

It is difficult to distinguish between cerebral tumor and radiation necrosis with computed tomography (CT). The magnetic resonance (MR) findings were reviewed in 55 irradiated patients (30 male and 25 female subjects, aged 5–91 years), who also had CT examination. Eight patients had radiation lesions, 5 diffusely in the deep white matter and 3 focally. Nine patients had recurrent or residual brain tumor, and 1 had radiation necrosis confirmed by surgery and/or biopsy. The findings in 25 other patients with various white matter disorders were reviewed. A multisection double-spin-echo imaging technique was utilized.

Radiation lesions were characterized by increased signal intensity in the deep periventricular white matter on T2-weighted images and decreased attenuation in the deep white matter on postcontrast CT scans. Signal intensity consistently was less than in normal white matter; however, this was difficult to recognize visually. The T1 and T2 relaxation times were significantly longer than in normal white matter. Relative spin density was greater in radiation lesions; however, this also was nonspecific for radiation lesions. Recurrent and residual brain tumor and radiation necrosis both appeared as slightly less intense lesions on images obtained with a short repetition time (TR), and a bright signal intensity lesions on long-TR images. Relaxation times did not differ significantly from those of radiation lesions.

Magnetic resonance imaging can depict cerebral radiation lesions with great sensitivity but has limitations; the findings are nonspecific and do not distinguish between radiation necrosis and recurrent or residual brain tumor. Radiation lesions can mask other lesions, e.g., subependymal spread.

▶ The differential diagnosis between recurrent brain tumor and radiation necrosis is often difficult. This study indicates that MR cannot reliably differentiate between the two. Positron emission tomography studies can discriminate between the two conditions (Patronas, N. J., et al.: *Radiology* 144:885–889, 1982), but this research instrument is not widely available. In many institutions, surgical biopsy remains the most practical way to make one diagnosis. There are some data from Hugo Rizzoli and colleagues to suggest that anticoagulation may help patients with radiation necrosis.—Robert M. Crowell, M.D.

Magnetic Resonance Imaging of Meningiomas
Robert D. Zimmerman, Cynthia A. Fleming, Leslie A. Saint-Louis, Benjamin C. P. Lee, John J. Manning, and Michael D. F. Deck (New York Hosp.–Cornell Med. Center)
AJNR 6:149–157, Mar.–Apr. 1985   19–6

Magnetic resonance (MR) imaging was performed in 28 patients with 32 meningiomas. Either a single-slice, three-dimensional anisotropic or a two-dimensional Fourier transformation multislice single-echo technique was used. Images were obtained in the axial plane and, where indicated, in the sagittal or coronal planes. Several pulse sequences were used in each case. Contrast-enhanced computed tomography (CT) also was performed.

Of the 18 women and 10 men (mean age, 68 years) in the study, 3 patients had multiple meningiomas and 7 had recurrent lesions; basal tumors predominated.

Contrast CT showed about half the meningomas more clearly than did MR imaging, and in no case was the latter method superior in detecting or characterizing a lesion or showing its extent. Three small lesions were not identified by MR imaging despite prior knowledge of their location. An absence of contrast between the tumor and adjacent cortex on MR imaging was noted with virtually all pulse sequences (Fig 19–4). Increasing the number of sequences was not helpful. Tumor identification depended on finding anatomic distortion. A hypointense rim, when present, helped delineate the periphery of the tumor. Inhomogeneity or mottling of the

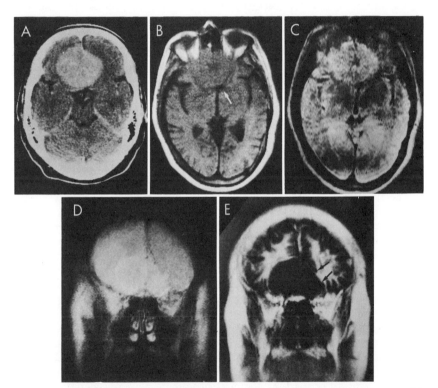

Fig 19–4.—Subfrontal meningioma, typical appearance. **A,** contrast-enhanced computed tomographic (CT) scan showing a typical homogeneously enhanced bilateral subfrontal tumor. **B,** spin-echo (SE) 30/500 scan. The tumor is isointense and is identified only because of its effects, such as obliteration of sulci and displacement of anterior third ventricle *(arrow.)* **C,** SE 90/1500 scan. Lesion is minimally hyperintense and slightly mottled. A thin halo of hyperintensity (correlating with edema identified on CT) surrounds and helps demarcate the tumor. **D,** coronal SE 120/1500 scan. The tumor is a poorly defined, slightly hyperintense mass. The lack of detail can be noted (relative to C) caused by low signal-to-noise ratio. **E,** coronal inversion-recovery 450/1500 scan. The tumor is a discrete hypointense mass (relative to nearby white matter) with the same intensity as adjacent cortex *(arrows)*, from which it is difficult to distinguish. The excellent visualization of the flat inferior dural base of the meningioma and demonstration of bilateral displacement of white matter and distortion of corticomedullary junction (buckling) can be seen, indicative of extra-axial mass effect. (Courtesy of Zimmerman, R.D., et al.: AJNR 6:149–157, Mar.–Apr. 1985.)

tumor also was a useful feature in some cases. Bony abnormalities were visualized in 11 of 16 patients with such changes seen on CT. The MR images did not demonstrate tumor calcification.

Image contrast could be improved in the MR evaluation of meningiomas. Calcification is not well shown by MR imaging. Digital intravenous angiography can sometimes be avoided, but angiography may be necessary when a venous sinus is involved to distinguish between partial and complete sinus occlusion.

▶ Meningiomas continue to be a bugaboo for diagnosis by MR imaging. In this series, which was evaluated by a very experienced neuroradiologic team, contrast CT showed up the meningiomas more clearly than did MR in half the cases. Three small lesions were missed by MR. Contrast enhancement or new pulse sequences may be able to overcome these problems. Recently, in the case of acute hematoma, it has been shown at Massachusetts General Hospital that special pulse sequences can show up acute hematomas. It is hoped that a similar approach, utilizing knowledge of the basic physics of the problem, can be used to remedy this imaging deficit.—Robert M. Crowell, M.D.

Magnetic Resonance Imaging of the Cavernous Sinus
David L. Daniels, Peter Pech, Leighton Mark, Kathleen Pojunas, Alan L. Williams, and Victor M. Haughton (Med. College of Wisconsin)
AJR 144:1009–1014, May 1985   19–7

The normal magnetic resonance (MR) appearances of the cavernous sinus were studied by correlating images from 7 normal subjects with cryomicrotomic sections of 6 cadaver heads. Imaging was performed on 15 patients, including 2 with pituitary adenomas and 1 with a parasellar aneurysm.

Coronal cryomicrotomic sections showed the cranial nerves in the cavernous sinuses to have a constant position with respect to the internal carotid artery. Coronal partial saturation and inversion recovery images with a slice thickness of 3 or 5 mm showed small foci of high-intensity signals representing cranial nerves III, V, and VI in the cavernous sinuses. The intensity of the signals was about equal to that of the corpus callosum. The Meckel cave had an intense signal in T2-weighted images and a low-intensity signal in T1-weighted images. Masses in the cavernous sinus were clearly visualized (Fig 19–5). Tumors producing a greater signal intensity than blood in the cavernous sinus or internal carotid artery were readily detected when they encroached on these structures.

The cranial nerves are effectively demonstrated in the cavernous sinuses by MR imaging. The sinus contents are better demonstrated than by computed tomography (CT), which often fails to show vascular structures unless dynamic techniques are used. Masses encroaching on the cavernous sinuses and those encasing or displacing the carotid artery may be detected better by MR imaging than by CT.

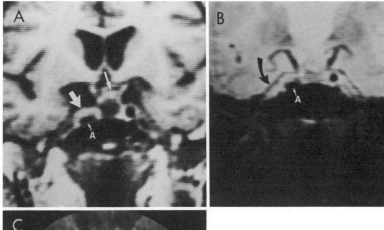

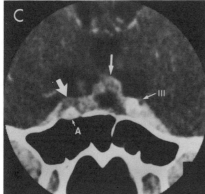

Fig 19–5.—A partly cystic pituitary adenoma *(thin arrow)* extending to the right cavernous sinus *(thick arrow)*. **A,** 5-mm-thick partial saturation image, 128 × 256 matrix, two averages; **B,** spin-echo image, 128 × 256 matrix, one average; and **C,** enhanced CT scan. Tumor displaces right internal carotid artery *(A)* but not lateral cavernous sinus wall *(curved arrow)*. (Courtesy of Daniels, D.L., et al.: *AJR* 144:1009–1014, May 1985. Copyright 1985, by the American Roentgen Ray Society.)

▶ Magnetic resonance (MR) imaging is more effective than computed tomography (CT) in delineating the parts of the cavernous sinus (Daniels et al.: *AJNR* 6:187–192, 1985). Cranial nerves in the cavernous sinus can be seen as well as signs of parasellar mass, including obliteration of venous spaces, displacement of the internal carotid artery, and bulging of the lateral wall.

Comparative data on MR imaging are not available, but CT and angiography gives specific diagnosis of extradural juxtacellar tumors (Moore et al.: *AJR* 145:491–496, 1985). Amongst 15 histologically proven tumors, 5 chordomas showed bony erosion and a posterior fossa component. Four trigeminal neuromas showed bony erosion at Meckel's cave and moderate contrast enhancement. Two cavernous meningiomas showed enhancement, expansion of cavernous sinus, and angiographic stain. Two cavernous hemangiomas of the cavernous sinus were intensely enhancing with angiographic stain. Sphenoid sinus mucocele showed bony destruction and lack of enhancement.—Robert M. Crowell, M.D.

Notes on Magnetic Resonance Imaging

▶ Magnetic resonance effectively recognizes supratentorial tumors (Lee et al.: *AJNR* 6:871–878, 1985). Of 80 cases studied with a 0.5-Tesla super-conducting system, 28 patients had verified gliomas, 34 were presumed to have primary tumors on clinical grounds, 13 had metastases, and 5 were postoperative. Lesions demonstrated on CT were equally well seen by MR. More metastases were shown on MR than CT. Magnetic resonance imaging revealed abnormal signals in 10 cases in which CT was equivocal. MR could not differentiate edemas from tumors, nor could it determine the histologic type of the tumors.

Magnetic resonance sometimes misses calcified intracranial lesions (Holland et al.: *Radiology* 157:353–356, 1985). MR demonstrated 41 of 50 lesions seen as calcified on CT scans, including 29 of 30 neoplasms and 10 of 10 arteriovenous malformations. Calcification was suspected in about 60% of the calcified lesions but was also suspected in 45% of the uncalcified lesions. In the 9 lesions undetected by MR, calcification was the only abnormal CT finding. Calcification findings on MR images included signal void, dampening, or diminution.

Small orbital lesions can be imaged with superior results using surface coil magnetic resonance imaging (Bilaniuk et al.: *Radiology* 156:669–674, 1985).

Magnetic resonance, particularly in sagittal images with the surface coil technique, depicts the anatomic relations of the jugular foramen with good resolution (Daniels et al.: *AJNR* 6:699–703, 1985).

Magnetic resonance imaging shows increased signal intensity on T1-weighted sequences after radiation treatment of the vertebral bodies (Ramsey and Zacharias: *AJR* 144:1131–1135, 1985).

According to Lee and Deck (*Radiology* 157:143–147, 1985), MR imaging is superior to CT in demonstrating distortion of optic chiasm and suprasellar carotid arteries. Magnetic resonance imaging can differentiate many pathologic features of juxtasellar lesions but does not demonstrate microadenomas.

Mikhael et al. (*J. Comput. Assist. Tomogr.* 9:852–856, 1985) report that MR imaging detected 11 verified tumors in the cerebellopontine angle. The authors believe that MR imaging can replace contrast cisternography in the detection of small lesions.

Rinck et al. (*Radiology* 157:103–106, 1985) did not find spin echo sequences effective in discriminating specific tumor types during MR imaging evaluation.

Magnetic resonance imaging depicts cavernous sinus better than CT, according to Daniels et al. (*AJR* 144:1009–1014, 1985).

Gadolinium-DPTA improves tumor delineation for almost all lesions, particularly for glioma and metastases, according to Felix et al. (*Radiology* 156:681–688, 1985).

Hyman et al. (*AJNR* 6:229–236, 1985) studied 50 cervical spines with 0.6-tesla MR imaging, using multislice and multiecho techniques. Diagnostic information was as good as or better than that derived from myelography, an invasive test. After plain radiographs, MR imaging is the investigative study of choice for cervical spine lesions.

Magnetic resonance imaging depicts tumors and arteriovenous malformations of the spinal cord (Di Chiro et al.: *Radiology* 156:689–697, 1985). In 25 of 38 examinations, MR imaging provided more information than other studies, but MR cannot be used in some patients and has drawbacks in others. Thus, MR imaging is not often the sole study for spinal cord lesions.

Gadolinium-DTPA can produce enhancement of cervical intraspinal tumors on MR imaging (Bydder et al.: *J. Comput. Assist. Tomogr.* 9:847–851, 1985).

Magnetic resonance imaging shows syringomyelia very well when cord diameter is enlarged, but may miss the lesion in normal-sized or small cords (Lee et al.: *AJNR* 6:221–228, 1985).

According to Holman et al. (*Invest. Radiol.* 4:370–373, 1985), MR imaging spectroscopy can detect cerebral infarction in gerbils at 3 hours.—Robert M. Crowell, M.D.

Other Intracranial Diagnostics

Dexamethasone Treatment of Brain Tumor Patients: Effects on Regional Cerebral Blood Flow, Blood Volume, and Oxygen Utilization

K. L. Leenders, R. P. Beaney, D. J. Brooks, A. A. Lammertsma, J. D. Heather, and C. G. McKenzie (Hammersmith Hosp., London)
Neurology 35:1610–1616, November 1985   19–8

Computed tomography evidence of peritumoral edema is reduced by the administration of dexamethasone. Positron emission tomography (PET) now has been used to determine whether such treatment consistently produces changes in brain physiology. PET was done by the ^{15}O steady-state inhalation technique in 10 patients with cerebral tumors (mean age, 53.5 years). Studies were repeated after treatment with dexamethasone. Administration of an intravenous dose of 20 mg was followed by oral therapy with 4 mg 4 times daily, over 1–5 days.

Regional cerebral blood flow decreased except in edematous areas after dexamethasone treatment. Regional cerebral blood volume decreased in all regions, but the regional cerebral metabolic rate of oxygen did not change significantly. The fractional extraction of oxygen was increased throughout the brain, with no change in oxygen utilization.

The effects of dexamethasone in these patients with brain tumor probably reflect direct constriction of cerebral vessels. Dexamethasone theoretically could artifactually alter regional cerebral blood flow by an effect on the size of any nonexchangeable water pool. Dexamethasone reduces the water content of the edematous brain, but no change in water content has been found in the normal brain.

▶ Dexamethasone evidently reduces water in brain tumors and diminishes local cerebral blood volume, probably through direct constriction of cerebral vessels. Positron emission tomography scanning distinguishes recurrent brain tumor from radiation necrosis, a useful clinical application. Regional PET scanners may have both research and clinical use (Digest 19–9).

Positron emission tomography discloses abnormalities in blood flow and oxygen utilization in the hemisphere contralateral to intracranial tumors, with improvement after decompressive surgery (Beaney et al.: *Psychiatry* 48:310–319, 1985).—Robert M. Crowell, M.D.

Prediction of Survival in Glioma Patients by Means of Positron Emission Tomography

Nicholas J. Patronas, Giovanni Di Chiro, Conrad Kufta, Dikran Bairamian, Paul L. Kornblith, Richard Simon, and Steven M. Larson (Nat. Insts. of Health, Bethesda, Md.)
J. Neurosurg. 62:816–822, June 1985   19–9

Differences in the biologic behavior of high-grade gliomas are not always apparent on angiograms or computed tomography (CT) scans. The prognostic usefulness of positron emission tomography (PET) with ^{18}F-2-deoxyglucose (FDG) was examined in 45 consecutive patients with grade III and IV astrocytomas, 33 men and 12 women aged 18–69 years. Most had been treated elsewhere, and 42 patients had had partial resection of disease. Eight tumors involved both hemispheres at admission. The studies were done with 3–5 mCi of FDG and either an ECAT II scanner or the multi-slice Neuro-PET scanner.

Contrast enhancement was present on the CT scans in the great majority of cases. No CT features consistently distinguished between tumors leading rapidly to death and those allowing survival for many months. In 36 cases the rate of glucose utilization was higher on the side of tumor (Fig 19–6). Most patients with a high ratio died within a few months, while some with low ratios lived much longer. The distribution of glucose utilization ratios above and below the median of 1.4:1 correlated significantly with the duration of survival. The ratio was more accurate than histologic grade in the determining of the duration of survival. Useful prognostic information in patients with high-grade gliomas can be provided by PET with FDG. It is better than CT or angiography for this purpose, and is superior to histologic typing in making a prognosis. It also can be used to monitor the short-term response to treatment.

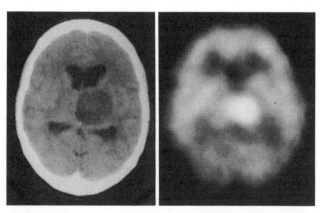

Fig 19–6.—Left: Computerized tomography (CT) scan after administration of contrast material showing a hypodense nonenhancing mass in the left thalamus. The lack of contrast enhancement is a feature most commonly found in relatively benign gliomas. Right: Positron emission tomography (PET) scan showing markedly increased glucose utilization activity in the tumor, indicating poor prognosis. The patient died 5 months after these studies. Thus, the PET scan was superior to CT in predicting tumor aggressiveness. (Courtesy of Patronas, N.J., et al.: J. Neurosurg. 62:816–822, June 1985.)

▶ This is an exciting report. The utilization of PET metabolic data to predict outcome represents a real advance and is apparently superior to other parameters for prognosis. If this article's finding can be confirmed, this type of evaluation could become of clinical importance. Spectroscopy studies of metabolism done with magnetic resonance can theoretically provide similar information.

Dynamic study of gliomas with L-methyl-11C-methionine and PET permit better evaluation of tumor extent and may affect preoperative grading (Lilja et al.: *AJNR* 6:505–514, 1985).—Robert M. Crowell, M.D.

Direct Coronal Computed Tomography for Presurgical Evaluation of Posterior Fossa Tumors
Thomas P. Naidich, Tadinori Tomita, Peter Pech, and Victor Haughton (Children's Mem. Hosp., Chicago; Univ. of Uppsala, Sweden; Med. Colege of Wisconsin, Milwaukee)
J. Comput. Assist. Tomogr. 9:1065–1072, Nov.–Dec. 1985   19–10

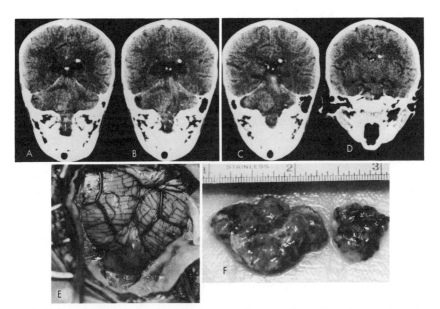

Fig 19–7.—Exophytic tumor in cisterna magna, spinal canal, and cerebellopontine angle in a 19-month-old girl with ependymoma. A to D, direct coronal, contrast-enhanced CT scans show a large, markedly asymmetric, inhomogeneously and predominantly faintly enhancing mass that bows the brain stem *(arrowheads,* **B** and **C**) across the midline, fills the cisterna magna, and extends downward *(white arrows,* **A** and **B**) through foramen magnum to C1 *(1).* Asymmetric elevation and compression of the ipsilateral cerebellar white matter indicates extra-axial, subcerebellar position of mass. Deviation of the brain stem confirms the extra-axial growth of tumor *(black arrow,* **D**) within the cerebellopontine angle. **E,** surgical exposure: wide suboccipital craniotomy and durotomy with patient sitting with head flexed. The cisterna magna was partially obliterated and filled by a grayish pink, gelatinous tumor mass *(arrowhead)* that grew out from the vallecula. The tumor extended to the cerebellopontine angle cistern and elevated the hemisphere asymmetrically. The tumor also extended under the cerebellar hemisphere through foramen magnum *(arrow)* into spinal canal. The great bulk of the tumor lay within the fourth ventricle and below the cerebellar hemisphere in the subcerebellar and cerebellopontine angle cisterns. **F,** small portion of surgical specimen. Gelatinous tumor packed the cisterns and surrounded the cranial nerves. (Courtesy of Naidich, T.P., et al.: J. Comput. Assist. Tomogr. 9:1065–1072, Nov.–Dec. 1985.)

Available computed tomographic (CT) methods have failed to precisely demonstrate surgically significant pathologic changes in cases of posterior fossa tumor. Direct coronal CT was evaluated as an alternative to axial CT in six patients with posterior fossa lesions on axial views. Serial, contiguous, 5-mm-thick, direct CT sections were obtained through the posterior fossa in a plane nearly perpendicular to the hard palate. One patient was studied both with and without intravenous contrast enhancement. The "hanging-head" position was used for coronal scanning.

Direct coronal CT demonstrated the anatomical features needed to plan surgery in these patients. The structures or tumor parts to be found immediately under the dura were seen, as well as anatomical relations among significant structures in the posterior fossa. The demonstration of extensive exophytic tumor growth into the cisterna magna and cerebellopontine angle is shown in Figure 19–7. Direct coronal CT was superior to axial CT in predicting the nature of tissue occupying the cisterna magna, and it was as good as or better than axial CT in detecting extensions to the cerebellopontine angle cistern.

Direct coronal CT displays all significant anatomical relations in the posterior fossa in the orientation found at surgical dissection. Greater patient discomfort is entailed, but the images are useful enough to warrant the increased time and radiation exposure required.

▶ Neurosurgeons must communicate with neuroradiologic colleagues to obtain optimum studies with which to guide surgical procedure. This need is particularly evident in the selection of further studies once a lesion has been identified. Often the choice will include reformatting of CT images or direct coronal images for depiction of a pathologic condition in the posterior fossa or near the sella.—Robert M. Crowell, M.D.

Confirmation of Brain Death With Portable Isotope Angiography: A Review of 204 Consecutive Cases

Julius M. Goodman, Larry L. Heck, and Brian D. Moore (Indianapolis Neurosurgical Group and Indiana Univ.)
Neurosurgery 16:492–497, April 1985   19–11

Using intravenous isotope cerebral angiography to demonstrate a critical cerebral blood deficit has been recommended as a means of confirming brain death. An attempt was made to determine the adequacy of a single angiogram showing termination of carotid flow at the skull base and a definite absence of uptake in the intracranial arteries. Two hundred four consecutively seen cases of suspected brain death were reviewed; all had been studied by isotope angiography. Scan results were considered consistent with brain death when all arterial and venous flow was absent on the dynamic study and the dural sinuses were not visualized on the static scan (Fig 19–8). Studies were done with 20–30 mCi of ^{99m}Tc-labeled human serum albumin.

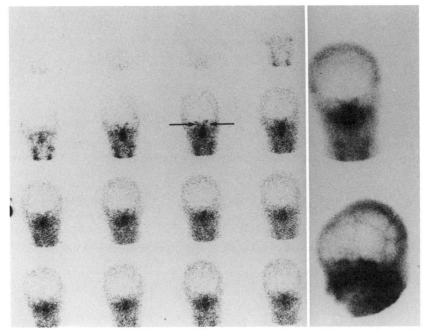

Fig 19–8.—This isotope angiogram confirms the clinical diagnosis of brain death. On the dynamic study *(left)*, flow in the carotid arteries appears to be arrested at the siphons *(arrows)*, and there is no intracranial vascular filling. Only scalp flow is noted above the base of the skull. Anterior and lateral static images *(right)* taken after the dynamic flow study show nonfilling of the dural sinuses. (Courtesy of Goodman, J.M., et al.: Neurosurgery 16:492–497, April 1985; Berlin-Heidelberg-New York; Springer.)

Arrest of the carotid circulation and absence of intracranial arterial circulation provided adequate confirmation of brain death when these were carefully established clinically—even if there was some visualization of the intracranial venous sinuses. Sequential scanning showed that, once intraranial arterial circulation was definitely absent, arterial flow never reappeared. Normal flow studies revealed three physician errors in diagnosing brain death clinically. Monitoring of intra-cranial pressure in barbiturate-treated patients showed a lack of isotope above the skull base following a pronounced terminal rise in pressure and fixation of the pupils. All 14 autopsies showed autolysis consistent with a diagnosis of respiratory brain death.

Laboratory confirmation of brain death can be used to reveal occasional clinical errors and to reassure anxious families that a treatable state has not been overlooked. An arbitrary waiting period and withdrawal of sedatives are not necessary when intravenous isotope angiography is used to confirm brain death.

▶ Goodman and colleagues have made an important contribution: portable isotope angiography is a reliable, available, and understandable method for confirmation of brain death. The method can confidently be recommended to confirm the clinical diagnosis of brain death, without an arbitrary waiting period, withdrawal of sedatives, normalization of brain temperature, etc. This approach is helpful to the care of the patient, for the doctor, the family, and for organ transplantation.—Robert M. Crowell, M.D.

CT Findings in Eclampsia

C. Colosimo, Jr., A. Fileni, M. Moschini, P. Guerrini (Catholic Univ., Rome)
Neuroradiology 27:313–317, July 1985   19–12

Computed tomography (CT) findings were reviewed in five patients seen between 1980 and 1984 with eclampsia. Four presented with episodes of seizures in the third trimester, while one was hospitalized with scleroderma and pre-eclampsia. All patients had arterial hypertension, edema with excessive weight gain, and proteinuria. A CT scan was done just after cesarean section while the patient was still sedated. Four patients improved rapidly after delivery, but the patient with scleroderma died with brain

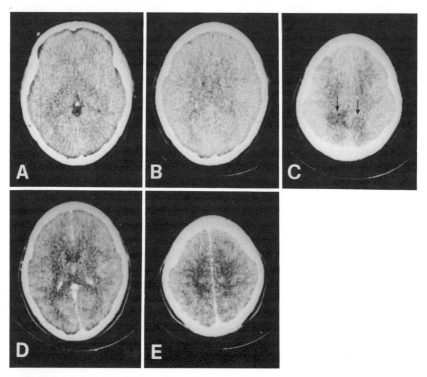

Fig 19–9.—A-E Case 2. A-C, unenhanced CT immediately after cesarian section shows bilateral hypodensities in the white matter of both posterior parietal lobes *(arrows)*. There is marked mass effect and edema and ventricular size is reduced. E-F, enhanced CT, 9 days after, reveals complete return to normal. (Courtesy of Colosimo Jr. C., et al.: Neuroradiology 27:313–317, July 1985. Berlin-Heidelberg-New York; Springer.)

hemorrhage and cardiorespiratory failure. Intravenous contrast was used for CT in three of the cases.

Focal densitometric changes were seen in all cases, usually as hypodensities without enhancement. In three cases the hypodense areas were bilateral and fairly symmetric (Fig 19–9). Marked cerebral edema was present in the patient with scleroderma. Follow-up studies of the other patients showed nearly complete disappearance of the densitometric changes after 7 to 14 days, accompanying the resolution of symptoms.

Bilateral hypodensities without enhancement are characteristic of eclampsia. The CT abnormalities are completely reversible. The lesions involve chiefly white matter and are associated with cerebral edema. Computed tomography is useful both in monitoring brain edema in relation to the neurologic course of eclampsia and in ruling out cerebral hemorrhage.

Notes on Other Intracranial Diagnostics

▶ A number of studies suggest that ultrasound may deserve wider application than digital subtraction angiography (DSA) for study of the carotid bifurcation:

Ball et al. studied complications of standard angiography and DSA (*Arch. Neurol.* 42:969–972, 1985). In 500 DSA tests, there were serious complications in 8.2%, with one permanent neurologic deficit. This is hard to understand; note that antecubital hematoma was deemed "serious." In 150 standard angiograms, there were serious complications in 2.7%, with no permanent neurologic deficits.

Zwiebel et al. (*Stroke* 16:633–642, 1985) found ultrasound and intravenous DSA quite similar in accuracy for evaluation of the carotid bifurcation. Since there is risk to DSA, ultrasound is preferred.

Doppler sonography detected complete or nearly complete vertebral occlusion in eight angiographically verified cases (Biedert et al.: *Neuroradiology* 27:430–433, 1985).

Ringelstein et al. describe Doppler monitoring of middle cerebral artery blood flow during carotid endarterectomy (*Nervenarzt* 56:423–430, 1985).

Kenaghy reports that duplex scanning detects carotid stenosis in over 50%, with 95% sensitivity and specificity, and detects carotid occlusion in 93%, compared with results of angiography (*J. Vasc. Surg.* 2:591–593, 1985).

Sekiya et al. (*J. Neurosurg.* 63:598–607, 1985) found that for monitoring of brainstem auditory evoked responses (BAERs) in dogs, delay of interpeak latency of waves I-V was caused by conduction block (temporary or permanent) in the cochlear nerve. Obliteration of BAERs, including wave I, was caused by occlusion of the internal auditory artery.

Drummond et al. report that high-dose sodium thiopental does not affect somatosensory evoked potentials and BAERs (*Anesthesiology* 63:249–254, 1985).

Single photon emission tomography detects infarction as well as computed tomography (CT) (Brott, T. G., et al.: *Radiology* 158:729–734, 1986). Regional CBF can also be measured with SPECT.

Schubert et al. report that SSEPs may be lost because of intracranial gas (*Anesth. Analg.* 65:203–206, 1986).—Robert M. Crowell, M.D.

Spinal Diagnostics

Somatosensory Evoked Potentials in Hysterical Paraplegia

Barry J. Kaplan, William A. Friedman, and Dietrich Gravenstein (Univ. of Florida)

Surg. Neurol. 23:502–506, November 1985   19–13

Hysterical neurologic deficit is a rare finding in which weakness and sensory loss are usually paradoxical, but the physician must exclude structural abnormality. Three patients seen in the past year had somatosensory evoked potential (SEP) recording after stimulation of the affected extremities as a possible alternative to invasive testing. Thalamocortical potentials were recorded from scalp electrodes on stimulation of the posterior tibial nerve.

Man, 29·years old, a prisoner, reported immediate low back pain and lower limb paralysis after having jumped from a top bunk to the floor and landing on his feet. Straight-leg raising was normal, but all muscle groups in the lower extremities were paralyzed. Examination of the upper limbs yielded normal findings. Reflexes were 2+ throughout. A T10 sensory level was present bilaterally, and proprioception and vibratory sense were absent in the lower extremities. A thoracolumbar metrizamide myelogram was normal, as were the cerebrospinal fluid findings. Recording of SEPs showed thalamocortical potentials of normal amplitude and latency (Fig 19–10). A psychiatric consultant concurred in the diagnosis of

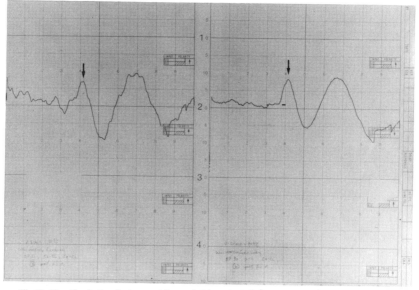

Fig 19–10.—Cortical evoked potential recorded from frontal midline-vertex midline electrode montage during stimulation of posterior tibial nerve in right leg (**left**) and left leg (**right**). The sweep time was 100 msec, the latency of first peak, 21 msec bilaterally (*arrows*). (Courtesy of Kaplan, B.J., et al.: Surg. Neurol. 23:502–506, November 1985. Reprinted by permission of the publisher. Copyright 1985, Elsevier Science Publishing Co., Inc.)

conversion reaction. Lower limb strength and sensation returned gradually over the next 24 hours.

Hysterical paralysis is typically seen in young, working class males with previous psychiatric illness and with minimal craniovertebral trauma. The finding of normal SEPs in a patient who denies sensation of the stimulus provides objective evidence of the hysterical nature of a deficit. Rehabilitation should include physical therapy and reassurance. Psychiatric consultation is indicated to define any underlying psychopathologic condition and provide support.

▶ Objective data from SEPs can be useful in the evaluation of hysterical paraplegia. This is helpful in our litigious society and certainly makes the treating physician more comfortable about the solidity of his diagnosis. In questionable cases, however, myelography or magnetic resonance imaging will exclude a surgical lesion.

Somatosensory evoked responses gave misleading information in 10 cases of 19 with unilateral lumbosacral radiculopathy (Aminoff: *Ann. Neurol.* 17:171–176, 1985).—Robert M. Crowell, M.D.

High-Resolution Surface-Coil Imaging of Lumbar Disk Disease
Robert R. Edelman, Gregory M. Shoukimas, David D. Stark, Kenneth R. Davis, Paul F. J. New, Sanjay Sanini, Daniel I. Rosenthal, Gary L. Wismer, and Thomas J. Brady (Massachusetts Gen. Hosp., Boston)
AJNR 6:479–485, July–August 1985   19–14

Magnetic resonance (MR) imaging may have several advantages over computed tomography (CT) and myelography in the evaluation of lumbar disk disease. The use of plane selection oriented parallel to the disk with multiplanar imaging allows MR imaging of the lumbar spine in a routine clinical setting. Seventeen patients aged 21–60 years were examined, 14 after CT or myelography within the past 2 weeks had shown lumbar disk disease and 3 because of symptoms. Subsequent surgery confirmed the CT and myelographic findings in 10 cases. A spin-echo technique was utilized. Eleven multislice sagittal images were obtained in 18 minutes.

Twenty-nine disk herniations or bulges were detected in the 17 patients. All abnormal disks were seen on initial sagittal MR images, and all disks seen as normal on MR were normal on CT and/or myelography. Cortical bone and epidural fat were distinguished by MR imaging. The nerve roots and root sheaths appeared as low-intensity structures on both T1- and T2-weighted images. The normal nucleus pulposus had intermediate signal intensity on T1-weighted images; herniated disk material had a similar or slightly lower intensity in most cases but occasionally was higher in intensity. Whereas T1-weighted images generally provided optimal anatomical detail and excellent contrast betwen the herniation, epidural fat, and nerve roots, T2-weighted images sometimes were better in delineating the disk from the thecal sac, especially when little epidural fat was present.

High-resolution surface-coil MR imaging of the lumbar spine can demonstrate risk herniation as well as can CT or myelography and is a practical alternative method. It may become the procedure of choice for MR imaging of lumbar disk disease as further technical improvements are made.

▶ In this study of 17 patients, high-resolution surface-coil MR imaging of lumbar disk disease was just as effective as CT or myelography. If these results can be confirmed in larger series, then this approach may become the method of choice for the diagnosis of lumbar disc disease. Since MR is not invasive and can be done on an outpatient basis, this would have great impact on the patterns of referral and economics in the evaluation of patients with low back pain. Indications for evaluation could be broadened and the cost of individual studies reduced.—Robert M. Crowell, M.D.

CT Myelography for Outpatients: An Inpatient/Outpatient Pilot Study to Assess Methodology
S. James Zinreich, Henry Wang, Marcia L. Updike, Ashok J. Kumar, Hyo S. Ahn, Richard B. North, and Arthur E. Rosenbaum (Johns Hopkins Med. Institutions, Baltimore)
Radiology 157:387–390, November 1985   19–15

Myelography, which must have a low risk if used broadly in the outpatient setting, was evaluated in terms of its diagnostic utility and safety by use of a preparation of 100 mg I/ml and volumes of 5–6 ml. Thirty-eight inpatients were initially examined by use of a 25-gauge needle and then managed as if they were outpatients. The procedure then was extended to 42 outpatients, and 25 other outpatients were examined with a preparation of 170 mg I/ml.

Eighty-nine percent of inpatients were free of side effects after myelography. Only 9.5% of outpatients having low-dose studies had headache or nausea, while 36% of those given the higher-iodine preparation were symptomatic. Two of these patients were moderately distressed and had to return to the hospital emergency room for symptomatic therapy.

Side effects are infrequent and usually mild with lower intrathecal doses of metrizamide for myelography. Outpatient myelography can be safely carried out by use of low-dose metrizamide, and even greater safety is expected as second-and third-generation contrast agents come into use. The economic benefits of outpatient examination will be considerable.

▶ Data from Johns Hopkins indicate effectiveness and safety for outpatient myelography using low-dose metrizamide and computed tomography. These results parallel those from other institutions. For example, among 79 patients undergoing outpatient myelography with 3.75 gm of metrizamide via a 25-gauge spinal needle, results were encouraging (Tate et al.: *Radiology* 157:391–393, 1985). None of the patients had significant neurotoxicity after the exam; 71% had minimal or no side effects. Three patients were admitted to the hospital for headache, nausea, vomiting, and back pain.

On the other hand, severe reactions, including death, can occur after positive contrast myelography (Baessler & Lahl: *Zeitblatt für Neururochurigie* 46:141–150, 1985). Such reactions are probably best managed in the hospital. Because of such cases, there may be malpractice liability in outpatient myelography. Surface-coil magnetic resonance imaging could avoid much liability if its diagnostic accuracy is sufficient (Digest 19–14).—Robert M. Crowell, M.D.

Myelography in Cancer Patients: Modified Technique
Ya-Yan Lee, J. Peter Glass, and Sidney Wallace (Univ. of Texas at Houston)
AJR 145:791–795, October 1985   19–16

Spinal cord and cauda equina compression in patients with cancer most often are due to epidural and/or leptomeningeal metastases. An accurate and safe means is needed of evaluating the entire spinal canal when spinal compression is a possibility. A total of 240 cancer patients had myelography for possible spinal compression in an 18-month period. A small volume of Pantopaque was injected at the L2–3 level, or at L4–5 if the higher level was the area of major concern. More contrast was introduced if a complete block was found. Air then was injected in a closed system and fluoroscopic spot myelographs obtained.

No serious complications occurred. Squeezing of dye by air successfully demonstrated a complete block in all 39 attempts, without worsening the existing neurologic deficit. Six of these patients had multiple blocks. Myelographic quality was satisfactory or better in 94% of cases. Twelve patients had a supplemental metrizamide computed tomography (CT) study. The findings in one case in which the "squeezing" maneuver was used are shown in Figure 19–11.

Pantopaque myelography remains useful in selected cases with possible spinal block. A squeezing technique can safely demonstrate the cephalad end of a block. High cervical puncture is more dangerous and will not adequately demonstrate multiple blocks. Use of a limited amount of Pantopaque does not compromise subsequent metrizamide myelography or CT. Retained Pantopaque can be used for follow-up evaluation of spinal-canal patency after treatment.

▶ Although the authors suggest safety and improved visualization, I am concerned about possible neurologic deterioration when intraspinal pressure is increased by injection of contrast and gas. I personally will await further confirmatory studies of safety and efficacy before switching from the more conventional procedure of placement of additional contrast material via a C1–2 puncture.—Robert M. Crowell, M.D.

Notes on Spinal Diagnostics

▶ Magnetic resonance (MR) imaging of the inter-vertebral disc indicates that T-1 and T-2 values of the normal nucleus pulposus decrease with age. Quantitative studies of MR images may assist in the diagnosis of intervertebral disk degeneration (Jenkins et al.: *Br. J. Radiol.* 58:705–709, 1985).

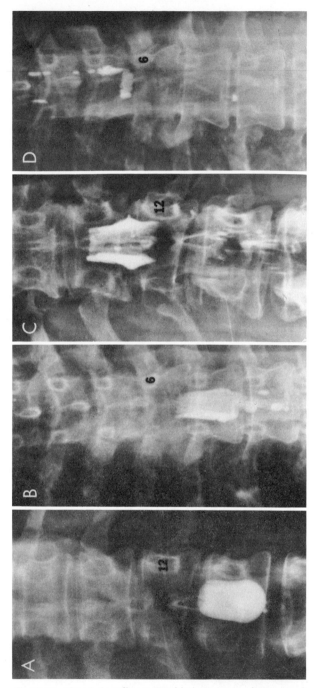

Fig 19–11.—Case 2. Spot films in Trendelenburg position during squeezing. The caudal ends of lower complete block at T12-L1 (**A**) and of higher complete block are at T6-T7 (**B**). Spot films in upright position after squeezing. Cephalad ends of lower complete block at T11-T12 (**C**) and higher complete block at T5-T6 (**D**). (Courtesy of Lee, Y., et al.: AJR 145:791–795, October 1985. Copyright 1985 by the American Roentgen Ray Society.)

A randomized, double-blind trial of iohexol and iopamidol for myelography showed equivalent side effects and quality of examination with the two agents: (Mac Pherson, et al.: *J. Radiol.* 58:849–851, 1985).

For lumbar myelography, iohexol is associated with fewer side effects than is metrizamide (Laasonen: *Acta Radiol Diagn (Stockh)* 26:761–765, 1985).

Badami et al. compared conventional myelography and computed tomographic (CT) myelography involving metrizamide as contrast agent with surgical findings in 30 patients with cervical radiculopathy and/or myelopathy. (*AJNR* 144:675–680, 1985). In 60% of the patients, metrizamide CT myelography provided significant additional information. In no case was a myelographic abnormality not detected by metrizamide CT myelography. In cervical myelopathy, a cross-section diameter of the cord of less than 50% of the subarachnoid space predicted a poor patient response to surgical intervention.

Postoperative fracture of the lumbar articular facet is a potential cause of postoperative pain and can be recognized by CT scanning (Rothman et al.: *AJNR* 6:623–628, 1985).

In patients with sciatica, CT can be used to identify compression or deformity of the sciatic nerve by pelvic lesions (Pech and Haughton: *AJR* 144:1037–1041, 1985).

Transabdominal ultrasound can diagnose intervertebral disks in up to 86% of the cases (Tolly: *Fortschritte der Rondgenstrahlen* 141:546–555, 1984).

Unfused ossicles of the lumbar spine may be diagnosed by CT (Pech and Haughton: *AJNR* 6:629–631, 1985).—Robert M. Crowell, M.D.

20 Techniques

Introduction

In the field of brain tumor management, a host of advances have been reported. Several new methods of radiation treatment command attention. According to Manaka et al. (Digest 20–1), standard radiotherapy is a very useful means of improving survival and quality of life in patients with craniopharyngioma, especially when subtotal resection has been carried out. Instillation of phosphorous-32 into cystic tumors, including astrocytomas and craniopharyngiomas, reduces cyst size and fluid reaccummulation while sparing normal brain tissue (Digest 20–2) interstitial irradiation of skull base tumors has given encouraging results, but significant cranial nerve complications may occur (Digest 20–4). Ultrasound may be used to guide implantation of radiation sources into brain tumors (Digest 20–5). Heavy particle beam therapy gives good results in the treatment of sacral chordoma (Digest 20–6).

Stereotaxic surgery for brain tumors has made recent gains. Coffee and Lunsford (Digest 20–7) report that stereotaxic biopsy can be safely carried out even for lesions of the midbrain and pons. (Digest 20–7). Kelly and colleagues (Digest 20–8) have described a "Star Wars" approach to brain tumors in which computer technique guides a microsurgically directed laser in the obliteration of deep-seated tumors through a small craniotomy.

Other brain tumor treatments include the neodymium: yttrium-aluminum-garnet laser, which has promise for neurosurgery (Digest 20–9), and microwave hyperthermia, also a promising treatment method (Digest 20–10).

Robert M. Crowell, M.D.

Radiotherapies

The Efficacy of Radiotherapy for Craniopharyngioma

Shinya Manaka, Akira Teramoto, and Kintomo Takakura (Univ. of Tokyo)
J. Neurosurg. 62:648–656, May 1985   20–1

The value of radiotherapy in the treatment of craniopharyngioma was studied in 125 surgical patients, 45 of whom had received radiotherapy. The series included all survivors surgically treated in 1950–1979 except those who underwent total tumor removal. More than one third of the patients were children. The mean follow-up was nearly 9½ years. Cobalt irradiation was given to study patients in an average total dose of 5,000 rads. No significant complications resulted.

Survival rates at 5 years were 89% and 35% for irradiated and control patients, respectively; 10-year rates were 76% and 27%. Median survival exceeded 10 years for irradiated patients, compared with only 3 years for control patients. Statistical analysis confirmed a much better outcome for irradiated patients in terms of survival time. Both children and adults had long-term survival after radiotherapy. Even patients who underwent minimal surgery, such as biopsy or cyst evacuation, had long survival times when irradiated. All irradiated patients with tumors less than 2 cm in diameter survived 10 years, as did three fourths of those with tumors 2–5 cm in diameter.

Radiotherapy is a very useful means of improving survival and the quality of life in patients with craniopharyngioma. Survival after subtotal resection and radiotherapy is comparable with that after putative total tumor resection. It seems best to attempt total removal or, if this is not feasible, to remove as much of the tumor as possible and administer radiotherapy.

▶ These results indicate a useful means of improving survival and quality of life by radiotherapy for patients with craniopharyngioma. Because of the very substantial morbidity and even mortality associated with attempts at total removal of these lesions, the surgeon should keep in mind that there is an alternative with lower immediate risk. When the cleavage plane becomes obscure or adhesions are intense, it is probably better to settle for a subtotal removal and radiate the lesion. Early results with proton beam irradiation suggest that this modality may be even more useful.—Robert M. Crowell, M.D.

Phosphorus-32 Therapy of Cystic Grade IV Astrocytomas: Technique and Preliminary Application

Vicente Taasan, Brahm Shapiro, James A. Taren, William H. Beierwaltes, Paul McKeever, Richard L. Wahl, James E. Carey, Neil Petry, and Shirley Mallette (Univ. of Michigan)

J. Nucl. Med. 26:1335–1338, November 1985   20–2

Intracavitary radiophosphorus instillation is a means of delivering relatively large doses of radiation to a focal brain region. Eleven intracavitary ^{32}P treatments were given to six patients with cystic brain tumors, including three with craniopharyngioma, two with grade IV astrocytoma, and one with grade II astrocytoma. Most instillations were done stereotactically. The desired dose to the target cyst wall was 20,000 rads. Cyst volumes ranged from 2 to 44 ml, and actual delivered doses of ^{32}P ranged from 0.11 to 2.5 mCi.

Cyst instillation was successful in all cases, by use of either stereotactic methods or an indwelling catheter. No leakage of activity outside the target cyst was observed. Bremsstrahlung scanning of the upper abdomen was negative for reticuloendothelial system activity. No anemia, leukopenia, or thrombocytopenia resulted. Cyst fluid aspiration was necessary less often in the patients with craniopharyngioma. Both cyst size and the frequency of aspiration were reduced in the patients with grade IV astrocytoma.

Stereotactic instillation of ^{32}P chromic phosphate is a potentially useful means of delivering large tumoricidal doses of radiation to cystic brain tumors, with minimal risk. The rate of cyst fluid reaccumulation can be reduced and cyst size decreased. Normal brain tissue is spared from damaging radiation.

▶ The authors present encouraging results after instillation of ^{32}P in cystic astrocytomas and craniopharyngiomas. Complications of the stereotaxic procedure were negligible. Further data are needed to establish the indications for application of this promising modality (see Digest 20–3).—Robert M. Crowell, M.D.

Stereotactic Treatment for Expanding Cysts of Craniopharyngiomas by Endocavitary Beta Irradiation
A. Musolino, C. Munari, S. Blond, O. Betti, Y. Lajat, C. Schaub, S. Askienazy, and J. P. Chodkiewicz (Centre Hospitalier Sainte-Anne and Institut National de la Santé et de la Recherche Médicale, Paris; Centre Hospitalier Régional, Nantes, France; and Institutos Medicos Antartida, Buenos Aires)
Neurochirurgie 31:169–178, 1985   20–3

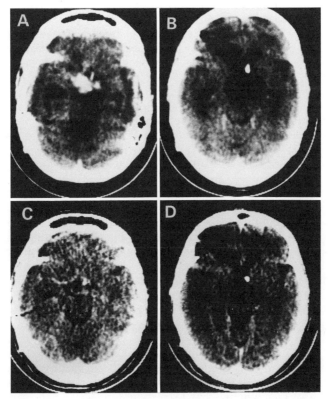

Fig 20–1.—Solid and cystic craniopharyngioma in a 32-year-old woman. **A** and **B**, before cavitary irradiation. **C** and **D**, 15 months after intracystic injection of collodial [198] Au (15 mCi; 10,000 rads). There is disappearance of solid tumor and partial shrinkage of cyst. (Courtesy of Musolino, A., et al.: Neurochirurgie 31:169–178, 1985.)

Eighteen cystic craniopharyngiomas were treated in 16 patients between January 1975 and July 1982 by endocavitary injection of radioactive pharmaceuticals. Colloidal [186]Re was used for 17 injections. Two were made with colloidal [198]Au, and one was made with colloidal [90]Y.

Follow-up for a mean of 3 years showed that all lesions were effectively treated. The formerly expansive cysts were shrunken (Fig 20–1), and obliteration was achieved in three fourths of the cases. Formation of fluid ceased. There were no early or late side effects. Late reexpansion of 1 lesion after 11 months was effectively treated by a second injection. Colloid isotope leaked into the spaces of the cerebrospinal fluid in 18% of injections, but no clinical sequelae were noted.

Cystic craniopharyngiomas have consistently been effectively treated by intracystic injection of a β-emitting radionuclide in colloidal form. A wall dose of 30,000 rads is safest; the dose should not exceed 40,000 rads.

▶ The results of endocavitary β irradiation in craniopharyngiomas of cystic type are striking. It is important to note that the technique is not without complications, however: a unit in Stockholm has reported one case of blindness, evidently due to layering of the colloidal suspension of [32]P. Barbotage performed up to eight times probably can effect mixing to the point of avoiding such layering. Direct injection into a catheter placed within the cyst obviates the difficulties of dose calculation when one uses an Ommaya device, with its relatively large volume and difficulty of dosage calculation.—Robert M. Crowell, M.D.

Interstitial Irradiation of Skull Base Tumors
Mark Bernstein and Philip H. Gutin (Univ. of Toronto and Univ. of California at San Francisco)
Can. J. Neurol. Sci. 12:366–370, November 1985   20–4

Some extra-arachnoidal, histologically low-grade neoplasms cannot be totally removed grossly, and adjuvant irradiation may prevent or delay recurrent disease in these cases. The relative radioresistance of slow-growing, mitotically inactive tumors necessitates high tumor radiation doses to obtain maximum benefit, but brain tolerance of radiation must be considered.

The endocrinologic results of local radiation of pituitary adenomas with various isotopes such as ^{90}Y have been encouraging, especially in acromegaly. Visual impairment has lessened after brachytherapy. Stereotactic gamma radiosurgery has been used successfully to treat endocrine-inactive adenomas and prolactinomas. Intracystic irradiation is an effective and relatively safe means of controlling craniopharyngioma cysts, especially if symptoms recur after conventional external beam therapy. Solid tumors have been treated with radioactive implants. Experience with interstitial irradiation of meningiomas has been quite limited, and the same is true of chordoma. Radioactive implants have given encouraging results in cases of acoustic schwannoma, but significant cranial nerve complications may occur.

Interstitial brachytherapy provides an improved therapeutic ratio between tumor and normal brain tissue. It may be most useful for treating invasive, aggressive adenomas that recur after surgery and external beam teletherapy. Intracystic isotope therapy can control recurrent craniopharyngioma cysts. Damage to normal tissues in the skull base has limited the use of interstitial irradiation in treating basal meningiomas and chordomas.

▶ In the age of widespread use of computed tomography (CT) scanners, patients with little or no neurologic deficit frequently present with evidence of substantial benign intracranial neoplasms. Often such lesions may pose substantial risk for total removal, even in the age of microsurgery and lasers. In this setting, there is little hurry for treatment, and were an effective nonsurgical therapy available it would become quite popular. High-intensity radiation may be such a modality. Such dosage may be delivered by interstitial radiotherapy or externally by the penetration of heavy particle (proton) beam therapy. Further experience will be needed to establish indications for utilization of these special radiation strategies. It seems likely that a marriage of surgical and radiation techniques will prove even more useful than at present. The close collaboration of the neurosurgeon with the radiation medicine specialist is obviously crucial.—Robert M. Crowell, M.D.

New Technique for Removable Implantation of Radionuclides in Central Nervous System Neoplasm by Ultrasonic Guidance

Yutaka Tsutsumi, Yukihiko Andoh, Masao Matsutani, and Akio Asai (Teishin and Komagome Metropolitan Hosps., Tokyo)
Surg. Neurol. 23:520–524, November 1985   20–5

A technique has been devised for inserting removable tubes into a brain tumor under real-time ultrasonic B mode guidance as a preliminary to interstitial brachytherapy. Observation of tube insertion in real time permits free selection of tube-positioning sites for insertion into the tumor. The length of tube that remains within the tumor mass is readily measured during the procedure. The procedure can be carried out in the operating room. A craniotomy 4 cm in diameter is used. The tubes are arranged in parallel for proper dose distribution. A trocar 3 mm in diameter is inserted to provide a route for the silicon tubing. The transducer is fixed on the dura to monitor tube insertion.

Woman, 52 years old, was seen 7 months after nearly total removal of a glioblastoma multiforme of the left temporal lobe. A mass had appeared on computed tomography at the head of the right caudate nucleus. Three silicon tubes were inserted into the tumor as shown in Figure 20–2. Computed tomography performed on the next day confirmed correct tube placement. A biopsy confirmed glioblastoma multiforme. Seeds of ^{192}Ir were introduced 6 days after the tube placement. Isodose curves indicated a satisfactory dose distribution.

Interstitial brachytherapy avoids radioactive effects on normal tissues while massively treating the tumor bulk. Tube placement is reliably carried out under ultrasonic real-time guidance. Image resolution is suboptimal

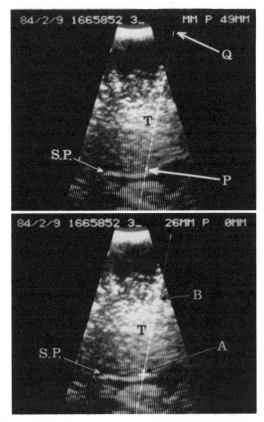

Fig 20–2.—Epidural real-time sonograms just before insertion of the silicon tube. **Top,** the length from the dural level to the deepest surface of the tumor as measured on the puncture guideline. Point Q denotes the level of duramater, whereas point P indicates that the luminous point as measuring mark stays at intersection of the deepest surface of the tumor echo and puncture guideline. The length between these two points is indicated as 49 mm at upper right corner. **Bottom,** the length of that portion of puncture guideline that penetrates the tumor. Large and small white crosses are placed at the intersections of the tumor echo border and the puncture guideline, and the length (26 mm) between them is displayed at upper right corner. T, tumor; and S.P., echo of septum pellucidum. (Courtesy of Tsutsumi, Y., et al.: Surg. Neurol. 23:520–524, November 1985. Reprinted by permission of the publisher, Copyright 1985, Elsevier Science Publishing Co., Inc.)

at deeper levels of observation with present equipment. A single burr hole is insufficient; a small craniotomy is necessary.

Early Results of Ion Beam Radiation Therapy for Sacral Chordoma: A Northern California Oncology Group Study

William M. Saunders, Joseph R. Castro, George T. Y. Chen, Philip H. Gutin, J. Michael Collier, Sandra R. Zink, Theodore L. Phillips, and Grant E. Gauger (Univ. of California at San Francisco and Berkely and Northern California Oncology Group, Palo Alto)

J. Neurosurg. 64:243–247, February 1986   20–6

RESULTS OF TREATMENT OF SACRAL CHORDOMAS

Case No.	Type of Surgery*	Current Status	Survival Time (mos)
1	partial	no evidence of primary tumor, but distant metastasis	88
2	biopsy	died from persistent tumor	22
3	total	no evidence of tumor	63
4	biopsy	tumor shrinking	47
5	biopsy	stable	19
6	total	no evidence of tumor	12
7	total	no evidence of tumor	6
8	partial	stable	6

*Total: removal of all gross tumor, microscopic tumor left or suspected; partial: debulking of tumor, gross tumor left; biopsy: biopsy only, with no attempt at tumor debulking.
(Courtesy of Saunders, W.M., et al.: J. Neurosurg. 64:243–247, February 1986.)

Chordomas are malignant neoplasms arising from remnants of the embryonal notochord; they can metastasize. A pilot study of helium and neon ion beam therapy was undertaken in eight patients with sacral chordoma who were seen between 1977 and 1984. The six men and two women (mean age at presentation, 60 years) were administered daily doses of 2.0–2.25 "Gray Equivalent" (GyE). Four patients were initially treated conventionally.

The results on follow-up for an average of 33 months are given in the table. Only one patient had had a local recurrence of tumor and died of the disease 22 months after radiotherapy. Another patient with control of the primary tumor is doing well after resection and irradiation of a mandibular metastasis. Three other patients had gross total excision of disease. No serious complications occurred. Total tumor doses ranged from 70 to 80.5 GyE.

Ion therapy beams have been used to deliver safely potentially curative doses of radiation to chordomas in the skull base, spine, and sacral regions. Radiation doses higher than those usually given have been administered. Seven of eight patients have had no sign of tumor progression during a short follow-up.

▶ Heavy particle therapy (with protons, helium, or neon ions) seems particularly attractive for lesions in or near the CNS. A very large dose of ionizing radiation can be focused quite precisely with very little radiation to nearby neural structures. Kjellberg has reported the safety and probable effectiveness of such treatment for brain arteriovenous malformations (AVMs) (*N. Engl. J. Med.* 309:269–273, 1983). Hosobuchi and colleagues recently presented similar data on AVMs but observed occasional complications related to thrombosis or radiation necrosis (American Association of Neurological Surgeons meeting, Denver, April 13–17, 1986).

Heavy particle therapy can also be used for tumors, as indicated in the present report from the University of California. In a small series of sacral chordomas, safety is evident; however, the follow-up is short, precluding meaningful comment on effectiveness. Although the authors used fractionated therapy, which is routine in orthovoltage radiation therapy, there is a theoretical reason to expect that data will indicate that one-shot treatment causes similar biologic effects and avoids problems of uneven dosage.

It seems highly likely that a combination of radical subtotal resection for decompression and heavy particle therapy for long-term control will become a mainstay in the management of sacral chordoma and other lesions in or near CNS, which are difficult to resect with low morbidity.—Robert M. Crowell, M.D.

Other Tumor Adjuncts

Stereotactic Surgery For Mass Lesions of the Midbrain and Pons
Robert J. Coffey and L. Dade Lunsford (Univ. of Pittsburgh and Univ. of Florida)
Neurosurgery 17:12–18, July 1985   20–7

Stereotactic biopsy of deep supratentorial lesions guided by computed tomography (CT) is an established approach. The same method holds promise for evaluating mass lesions of the midbrain and pons, where open operative approaches are a major undertaking. A transparenchymal trajectory to the midbrain and rostral pons via a frontal approach, and to the caudal lateral pons via a suboccipital transcerebellar approach, provide ready access while avoiding major vessels and cranial nerves. Twelve patients with mass lesions in these regions underwent CT-guided stereotactic surgery between 1982 and 1984. All patients preoperatively had contrast-enhanced CT and 6 had cerebral angiography. General anesthesia was

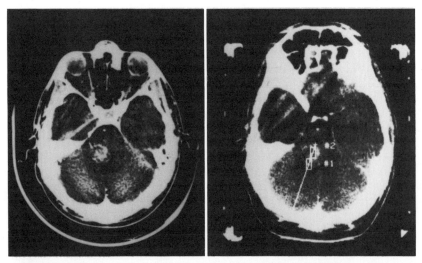

Fig 20–3.—**Left,** preoperative intravenous contrast-enhanced CT scan demonstrates a mass in the right lateral pons and the middle cerebellar peduncle. **Right,** intraoperative stereotactic CT scan demonstrates the target selected for aspiration and biopsy *(plus marks)*. The probe trajectory is indicated, as are two spiral biopsy sites within the lesion, which proved to be apontine hematoma. (Courtesy of Coffey, R.J., and Lunsford, L.D.: Neurosurgery 17:12–18, July 1985.)

used in 3 patients with lateral pontine biopsy targets near the middle cerebellar peduncle.

Adequate specimens were obtained in all cases. Treatment included ventriculostomy placement in 2 patients, cyst aspiration in 2, removal of hematoma in 2, and removal of necrotic tumor in 3. No neurologic deficit resulted from the procedures. Six patients experienced improvement after removal of fluid from cystic lesions. All 5 patients with non-neoplastic diagnoses and 2 with metastatic cancer were well at follow-up examination 6–20 months later. The CT findings in a patient having a transcerebellar procedure are shown in Figure 20–3.

Accurate histologic diagnosis altered the course of management in half of these cases. No neurologic deficit or death resulted from CT-guided stereotactic surgery. Treatment was possible in cases of hematoma or other cystic lesions that were amenable to aspiration or drainage. This approach is potentially the safest and most reliable means of diagnosing and treating lesions in the mesencephalon and pons.

▶ Biopsy material is needed for optimum planning of management of brain tumors. Now such biopsy is possible even within the pontomesencephalic area, as demonstrated in this trail-blazing report by Coffey and Lunsford. Similar results have been reported by Apuzzo, using an entry point 2 cm posterior to the coronal suture for target points in the pontomesencephalic region. Such procedures can be done with local anesthesia. Use of ventriculostomy for tumors in this region should be considered because of the possibility of biopsy-induced hydrocephalus.

Stereotaxic surgery has reached the point where it may be recommended for biopsy of even the deepest brain lesions.—Robert M. Crowell, M.D.

Computer-Assisted Stereotaxic Laser Resection of Intra-Axial Brain Neoplasms

Patrick J. Kelly, Bruce A. Kall, Stephan Goerss, and Franklin Earnest IV (Mayo Clinic)

J. Neurosurg. 64:427–439, March 1986   20–8

Deep-seated subcortical intra-axial tumors present special problems to the neurosurgeon who is attempting to preserve neurologic function while removing the tumor. A computer-interactive stereotaxic system (Fig 20–4) has been developed to transpose a tumor volume in stereotaxic space. A stereotaxically directed, computer-monitored CO_2 laser is then used to vaporize the volume as the surgeon monitors the position of a cursor representing the laser beam against planar contours of the tumor displayed on a monitor in the operating room. The tumor is approached through a cranial trephination and circumferential dural opening and vaporized slice by slice with the use of 65–85 W of defocused laser power in continuous mode.

Seventy-eight patients (45 male and 33 female, aged 2–76 years) underwent 83 computer-assisted stereotaxic laser resections of subcortical

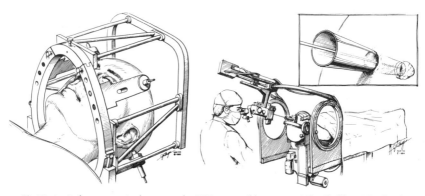

Fig 20–4.—Left, computerized tomography (CT)-compatible stereotaxic headholder with a localization system that consists of nine rods arranged in the shape of the letter "N" located bilaterally and anteriorly. This produces nine reference marks on each CT slice from which the position and orientation of the slice in stereotaxic space may be determined. **Right,** computer-interactive stereotaxic 400-mm arc-quadrant that directs the operating microscope and laser beam to the target point. A small internal arc-quadrant holds a stereotaxic retractor (inset). (Courtesy of Kelly, P.J., et al.: J. Neurosurg. 64:427–439, March 1986.)

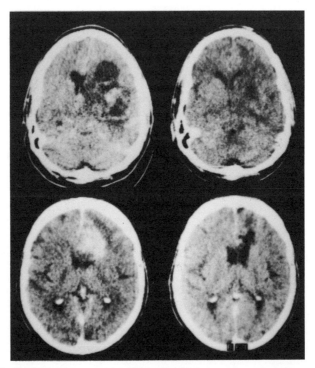

Fig 20–5.—Pre (left) and postoperative **(right)** CT scans in 2 patients with grade III astrocytomas. (Courtesy of Kelly, P.J., et al.: J. Neurosurg. 64:427–439, March 1986.)

intra-axial lesions between 1980 and 1985. Fifty-one lesions were located deep and centrally in the hemispheres. Glioblastomas, grades II and III astrocytomas, and metastatic tumors were most frequent. Neurologic examination 1 week after the 83 procedures revealed that 48 patients improved from their preoperative level, whereas 23 were unchanged. After surgery 12 patients had an increased neurologic deficit, 3 of whom died, 1 from brain stem edema, 1 from infection, and 1 from pulmonary emboli. Patients with glioblastoma survived for an average of 38 weeks. Patients with lower-grade circumscribed astrocytomas did better in terms of morbidity and completeness of resection than those with infiltrative neoplasms (Fig 20–5).

Computer-assisted stereotaxic laser microsurgery is an effective approach to intracranial intra-axial lesions in subcortical locations, especially circumscribed deep-seated lesions. Although there is no appreciable prolongation of survival times in patients with glioblastomas treated by the stereotaxic method in comparison with those operated on with the use of conventional techniques, survival rates remained the same for patients with lesions in locations previously associated with poorer survival when treated by conventional techniques.

▶ Kelly and colleagues present a dazzling, high-tech approach to deep brain neoplasms. The fusion of microsurgery, stereotaxis, computed tomography, and laser appears relatively safe and effective in the vaporizing of deep lesions. Nonetheless, survival results so far are no different than those with conventional treatment modalities. The approach is promising, especially in relation to adjunctive therapies, but more data will be needed to establish a role for this type of surgery.—Robert M. Crowell, M.D.

Time Course and Spatial Distribution of Neodymium:Yttrium-Aluminum-Garnet (Nd:YAG) Laser-Induced Lesions in the Rat Brain

Hans R. Eggert, Marika Kiessling, and Paul Kleihues (Univ. of Freiburg, Federal Republic of Germany)
Neurosurgery 16:443–448, April 1985   20–9

The deep coagulation necrosis produced by the Nd:YAG laser should be useful in the shrinking of brain tumors and the coagulating of vessels. The effects of Nd:YAG laser irradiation were examined in adult Wistar rats. A constant energy density of 461 joules per sq cm was used to irradiate the brains of 28 rats, and the brains were examined after intervals of 30 minutes to 80 days. In a second series, 84 rats were allowed to survive 48 hours after irradiation with 231–3,077 joules per sq cm.

An area of edema containing thrombosed vessels resulted from irradiation at energy levels of more than 30 joules. Central coagulation necrosis was surrounded by a zone of delayed colliquation necrosis and in turn by perifocal edema (Fig 20–6). Eventually the cortical defect became covered by a pial membrane. Perifocal edema in the hemispheric white matter

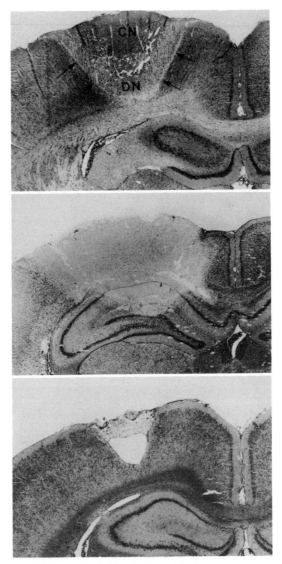

Fig 20–6.—**Top,** at 30 minutes after irradiation (30 joules), the central coagulation necrosis (CN) is surrounded by a zone of delayed colliquation necrosis (DN) and a small rim of perifocal edema *(arrows)*. **Center,** at 48 hours (100 joules), the entire lesion is necrobiotic, with marked perifocal edema spreading into the white matter, including the corpus callosum. **Bottom,** after 80 days (30 joules), the necrotic tissue has been absorbed, and the defect is covered by a pial membrane containing macrophages. (Courtesy of Eggert, H.R., et al.: Neurosurgery 16:443–448, April 1985.)

resolved within 5 days after irradiation. Lesion size varied with the level of applied energy, but lesion depth varied less than the diameter at the brain surface. Relatively narrow, deep lesions were seen at low energy levels and comparatively shallow, wide lesions at high energy levels.

Irradiation of rat brain with the Nd:YAG laser can serve as a model of defined brain lesions in studies of brain edema and other postinjury changes. Accidental exposure of normal brain tissue during laser coagulation of a tumor or of blood vessels apparently produces lesions of a size that may be acceptable in most brain regions.

▶ As Michael Edwards states in a comment that follows the article, the Nd:YAG laser is taking its place in neurologic surgery, primarily in the treatment of vascular tumors that cannot be embolized preoperatively, but not for "eloquent brain," because of the depth of penetration and injury.—Robert M. Crowell, M.D.

Microwave Hyperthermia for Brain Tumors

Arthur Winter, Joy Laing, Robert Paglione, and Fred Sterzer (Hosp. Ctr. at Orange and RCA Labs., Princeton, N.J.)
Neurosurgery 17:387–399, September 1985   20–10

Localized thermotherapy is being increasingly used to treat solid malignant tumors. Malignant brain tumors may be especially suitable, since they do not metastasize, and conventional methods generally have produced discouraging results. Twelve patients whose conditions failed to respond to standard treatments received thermotherapy. Hyperthermia of about 43 C was induced using microwaves at a frequency of 2450 MHz that were guided into the tumor by one or more semirigid coaxial applicators

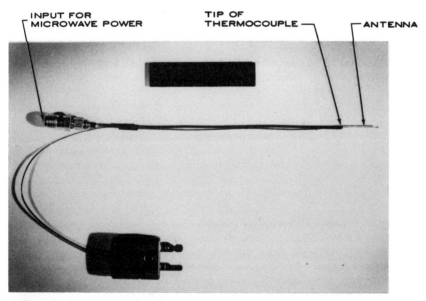

Fig 20–7.—Miniature coaxial applicator with integral thermocouple. (Courtesy of Winter, A., et al.: Neurosurgery 17:387–399, September 1985.)

within 16-gauge tubes or needles (Fig 20–7). Heating patterns first were examined in phantom materials and in dogs. The clinical tumors were treated for 1 hour on several occasions, a few days apart.

Intractable headache was relieved in five patients, and recurrent headaches were less severe and required less medication. Neurologic function improved in five of the 12 patients, speech in 2, and 2 others had less confusion than before. No adverse effects were observed with repeated microwave thermotherapy. Objective tumor responses were seen in three fourths of the cases, and the same proportion of patients benefited clinically. The microwave power needed to heat for a given time or a given volume declined during the course of treatment.

Microwave thermotherapy is a promising means of treating malignant brain tumors, either alone or in conjunction with radiotherapy and chemotherapy. Trials in patients with less advanced disease are warranted. Improvements are needed in the equipment used. Applicators that can be left in place for several months and receive external microwave energy noninvasively would be useful, as would sensory devices for measuring brain temperatures without damage to healthy tissues.

▶ This report indicates the feasibility and safety of using microwave-induced hypothermia in patients with brain tumors through multiple antennas during multiple treatment sessions. Utilization of temperature monitoring in nearby sites would be helpful. Despite drawbacks, the report indicates a potentially fruitful area of clinical research for tumors without proven effective therapy.

A phase-1 trial of thermochemotherapy for brain malignancy has yielded encouraging results and phase 2 trials are warranted (Silberman et al.: *Cancer* 56:48–56, 1985).—Robert M. Crowell, M.D.

Vascular Techniques

Mechanical and Metallurgical Properties of Carotid Artery Clamps
Manuel Dujovny, Nir Kossovsky, Ram Kossowsky, Ricardo Segal, Fernando G. Diaz, Howard Kaufman, Alfred Perlin, and Eugene E. Cook (Henry Ford Hosp., Detroit, and other American hospitals; Westinghouse Electric Corp., Pittsburgh; Metatech Corp., Skokie, Ill.; and West Virginia Univ.)
Neurosurgery 17:760–767, November 1985   20–11

Carotid artery occlusion is widely used in conjunction with extracranial-intracranial vascular bypass surgery for giant aneurysms. The mechanical, metallurgic, and biocompatibility properties of seven carotid artery clamps were evaluated. They included three Selverstone and two Salibi clamps, a Crutchfield clamp, and a Kindt clamp.

None of the clamps showed evidence of pressure plate retreat. The Crutchfield clamp, the only one made from an ASTM-ANSI-approved implantable stainless steel, was the only one with clean surfaces free from debris. Machining and surface debris consisting of aluminum, silicon, and sulfur was abundant on the Selverstone and Salibi clamps. The Salibi and Kindt clamps were sensitive to magnetic flux. The Crutchfield clamp ex-

PASSIVATION-REACTIVATION TEST; PITTING POTENTIAL TEST

Clamp Type	Free Oxidation Potential (mV)	Pitting Potential (mV)	Potential Difference (mV)	Corrosion	Pitting by SEM	Ferromagnetic Sensitivity
Crutchfield	−300	+310	610	0	0	Negative
Selverstone (Codman #19-1000) (all 304 ss)	−330	+200	530	2+	2+	Negative
Selverstone (access plate (403 ss) and frame)	−585	−75	510	1+	2+	Negative
				4+	4+	Plate is ferromagnetic
Selverstone (Codman #19-1003) (100% 304 ss)	−270	+445	715	3+	3+	Negative
Salibi (304 ss) (pressure plate from 1% Cr, 1% Mn steel)	−725	−525	200	2+	2+	Negative
Salibi (Codman)				4+	4+	Plate is ferromagnetic
Kindt (301 ss)	−160	+317	477	2+	2+	Ferromagnetic

(Courtesy of Dujovny, M., et al.: Neurosurgery 17:760–767, November 1985.)

hibited good corrosion resistance in the pitting potential test (table). No corrosion or pitting was seen on scanning electron microscopic (SEM) examination. The Selverstone clamp had lower pitting potentials and showed varying degrees of corrosion and surface pitting on SEM examination. The Salibi pressure plate had a low pitting potential and showed severe corrosion.

Only the Crutchfield clamp, among those evaluated, is suitable for long-term implantation on metallurgical criteria. Surgeons should insist on detailed information about the metallurgic aspects of devices and on the production of devices from biocompatible materials.

▶ A number of years ago, McFadden (*J. Neurosurg.* 36:598–603, 1972) pointed out that the metallurgic properties of implanted vascular clips deserved careful attention to avoid delayed complications. The present report focuses attention on the metallurgy of implanted cervical carotid clamps. Data are presented indicating metallurgic problems with several of the available clamps. The only readily available clamp to pass the authors' criteria was the Crutchfield clamp. This information will be useful to neurosurgeons who implant such devices. The exact relation between the described criteria and the occurrence of delayed complications is yet unknown. However, the potential relation will not be lost on those who are interested in medical-legal problems.

From the same laboratory, an important study of aneurysm clip motion during magnetic resonance imaging (MRI) has been reported (*Neurosurgery* 17:543–548, 1985). Yasargil, Sugita, Heifetz Elgiloy, and Vari-Angle McFadden clips do not deflect. Mayfield, Heifetz, Vari-Angle, Pivot, and Sundt-Kees Multi-Angle clips deflect or slip off aneurysms. Thus, this latter group should be avoided if MRI is to be used.

The Joint Committee on Devices and Drugs of the AANS and CNS develops standards for such devices that should be known to neurosurgeons who use these instruments. Only by careful attention to the design and monitoring of such devices can neurosurgeons expect to offer their patients optimum care.

This is just another area in which practicing neurosurgeons must continue to maintain their education.—Robert M. Crowell, M.D.

"Pre" Subclavian Steal Syndromes and Their Treatment by Angioplasty: Hemodynamic Classification of Subclavian Artery Stenoses
J. Theron, D. Melançon, and R. Ethier (Montreal Neurological Hosp.)
Neuroradiology 27:265–270, May 1985   20–12

Four patients with early modification of vertebral artery flow due to subclavian artery stenosis were successfully managed by subclavian artery angioplasty. A femoral approach was utilized, with an 8F or 9F catheter. No complications occurred. Heparin was not used, but patients received 600 mg of acetylsalicylic acid on alternate days for 1 week before the procedure.

Man, 65 years old, had had weakness of the left arm for several months that recently had become worse. The left radial pulse was very weak. The blood pressure was 120/70 mm Hg on the left and 150/90 mm Hg on the right. Digital arch angiography showed moderate stenosis of the right internal carotid artery and marked narrowing of the left subclavian artery. Good early filling of the left vertebral artery was noted. Conventional angiography confirmed the location of subclavian stenosis distal to the origin of the left vertebral artery. The subclavian artery was of normal caliber after angioplasty with an 8F catheter, and a good left radial pulse was present. The left arm was normally strong.

The "pre" subclavian steal syndromes are classified as follows: type I, stenosis proximal to the vertebral artery origin with interruption of flow only on head extension and rotation to the opposite side; type II, stenosis with stagnation of flow and lack of visualization of the vertebral artery on angiography; type III, the classic subclavian steal syndrome; type IV, stenosis distal to the vertebral artery origin. Angioplasty of the subclavian artery can effectively restore blood flow in the vertebral artery only in the first three groups of cases.

▶ Results of percutaneous angioplasty for prevertebral subclavian stenosis are excellent. Application of this approach to innominate stenosis can probably also produce satisfactory results. It behooves the neurosurgeon to keep abreast of these developments to recommend the appropriate treatment for patients with cerebrovascular occlusive disease.

Balloon dilatation of fibromuscular dysplasia in the internal carotid artery has been performed by open techniques successfully in two patients (Welch et al.: *N.Y. State J. Med.* 85:115–117, March 1985).—Robert M. Crowell, M.D.

Closure of Carotid-Cavernous Fistulas by Use of a Fibrin Adhesive System
Hiroshi Hasegawa, Shoji Bitoh, Jiro Obashi, and Motohiko Maruno (Osaka Koseinenkin Hosp., Japan)
Surg. Neurol. 24:23–26, July 1985   20–13

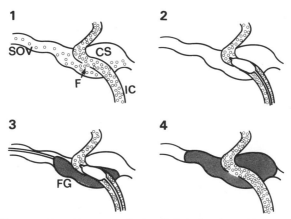

Fig 20–8.—Treatment of carotid-cavernous fistula with fibrin glue. **1,** carotid-cavernous fistula, direct type. IC, internal carotid artery; CS, cavernous sinus; SOV, superior ophthalmic vein; and F, fistula. **2,** nondetachable balloon is placed in the cavernous portion of the internal carotid artery to close fistula temporarily. **3,** fibrin glue (FG) is injected into cavernous sinus through a catheter in the superior ophthalmic vein. **4,** both balloon and intravenous catheter are removed, and fistula is closed with preservation of the carotid flow. (Courtesy of Hasegawa, H., et al.: Surg. Neurol. 24:23–26, July 1985. Reprinted by permission of the publisher, Copyright 1985, Elsevier Science Publishing Co., Inc.)

Injection of fibrin glue into the cavernous sinus through the dilated superior ophthalmic vein provides a new approach to the treatment of carotid-cavernous fistulas. The adhesive system consists of highly concentrated fibrinogen containing factor XIII, fibrin-stabilizing factor, and a solution of thrombin, calcium chloride, and aprotinin.

Woman, 24 years old, had severe proptosis and conjunctival injection in the left eye, which had been present for 3 months. A bruit was heard over the left retromastoid region, and carotid angiography showed a direct communication between the internal carotid artery and the cavernous sinus. An attempt to close the fistula with a polyurethane foam embolus failed, and the left internal carotid artery was ligated. The patient's condition improved, but she was worse 2½ years later, when a left carotid-cavernous fistula was documented, with the external carotid contributing to it. Placement of a copper wire into the cavernous sinus via the dilated superior ophthalmic vein did not reduce arterial flow in the vein, but injection of 6 ml of fibrin glue completely occluded the vein. Abnormal signs resolved within 3 months, and angiography confirmed complete occlusion of the fistula. Symptoms were still absent 6 months after the operation.

Fibrin adhesive solution is viscous and remains within a narrow channel, and it can mold itself to fit snugly in a complicated structure such as the cavernous sinus. Reflux of glue can be prevented by temporarily closing the fistula with an intra-arterial balloon when the glue is injected into the cavernous sinus (Fig 20–8). Further experience is needed for the effective and safe use of fibrin glue to close carotid-cavernous fistulas.

▶ The use of fibrin adhesive for the obliteration of carotid cavernous fistula appears to introduce a promising new adhesive into vascular neurosurgery. Attractive handling properties are described. Since it can be prepared from the patient's own blood products, the possibility of viral infection from other patients can thereby be precluded. It is possible that this material could be useful in the obliteration of arteriovenous malformations and aneurysms, hopefully by a percutaneous transvascular approach. In addition, this material has been utilized to close dural cerebrospinal fluid leaks even in such a confined space as a transoral exposure.—Robert M. Crowell, M.D.

Other Techniques

Percutaneous Lumbar Diskectomy Using a New Aspiration Probe

Gary Onik, Clyde A. Helms, Leonard Ginsburg, Franklin T. Hoaglund, and James Morris (Univ. of California at San Francisco and Medical Instrument Development Labs., Inc., San Leandro, Calif.)

AJR 144:1137–1140, June 1985   20–14

Percutaneous lumbar diskectomy is a relatively noninvasive alternative

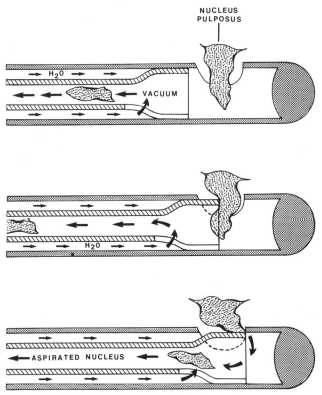

Fig 20–9.—Nucleotome aspiration probe. Diagram of distal end of needle in longitudinal section. Cutting sleeve within needle slices off any material sucked into port. Water for irrigation flows around cutting sleeve and is aspirated with disk material into center of hollow sleeve. (Courtesy of Onik, G., et al.: AJR 144:1137–1140, June 1985. Copyright 1985, by the American Roentgen Ray Society.)

to enzymatic disk decompression, but previous methods have involved large cannulas. A new, automated disk aspiration probe has been developed for percutaneous use. Its 2-mm diameter minimizes the risk of nerve root injury, and its automated action permits rapid removal of disk material. A trocar and a 2.5-mm cannula are inserted under fluoroscopic control. After a 22-gauge needle is inserted to the center of the disk, a hole is cut in the anulus with a 2-mm circular saw, and the Nucleotome probe (Fig 20–9) is inserted into the disk space and moved back and forth during section.

This method achieves disk decompression mechanically, avoiding anaphylaxis. A peripheral nerve could be injured, but the procedure is done with local anesthesia so that radicular pain can be reported. The device is designed so that it cannot leave the disk space; its tip cannot be inadvertently pushed through the anulus. No end point for the procedure has been standardized, but it seems best not to remove more disk than is necessary.

This procedure will be used only in patients whose chief symptom is sciatica and who have physical and computed tomographic findings consistent with disk herniation. At present it is limited to the L4-L5 level, but it should be possible to use curved cannulas to approach the L5-S1 level. Percutaneous lumbar diskectomy is a useful alternative to chymopapain injection and/or surgery in selected patients with herniated lumbar disk.

▶ Maroon, at the meeting of the Interurban Neurosurgical Society (Chicago, February 1986), presented clinical data from the application of this technique in approximately 50 patients. Up to 10 gm of disk were removed, and in general the clinical results were quite encouraging without major complications. A multicenter control study is now underway. Until reliable data are available, this method remains in the investigational phase.—Robert M. Crowell, M.D.

Pedicled Myocutaneous Flap or Latissimus Dorsi Muscle for Reconstruction of Anterior and Middle Skull Defects: An Alternative
Brooke R. Seckel, Joseph Upton, Stephen R. Freidberg, Kenneth P. Gilbert, and Joseph E. Murray (Lahey Clinic, Burlington, Mass., and Brigham and Women's Hosp. and Boston Univ.)
Head Neck Surg. 8:165–168, January–February 1986   20–15

Full-thickness defects of the anterior and middle parts of the skull after cancer resection present difficult problems in reconstruction. Free microsurgical transplantation of a flap is presently recommended when local flaps are not adequate. A pedicled myocutaneous flap of latissimus dorsi muscle, tunneled subpectorally, was used successfully to reconstruct large defects of the frontal, parietal, and temporal skull areas in 3 patients.

TECHNIQUE.—The defect is measured after resection of disease and confirmation of a clear margin. The initial incision is made from the axilla along the free border of the latissimus dorsi, and the muscle is elevated distally to proximally under

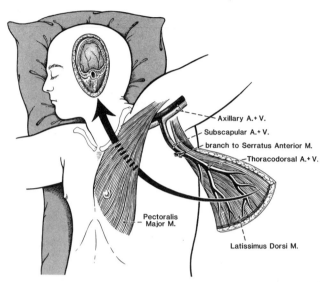

Fig 20–10.—Elevation and subpectoral course of the pedicled latissimus dorsi muscle flap. In some patients, the middle portion of the clavicle is removed. The flap may also be tunneled beneath the skin anterior to the clavicle. (Courtesy of Seckel, B.R., et al.: Head Neck Surg. 8:165–168, Jan.-Feb. 1986. Copyright © 1986. Reprinted by permission of John Wiley and Sons, Inc.)

direct vision. A distal myocutaneous flap then is elevated, and the proximal pedicle is dissected in order to rotate the flap superoanteriorly (Fig 20–10). A large subpectoral pocket is made, and the flap is tunneled beneath the pectoralis major muscle through the pocket into the skull defect (Fig 20–11). The neck flaps are

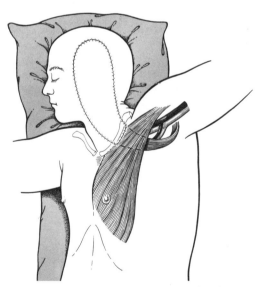

Fig 20–11.—Flap in place. (Courtesy of Seckel, B.R., et al.: Head Neck Surg. 8:165–168, Jan.-Feb. 1986. Copyright © 1986. Reprinted by permission of John Wiley and Sons, Inc.)

then closed over the pedicle, and the flap is sutured in place. The donor defect is covered with a split-thickness skin graft.

A 10 × 20-cm skin island flap reliably reaches the anterolateral skull surface up to 4–6 cm from the midline of the vertex. One patient had a 2-cm loss of the distal portion of the flap because of inadvertent surgical damage. Any excised dura should be replaced meticulously with a fascia lata graft. The present patients have lived 2–6 years after operation. One of them received irradiation after surgery.

► When there is a large scalp defect, the plastic surgeon can be a helpful resource. Often a rotation flap from the head and neck can be utilized. Sometimes a free flap with vascular pedicle can be used if there is a suitable scalp artery for anastomosis. When these established methods are unsuitable, the pedicled myocutaneous flap described in this article may be the best choice.— Robert M. Crowell, M.D.

Modified Halo Frame to Assist Omentum Transfer to the Scalp
M. J. Sandow, R. B. Hamilton, and P. G. Heden (Flinders Med. Centre, Bedford Park, Australia)
Br. J. Plast. Surg. 38:288–291, April 1985   20–16

The halo frame, developed for the management of spinal and facial injuries, was modified for scalp wound management. A patient undergoing replacement of the entire scalp with a free microvascular flap of greater omentum was treated with a modified Royal Berkshire Hospital halo frame with orthopedic external fixation apparatus added. Supporting legs and a transverse stabilizing bar were attached so that the frame could rest on any firm surface and hold the patient's head steady.

Man, 49 years old, was seen with recurrent basal cell cancer of the scalp after intracranial surgery and high-dose radiotherapy for cerebral astrocytoma at age 17 years. The entire scalp showed extensive radiation damage, with several areas of neoplastic damage. Excision of one neoplastic region had led to an area of exposed calvarium with osteomyelitis and dural pus. Irregular cortical thickening was present, and computed tomography showed encephalomalacia but no recurrent tumor. The scalp was excised from the supraorbital region to the occiput. The modified halo frame was applied, and the entire omentum was transferred to the scalp as an island flap. The gastroepiploic vessels were joined to the external carotid artery and external jugular vein. Split-skin grafting was performed next day. The patient was able to lie on the frame, without pressure being placed on the flap, and to walk about. The frame was removed 2 weeks after operation; the flap survived completely.

No known patient has had more of the electively excised scalp covered by a free omental flap. Avoidance of pressure on this sensitive flap is critical. Use of a modified halo frame provides wound access, completely avoids pressure on the flap, and allows patient mobility. The same method could be used in the management of scalp replantation or any occipital reconstruction involving microvascular transfer or even local flaps.

Pneumocephalus: Effects of Patient Position on the Incidence and Location of Aerocele After Posterior Fossa and Upper Cervical Cord Surgery
Thomas J. K. Toung, Robert W. McPherson, H. Ahn, Robert T. Donham, J. Alano, and Donlin Long (Johns Hopkins Med. Insts.)
Anesth. Analg. 65:65–70, January 1986   20–17

Tension pneumocephalus has been reported with increasing frequency after posterior fossa craniotomy; however, the true incidence of pneumocephalus (asymptomatic intracranial air) is unknown. A study was made of 100 consecutive patients, aged 1 month to 76 years, who underwent posterior fossa or intradural cervical cord surgery in the sitting, parkbench, and prone positions during 1983–1985. Supine, anteroposterior, and lateral skull radiographs were obtained 30–120 minutes after surgery.

All 32 patients operated on in the sitting position developed pneumocephalus, with a large amount of air in the frontoparietal subdural region. In 25 of the 32 patients, air was also found in the lateral and third ventricles; in 13, air was noted in the suprasella cistern; and in 4, in the pontine cistern. Twenty-two of the 32 patients had preoperative hydrocephalus, but only 8 had a ventriculoperitoneal shunt or intraoperative drainage procedures. Pneumocephalus developed in 73% of the patients operated on in the park-bench position and in 57% of those treated in the prone position. Both rates were significantly lower than that in the sitting group. Ten percent of patients in the park-bench group and 25% of those in the sitting group had intraventricular air.

Pneumocephalus is frequent after surgery on the posterior fossa or cervical spinal cord, particularly if performed in the sitting position. No single contributing factor can be identified. A large amount of intracranial air can be trapped if surgery is done in the sitting position on a patient with coexisting hydrocephalus.

▶ Postoperative pneumocephalus is clearly related to positioning, occurring in all patients operated on in the sitting position. Since tension pneumocephalus may cause mobidity and even mortality, this is another argument against the sitting position. The authors also note that avoidance of N_2O administration, especially during the final minutes before dural closure, may restrict the frequency and extent of postoperative pneumocephalus.—Robert M. Crowell, M.D.

Notes on Techniques

▶ Workers from M.D. Anderson report on 387 cancer patients treated with Ommaya reservoirs (*Neurology* 35:1274–1278, 1985). Complications included five intracranial hemorrhages, 15 malfunctions, and 15 meningitides; 10 patients had seizures, leukoencephalopathy, or pericatheter necrosis after intraventricular chemotherapy. The Ommaya reservoir enjoys an expanded role in neuro-oncology with recent advances in chemotherapy, according to Machado et al. (*Neurosurgery* 17:600–603, 1985). Indications include drug delivery, drug level monitoring, and tumor cyst drainage. The method is extremely safe, and technical failure tends to occur in the presence of mass lesions.

Yamagami et al. (*Surg. Neurol.* 24:421–427, 1985) report on neodymium-YAG laser application to rat cerebellum. They found 45 W (35.2 W/mm^2) to be safe. They have treated 109 tumor patients with this laser without reported complications.

Reinhardt et al. (*Eur. Surg. Res.* 17:333–340, 1985) report topographic localization of tumor tissue during surgery by use of intravenous ^{32}P and a local semiconduction probe. Further resection was guided by tumor localization.

Porous hydroxyapatite ceramics may be used as prostheses, for example, in anterior cervical fusion (Koyama, T., and Handa, J.: *Surg. Neurol.* 25:71–73, 1986).—Robert M. Crowell, M.D.

21 Tumors

Introduction

Understanding of primary brain tumors has advanced. Jennings and co-workers describe the natural history and pathogenesis of intracranial germ cell tumors in a review of 389 histologically confirmed neoplasms (Digest 21–1). A human medulloblastoma has been established and characterized in tissue culture (Digest 21–2). Bullard and Bigner (Digest 21–3) describe promising applications of monoclonal antibodies for the diagnosis and treatment of primary brain tumors. Radioactive monoclonal antibody has been used to irradiate glioma (Digest 21–4). Kornblith's group describes exciting results with interleukin-2-activated lymphocytes (killer cells) against human glioblastoma in tissue culture (Digest 21–5). Hemoperfusion of regional venous drainage may be used to reduce systemic exposure from interarterial chemotherapy (Digest 21–6). Radioactive agents that normally have little effect on cerebral blood flow have marked effects on flow to brain sarcomas in an animal model (Digest 21–7).

The important problem of cerebral metastases attracts attention. Sites of primary malignancies were described in a review of 120 cases of cerebral metastasis (Digest 21–8). Tummarello and colleagues describe resection of solitary intracranial metastases from non-small cell lung cancer (Digest 21–9). Weisberg has characterized clinical and computed tomographic correlation of solitary cerebellar metastases (Digest 21–10). Metastatic melanoma in the brain is little affected by radiation therapy (Digest 21–11).

Treatment of pituitary neoplasms shows evidence of progress, in terms of both medical and surgical management. Preliminary data with a somatostatin analogue provide encouraging results in the long-term treatment of acromegaly (Digest 21–12). Bromocriptine therapy can lead to remarkable improvement in visual function in patients with prolactinoma (Digest 21–13). On the other hand, bromocriptine is not likely to be helpful in the treatment of large, functionless pituitary tumors (Digest 21–14). Screening techniques have been established for rapid identification of pituitary adenomas at biopsy (Digest 21–15). Dural biopsy at transsphenoidal surgery shows invasion in 85% of patients with pituitary adenoma (Digest 21–16). Computed tomography (CT) can demonstrate cavernous sinus invasion by pituitary tumors and thus assist operative intervention (Digest 21–17). After transsphenoidal surgery for pituitary adenoma, visual recovery is noted in three quarters of the cases (Digest 21–19). The Glasgow group reports good long-term results for treatment of 77 patients with presumed prolactinoma by transsphenoidal operation (Digest 21–20). Analysis of 257 patients with large or invasive pituitary adenomas suggest that surgical removal and CT follow-up with reoperation where needed is superior to surgery and postoperative radiation therapy (Digest

21–21). Review of 120 patients at the Mayo Clinic documents CT findings after transsphenoidal resection of pituitary adenomas (Digest 21–22). Laws and colleagues report good success from transsphenoidal surgery after unsuccessful prior treatment (Digest 21–23).

Treatment for other benign neoplasms was described in a number of publications. Transventricular microsurgical excision of colloid cyst of the third ventricle produced excellent results in 36 cases (Digest 21–24). Acoustic neuromas can be removed totally with low mortality and morbidity by a posterior fossa approach (Digest 21–25). Cerebellopontine meningioma may be difficult to diagnose, but CT can identify most of the lesions (Digest 21–26). The most characteristic finding is a broad-based mass along the petrous ridge not centered over the porus acousticus (Digest 21–27). Pertuiset analyzed 353 of his own cases of meningiomas and found that major deficits were usually related to occlusion of large arteries at the base of the brain; some lesions should be judged inoperable when there is little chance the patient will come through surgery without new deficits (Digest 21–28). Schwannomas of the jugular foramen may be diagnosed by CT; total removal usually involves paralysis of the lower cranial nerves (Digest 21–29). Despite surgical reception and postoperative radiation, 11 of 26 patients with intracranial chordoma died in a mean follow-up of 5½ years (Digest 21–30). Results with sacral chordoma are also discouraging despite irradiation (Digest 21–31). Central nervous system sarcoidosis occasionally presents as an intracranial tumor (Digest 21–32).

Robert M. Crowell, M.D.

Gliomas

Intracranial Germ-Cell Tumors: Natural History and Pathogenesis

Mark T. Jennings, Rebecca Gelman, and Fred Hochberg (Memorial Sloan-Kettering Cancer Ctr., New York, and Harvard Univ., Dana-Farber Cancer Inst., and Massachusetts Gen. Hosp., Boston)
J. Neurosurg. 63:155–167, August 1985   21–1

Review was made of 119 reports that included 711 cases of diencephalic and pineal tumor, 389 of which were confirmed pathologically and were clinically informative. Sixty-five percent of these lesions were germinomas and 18% were teratomas. The remaining lesions were endodermal sinus tumors, embryonal carcinomas, and choriocarcinomas.

Most tumors arose along the midline from the suprasellar cistern to the pineal gland; 57% of germinomas arose in the suprasellar cistern; 68% of nongerminomatous tumors involved the pineal gland. About two thirds of the tumors were diagnosed between age 10 and 21 years. Parasellar germinomas tended to present with visual field defects, diabetes insipidus, and hypothalamic-pituitary disorders; nongerminomatous tumors presented as posterior third ventricular masses with hydrocephalus and midbrain compression. Germ cell tumors are disseminated both by infiltrating the hypothalamus and via the ventricular and subarachnoid pathways.

CHEMOTHERAPEUTIC EXPERIENCE WITH PRIMARY
INTRACRANIAL GERM CELL TUMORS*

Tumor Type & Chemotherapy	Survival Period & Outcome	References
germinoma		
MTX, CyP, ActD	13 days, dead	146
MTX, CyP, ActD	114 mos, alive	14
BCNU	1 mo, dead	57
CyP	12 mos, alive	3
Vbl, Pbz, CCNU	4 mos, alive	3
c-Pl, Ble, Vbl	12 mos, alive	92
c-Pl, Ble, Vbl	24 mos, alive	91
Vcr, NM	38 mos, alive	73
c-Pl, Ble, Vbl	8 mos, dead	68
embryonal carcinoma		
Ble	4 mos, dead	113
Ble	11 mos, dead	7
CyP, ActD, Vcr	9 mos, alive	85
endodermal sinus tumor		
CyP, ActD, Vcr	12 mos, alive	100
Pbz, Vcr, DHGC	9 mos, dead	142
CyP, ActD, c-Pl,		142
Chl, Vbl, Ble		
MTX, Ble, Vcr	8 mos, dead	6
choriocarcinoma		
Ble	1 mo, dead	55
MTX, BCNU, Vcr	30 mos, alive	3
MTX, ActD, Ble, Vbl	20 mos, alive	48
MTX, ActD	48 mos, alive	67
MTX	20 mos, alive	67
MTX	3 mos, dead	67

*ActD, actinomycin D; BCNU, 1,3-bis(2-chloroethyl)-1-nitrosourea; Ble, bleomycin; Chl, chlorambucil; c-Pl, cis-platinum; CyP, cyclo-phosphamide; CCNU, 1-(2-chloroethyl)-3-cyclohexyl-1-nitrosourea; DHGC, dianhydrogalactitol; MTX, methotrexate; NM, nitrogen mustard; Pbz, procarbazine; Vbl, vinblastine; and Vct, vincristine.

(Courtesy of Jennings, M.T., et al.: J. Neurosurg. 63:155–167, August 1985. Reproduced with permission from Jennings, M.T., et al.: *Diagnosis and Treatment of Pineal Region Tumors*. Baltimore: Williams & Wilkins, 1984, pp. 116–138.)

Surgical biopsy or resection was followed by radiotherapy in 203 cases. Forty-two other tumors were irradiated, and a histologic diagnosis was made at later surgery or at autopsy. Mortality at the time of initial reporting was 46%.

Germinomas were associated with longer survival times, but choriocarcinoma carried a poor prognosis. The extent of dissemination of disease was predictive of survival. Neoplastic involvement of the hypothalamus, third ventricle, and spinal cord was an adverse prognostic finding.

Reports of chemotherapy in cases of primary intracranial germ cell tumor are given in the table. Criteria are needed to determine which patients are at great enough risk to justify toxic drug therapy. Nongerminomatous tumor may itself be an indication for adjunctive chemotherapy in addition to surgery and aggressive radiotherapy.

High-risk patients can be identified by determining the full extent of disease at initial presentation. If gonadotropins are found to direct differentiation toward nongerminomatous elements, pharmacologic measures may help control disease.

▶ This report nicely reviews available information on germ cell tumors. Nongerminomatous tumor is probably itself an indication because of its bad risk for adjunctive chemotherapy in addition to surgery and aggressive radiotherapy.

Human chorionic gonadotropin (HCG) or alpha-fetoprotein levels in serum or cerebrospinal fluid have been correlated with nongerminomatous tumors. Elevations in HCG levels have been reported in germinomas as well. The presence of elevated markers may be an indication for chemotherapy. Dissemination of disease is also correlated with poor outcome. Neuroendocrinologic evaluation and computed tomography scanning (probably supplemented by magnetic resonance scanning) should provide the most effective evidence of spread. If there is evidence of dissemination, even in germinomatous tumor, chemotherapy is probably indicated. Neurosurgeons will want to monitor carefully further reports on the utilization of chemotherapy in this group of patients.—Robert M. Crowell, M.D.

Establishment and Characterization of the Human Medulloblastoma Cell Line and Transplantable Xenograft D283 Med
H. S. Friedman, P. C. Burger, S. H. Bigner, J. Q. Trojanowski, C. J. Wikstrand, E. C. Halperin, and D. D. Bigner (Duke Univ. and Univ. of Pennsylvania)
J. Neuropathol. Exp. Neurol. 44:592–605, November 1985   21–2

Medulloblastoma accounts for one fourth of pediatric brain tumors; current treatment is unsatisfactory. A new continuous cell line and transplantable xenograft, D283 Med, was derived from peritoneal implants and ascitic fluid of a child with metastatic medulloblastoma and grown in vitro in suspension culture. The patient was a 6-year-old child who received radiotherapy after subtotal tumor excision and shunt placement and developed ascites 7 months later. Death occurred 3 days after laparotomy.

The surgical specimen consisted of a cellular lesion with abundant mitoses. The cells grew in vitro with spontaneous macroscopic spheroid formation. The population doubling time was 53 hours. The mean colony-forming efficiency in an agarose medium was 1.8%. The cell line grew in athymic mice as serially transplantable intracranial and subcutaneous xenografts. The intracranial tumors grew as masses of small cells with many mitotic figures and prominent anuclear zones resembling neuroblastic rosettes; subcutaneous tumors lacked rosettes. The tumor cells expressed glutamine synthetase, neuron-specific enolase, and neurofilament protein, but not glial fibrillary acidic protein or S-100 protein. Xenografts at both sites retained the marker chromosomes found in stemline karyotypes of the peritoneal implant and ascitic fluid cells but lacked the additional copy of chromosome 11.

This cell line may permit further study of the biologic properties of human medulloblastoma and of its sensitivity to various treatments.

▶ The extensive studies of animal brain tumors in tissue culture have left a question regarding comparability with the clinical setting. Now Friedman and colleagues have established a metastatic medulloblastoma from patient tissue culture. This approach of utilizing clinical material for experimental studies seems promising with regard to overcoming species variation in tumors.—Robert M. Crowell, M.D.

Applications of Monoclonal Antibodies in the Diagnosis and Treatment of Primary Brain Tumors
Dennis E. Bullard and Darell D. Bigner (Duke Univ.)
J. Neurosurg. 63:2–16, July 1985   21–3

There is great potential for the use of monoclonal antibodies in neuro-oncology to increase the specificity of both diagnosis and treatment of CNS tumors. Preferential localization of a rabbit antiglioma serum (Fig 21–1) in human glioma tissue was reported in 1965. In addition to the uniformity and ease of producing large amounts of antibody, monoclonal

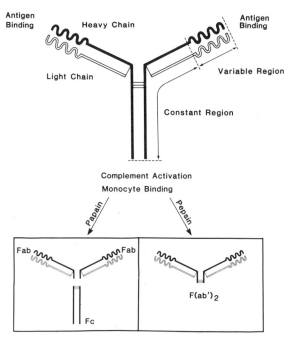

Fig 21–1.—Diagram of antibody, showing basic structure including light and heavy chains and constant and variable regions. Antigen-binding occurs in the variable region, whereas such biologically mediated events as complement activation and monocyte binding occur at the Fc portion of the constant region. When an antibody is digested by the enzyme papain, two Fab fragments and one Fc fragment are derived. The Fab fragments are capable of binding to antigens without the induction of such processes as complement activation. In contrast, digestion with pepsin results in destruction of the Fc part of the antibody, whereas the two Fab fragments are still attached at a disulfide bond producing F(ab')$_2$ fragment. (Courtesy of Bullard, D.E., and Bigner, D.D.: J. Neurosurg. 63:2–16, July 1985.)

antibodies have great potential for in vivo use because of their high specificity. Radioactively labeled monoclonal antibodies are useful for in vivo imaging because of their purity, and because indifferent antibodies of the same class can be used to subtract background interaction. High diagnostic specificity can be obtained by using immunohistochemical methods and monoclonal antibodies as reagents. The ability to distinguish between normal organ-specific and tumor-specific antigens will allow determination of the cell of origin of many CNS tumors.

Tumor vascularity, vascular permeability, and tumor blood flow are factors in the delivery of monoclonal antibodies to solid tumors. If problems in antibody localization and delivery are solved, monoclonal antibodies will be usable as carriers of drugs or radionuclides. Both polyclonal and monoclonal antibodies of varying specificity have been successfully coupled with a wide range of chemotherapeutic agents. Antibody-mediated immunologic reactions are also a possibility. Radionuclides bound to monoclonal antibodies can be used therapeutically as well as diagnostically. Radionuclides can be secondarily activated, providing high target specificity and local effect. Plant toxins bound to monoclonal antibody might be used for treatment of neoplasms.

▶ Physicians have long sought the "silver bullet" for brain tumors. This agent would have the necessary specificity to selectively seek out and destroy tumor cells, while not harming normal tissues. Monoclonal antibodies seem highly promising in this respect: they are highly specific and can carry cytotoxic substances. So far, problems with specificity of antibody localization and delivery have hindered effective clinical utilization of this approach. However, this report suggests that significant advances are being made in this area, an impression sustained by the next selection.—Robert M. Crowell, M.D.

Antibody Guided Irradiation of Brain Glioma by Arterial Infusion of Radioactive Monoclonal Antibody Against Epidermal Growth Factor Receptor and Blood Group A Antigen
A. A. Epenetos, N. Courtenay-Luck, D. Pickering, G. Hooker, H. Durbin, J. P. Lavender, and C. G. McKenzie (Hammersmith Hosp. and Imperial Cancer Research Fund, London)
Br. Med. J. 290:1463–1466, May 18, 1985   21–4

High radiation doses might sterilize advanced brain glioma, but at the expense of producing unacceptable brain damage. Antibody-guided irradiation theoretically could deliver a tumoricidal dose with a minimal dose to normal brain tissue. A patient with recurrent grade IV glioma resistant to conventional treatment exhibited uptake by the tumor of a monoclonal antibody against epidermal growth factor (EGF) receptor on antibody-guided radionuclide scanning. The antibody, 9A, cross-reacted with blood group A antigen. Antibody labeled with 45 mCi of ^{131}I was delivered to the tumor region by internal carotid artery infusion. Treatment began after partial tumor removal and conventional radiotherapy.

Computed tomography showed tumor regression after antibody administration, though cerebral edema persisted. Clinical improvement was appreciable and sustained, and no toxic effects of treatment were observed. The patient's quality of life was improved.

Antibody-guided irradiation using a monoclonal antibody against EGF receptor and blood group A antigen was associated with objective tumor shrinkage and clinical improvement in this case of grade IV glioma. This treatment may prove to be useful in the management of brain gliomas resistant to conventional measures. The duration of benefit from this treatment remains to be determined.

▶ Irradiation guided by antibody made against epidermal growth factor receptor appears to have caused tumor regression in this single case report. This is encouraging, but clearly further confirmatory experience will be needed to estabilsh a clinical role for this approach.—Robert M. Crowell, M.D.

In Vitro Killing of Human Glioblastoma By Interleukin-2-Activated Autologous Lymphocytes

Steven K. Jacobs, Debra J. Wilson, Paul L. Kornblith, and Elizabeth A. Grimm (Natl. Insts. of Health, Bethesda, Md.)
J. Neurosurg. 64:114–117, January 1986   21–5

Current treatment of malignant glioma is unsatisfactory, but culture of blood lymphocytes with the lymphokine interleukin-2 (IL-2) has led to the generation of lymphokine-activated killer lymphocytes (LAKs) that can lyse several types of nonglial tumors. Studies were done in patients with Karnovsky functional ratings greater than 50 who underwent operative tumor debulking in order to determine whether their lymphocytes, when activated, would kill autologous glioblastoma cells in vitro. Glioma target cell preparations were exposed to LAKs prepared by incubation of peripheral blood lymphocytes with purified recombinant IL-2.

Lymphocytes from all 8 patients produced marked lysis of autologous as well as allogeneic glioblastoma after being activated with IL-2. Significant lysis of autologous fresh tumor by patient LAKs was seen in 4 of 5 studies. The findings could not be related to patient age, previous treatment, or dexamethasone administration.

Lymphocytes from brain tumor patients consistently lyse autologous glioblastoma cells in vitro after being activated by IL-2. A clinical trial of LAKs in the intraoperative immunotherapy of malignant glioma is under way. No specificity for lysis of autologous glioblastoma was evident; the basis for the apparent broad specificity of LAKs for many types of tumor is unknown.

▶ These are very exciting results. In eight tumors studied in vitro interleukin-2 activated killer lymphocytes which lysed glioblastoma cells. We await with interest the results of clinical trials of activated killer lymphocytes in the treatment of glial tumors.—Robert M. Crowell, M.D.

Reduced Systemic Drug Exposure by Combining Intra-arterial Chemotherapy With Hemoperfusion of Regional Venous Drainage

Edward H. Oldfield, Robert L. Dedrick, Russell L. Yeager, W. Craig Clark, Hetty L. DeVroom, Dulal C. Chatterji, and John L. Doppman (Natl. Insts. of Health, Bethesda, Md.)
J. Neurosurg. 63:726–732, November 1985   21–6

Systemic toxicity frequently limits the dose of anticancer drug deliverable by the intra-arterial route. In monkeys, brain exposure has been markedly increased by combining intracarotid BCNU (1,3-bis[2-chloroethyl]-1-nitrosourea) infusion with drug removal from the ipsilateral jugular blood by hemoperfusion. Carotid infusion of BCNU was compared with a combined infusion-extracorporeal hemoperfusion technique in four patients with malignant cerebral gliomas. In the latter approach the ipsilateral jugular venous drainage was pumped extracorporeally through a hemoperfusion cartridge containing a nonionic adsorbent resin (Fig 21–2). A dose of 220 mg of BCNU/sq m was infused over 45 minutes, and jugular blood was passed through a catheter at 300 ml per minute. Infusions were given at 6-week intervals.

Hemoperfusion of jugular venous blood during intracarotid infusion of BCNU reduced systemic exposure by 56% to 87% and increased the total

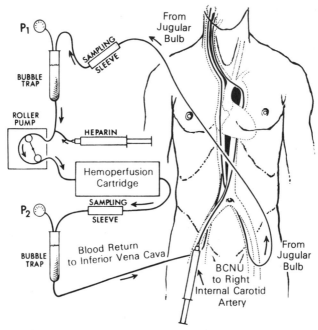

Fig 21–2.—Catheter placement and extracorporeal circuit in treatment combining hemoperfusion of jugular blood with intracarotid infusion of BCNU. Jugular blood was propelled through the hemoperfusion system at 300 ml per minute by a roller pump while 220 mg of BCNU per sq m was infused into the suprasellar segment of the internal carotid artery over 45 minutes. (Courtesy of Oldfield, E.H., et al.: J. Neurosurg. 63:726–732, November 1985.)

body clearance of drug two- to eightfold. The calculated pharmacokinetic advantage, expressed as the brain-body exposure ratio, ranged from 21:1 to 55:1 when the combined approach was used.

Hemoperfusion of jugular drainage is a useful adjunct to intracarotid chemotherapy in patients treated for malignant cerebral glioma. The approach may be applicable to tumors and other disorders at any site where arterial drug delivery and collection of venous blood for drug removal are feasible. One patient in this study had focal brain injury after the supraophthalmic infusion of BCNU. Cerebral injury is infrequent after infusion of comparable doses into the cervical segment of the internal carotid artery.

▶ The use of intra-arterial chemotherapy for brain tumors is supported by a solid rationale, with encouraging preliminary results. The addition of hemoperfusion of regional venous drainage to limit systemic toxicity is logical. However, these methods are as yet investigational and cannot be recommended for routine utilization.

In another article on chemotherapy, Mahaley et al. (*J. Neurosurg.* 63:719–725, 1985) report on the administration of interferon to 19 patients with recurrent glioma. Each patient had previously undergone surgical intervention and radiation therapy. Seven of 17 evaluatable patients showed tumor regression at 12 weeks and 10 showed tumor progression. Interferon appears to be efficacious in the treatment of gliomas. Further studies are needed to establish the method for general use.

Supraclinoid intercarotid chemotherapy is safe and effective with a new flow-directed soft-tip catheter (Charnsangavej et al.: *Radiology* 155:655–657, 1985).—Robert M. Crowell, M.D.

Vasoactive Drugs Produce Selective Changes in Flow to Experimental Brain Tumors
Lori A. Panther, Gary L. Baumbach, Darell D. Bigner, Donald Piegors, Dennis R. Groothuis, and Donald D. Heistad (VA Med. Ctr. and Univ. of Iowa, Duke Univ., and Northwestern Univ.)
Ann. Neurol. 18:712–715, December 1985   21–7

Most vasoactive drugs do not readily penetrate the blood-brain barrier or alter cerebral blood flow. The effects of such drugs on blood flow to brain tumors, with an abnormal barrier, were studied by the microsphere method by use of adenosine, a potent dilator in most vascular beds, and norepinephrine, a potent constrictor. Both drugs have little effect on cerebral blood flow when given intravenously. Studies were done in dogs with brain tumors induced by avian sarcoma virus. All tumors were in the left cerebral hemisphere and stained brightly with Evans blue dye, indicating an abnormal blood-brain barrier. Vascularity appeared to be increased on histologic study.

Control blood flow tended to be higher in the sarcomas than in normal cerebrum, but there was much variation among tumors. Infused adenosine consistently produced a marked increase in blood flow to the tumors, while flow to the peritumoral cerebrum and other brain areas did not increase.

Norepinephrine reduced tumor blood flow by about a third, and did not change flow to other brain areas. Hypercapnia increased blood flow to normal cerebrum more than twofold but did not increase tumor blood flow.

Vasoactive agents that normally have little effect on cerebral blood flow had marked effects of flow to brain sarcomas in this model. Both an abnormal blood-brain barrier and other differences between vessels in normal and tumorous brain may be responsible. The findings bear on the delivery of lipid-soluble chemotherapeutic agents such as 1-3-bis(2-chloroethyl)-1-nitrosourea (BCNU) and aziridinylbenzoquinone (AZQ) to brain tumors.

▶ The data suggest that blood flow and cerebral blood volume within brain tumors can be remarkably affected by exogenous drugs. These effects could have important implications in the delivery of chemotherapeutic agents. In addition, clinicians should be aware that the systemic administration of vasoactive drugs could have deleterious effects such as vasogenic edema, so that these drugs should be used only with caution.

In experimental rat brain tumor studies, intracarotid mannitol increased entry of chemotherapeutic agents into the brain rather than the tumor (Hiesiger et al.: *Ann. Neurol.* 19:50–59, 1986).

Combination chemotherapy in vitro exploiting glutamine metabolism of human glioma suggests that this approach might improve chemotherapy in clinical settings (Dranoff et al.: *Cancer Res.* 45:4082–4086, 1985).—Robert M. Crowell, M.D.

Notes on Primary Brain Tumors

▶ Extraneural metastasis of CNS tumor is more common than previously stated (Hoffman and Duffner: *Cancer* 56:1778–1782, 1985). Such lesions are universally fatal. This complication can be avoided by avoiding shunting or using a filter device if a shunt is needed.

Rapid treatment with radiation therapy is more important than large fraction size in treatment of metastatic melanoma in the brain. Complete excision increases mean survival time only 2 months, according to Chou et al. (*Cancer* 56:10–15, 1985). In our experience at the University of Illinois, surgical excision can lead to improved quality of life.

Osteogenic sarcoma of the skull may best be treated with wide surgical excision and chemotherapy, according to Sundaresan et al. (*J. Neurosurg.* 63:562–567, 1985).

According to Edwards et al. (*Cancer* 56:1773–1777, 1985), tumor markers in CSF are generally not useful in establishing a histologic diagnosis but can help to monitor therapy and predict recurrence.

Lammertsma et al. (*Brit. J. Radiol.* 58:725–734, 1985) describe diminished oxygen extraction ratio (OER) in tumors studied by positron emission tomograph scanning.

In 22 biopsy-proven supratentorial ependymomas, computed tomography showed intraparenchymal lesions larger than 4 cm in most cases, which are often cystic. Contrast enhancement was moderate to intense, with intratumoral calcification in one third of the cases and hydrocephalus and edema in 50% of the cases (Armington et al.: *Radiology* 157:367–372, 1985).

Tumor grading of oligodendrogliomas permitted significant prognostic statements to be made in a retrospective study of 554 cases from the Armed Forces Institutes of Pathology (Ludwig et al.: *Ann. Neurol.* 19:15–21, 1986).

Primary CNS lymphoma constitutes one of the criteria for diagnosis of acquired immune deficiency syndrome (AIDS). In six homosexual men with this lesion, computed tomography showed hypodense, contrast-enhancing lesions, whereas isodense or hyperdense lesions were seen in patients with such lymphomas who did not have underlying immunodeficiency. Immunologic abnormalities in the patients with primary CNS lymphoma were similar to those seen in patients with AIDS who present with Kaposi's sarcoma or opportunistic infections (Gill et al.: *Am. J. Med.* 78:742–748, 1985).

Non-Hodgkin's lymphoma of the brain can be correctly identified by computed tomography (deep white matter hypodensity) in about 50% of the cases. Pathologic confirmation by limited biopsy is essential for accurate diagnosis (Lerais et al.: *Sem. Hop. Paris* 61:1137–1142, 1985).

In 32 cases of primary CNS lymphoma certain radiographic features suggested the diagnosis (Jack et al.: *AJNR* 6:899–904, 1985). Most of the lesions showed increased density with enhancement that was homogenous. In 12 of 32 patients there was a homogenous vascular stain in the late arterial or early venous phase. Such an angiographic pattern and a dense, homogenously enhancing parenchymal lesion suggest primary lymphoma.

Primary intracranial lymphoma may occur even in infancy (Berry et al.: *Am. J. Pediatr. Hematol. Oncol.* 7:141–147, 1985).

Experience with radical excision of 34 brain stem gliomas in children led Epstein and McLeary to recommend radical excision for cervicomedullary lesions and radiation or chemotherapy for more rostral lesions (*J. Neurosurg.* 64:11–15, 1986).

The Kyoto University group advocates a conservative policy with radiation for most brain stem gliomas. (Tokuriki, Y., et al.: *Acta Neurochir.* 79:67–73, 1986).

Adult medulloblastoma appears to behave similarly to the childhood lesion (Pobereskin, L., and Treip, C.: *J. Neurol. Neurosurg. Psychiatry* 49:39–42, 1986).

A homogeneous vascular stain in a densely enhancing brain lesion suggests lymphoma (Jack, C. R., et al.: *AJNR* 146:271–276, 1986).

Surgical resection plus high-dose radiation therapy offers the best chance for prolonged survival in CNS chordoma (Amendola, B.E., et al.: *Radiology* 158:839–843, 1986).

Because of brain necrosis after radiotherapy for primary brain tumor, targeting therapy to the tumor is advocated instead of whole brain irradiation (Hohwieler, M. L., et al.: *Neurosurgery* 18:67–74, 1986).

Excision of a wide strip of dura around 14 meningiomas revealed multifocality in all 14 (Borovich, B., and Doron, Y.: *J. Neurosurg.* 64:58–63, 1986). This may explain some recurrences, and wide dural excision is suggested to prevent recurrence.

Depot-bromocriptine appears to be superior to the oral agent in terms of lessened side effects and increased compliance (Grossman, A., et al.: *Clin. Endocrinol.* 24:231–238, 1986).

Interstitial irradiation of a pituitary tumor can lead to visual improvement (Kermar, P. P., et al.: *Neurosurgery* 18:82–84, 1986).

Cerebellopontine angle lipoma can be followed on computed tomography, for excision is impossible and even biopsy carries substantial risk (Pensak, M. L., et al.: *Arch. Otolaryngol.* 112:99–101, 1986).

Laboratory Notes

▶ Thymidine kinase is present in tumor cysts but not in nonneoplastic cysts, according to Persson et al. (*J. Neurosurg.* 63:568–572, 1985).

Graham et al. (*Neurosurgery* 17:537–542, 1985) describe in vitro studies of hexokinase activity in gliomas. Malignant gliomas showed elevated hexokinase activity compared with lower grade astrocytomas, which may explain the differences in 18 fluoro-2-deoxyglucose uptake in positron emission tomography scans. Such studies may help expand understanding of the basic biochemistry of brain tumors, and such fundamental knowledge will be important to future diagnosis and treatment.

Yamasaki et al. (*J. Neurosurg.* 63:763–770, 1985) report on γ-interferon production by a glioma-specific, cytotoxic T lymphocyte clone. Investigations of T lymphocyte clones in culture suggest that the interferon did not have direct cytotoxic action on cells but may play a role in the process of antigen recognition of cells. These results may be compared with those of recent studies that demonstrate a remarkable tumoricidal sensitization of T lymphocyte "killer cells" to glioma cells in tissue culture.

Shinoda et al. report on immunohistochemical studies in intracranial germ cell tumors (*J. Neurosurg.* 63:733–739, 1985). Thirteen of 17 germinomas showed staining for placental alkaline phosphatase (PLAP). Since other primary nongerm cell tumors rarely showed PLAP staining, this test is a useful marker for intracranial germinoma. Positive α-fetoprotein staining was seen in several yolk sac tumors and a few embryonal carcinomas.

Cultured glioma cells may demonstrate resistance to natural killer cell attack, according to Yates et al. (*J. Neuropathol. Exp. Neurol.* 44:371–383, 1985). Such effects could blunt the impact of treatment with interferon or interleukin.—Robert M. Crowell, M.D.

Metastases

Sites of Primary Malignancies in Patients Presenting With Cerebral Metastases: A Review of 120 Cases
Thierry Le Chevalier, Frederick P. Smith, Philippe Caille, Jean Paul Constans, and Jacques G. Rouesse (Institut Gustave-Roussy, Villejuif, and Hôpital St. Anne, Paris, and Georgetown Univ.)
Cancer 56:880–882, Aug. 15, 1985   21–8

Review was made of the data on 120 consecutive patients seen in 1959–1979 who presented with brain lesions as the first sign of malignant disease. In the 89 male and 31 female patients (median age, 54 years), increased intracranial pressure and motor deficit were the most frequent presenting features. Nearly one third of the patients had seizures, and more than 40% had behavioral changes. Nearly 90% of brain metastases were in the

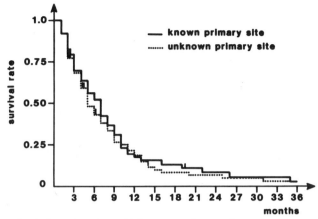

Fig 21–3.—Survival rates in patients with known vs. unknown primary sites. (Courtesy of Le Chevalier, T., et al.: Cancer 56:880–882, Aug. 15, 1985.)

cerebrum. Of 86 evaluable lesions, 44% were adenocarcinomas, and 30% were undifferentiated or small-cell carcinomas. Lung cancer accounted for 51% of primary tumors.

Solitary metastases were excised when feasible, and many patients had postoperative irradiation. Radiotherapy was used initially in 34 cases. Systemic treatments were used when indicated. Survival was 52% at 6 months, 18% at 1 year, and 5% at 2 years. Patients with a known primary site had survival rates of 20% at 1 year and 6% at 2 years (Fig 21–3).

A primary site was identified in about half the present cases. The lung has been the most frequent primary site in patients presenting with cerebral metastases. Gastrointestinal malignant conditions were more frequent than expected in the present series. There appears to be little reason to undertake extensive efforts to identify primary sites in these cases, since patients in whom a primary site was not identified have done no worse than the others.

► The results indicate that cerebral metastases emanate from the lung in about one half the cases and from the gastrointestinal tract more commonly than is generally accepted. The report adds weight to the concept that extensive evaluation for a primary tumor site is not valuable in that outcome does not appear to be affected by identification of the primary source.—Robert M. Crowell, M.D.

Non-Small Cell Lung Cancer: Neuroresection of the Solitary Intracranial Metastasis Followed by Radiochemotherapy

Diego Tummarello, Emilio Porfiri, Franco Rychlicki, Salvatore Miseria, and Riccardo Cellerino (Univ. of Ancona and Gen. Hosp. of Ancona, Italy)
Cancer 56:2569–2572, Dec. 1, 1985   21–9

Sporadic long-term survival has been reported in patients with brain metastases of non-small cell lung cancer after neurosurgery and control of systemic disease. Fifteen patients (median age, 49 years) with advanced intrathoracic disease and solitary metastases were managed by systemic chemotherapy, chest and brain irradiation, and craniotomy. Fourteen patients had adenocarcinoma, and 1 had squamous-cell carcinoma. Fourteen had a solitary intracranial metastasis, and 1 patient had a double resectable metastasis. Three patients were seen after pulmonary lobectomy, whereas 12 were untreated. Seven patients had a neurologic deficit as the first sign of disease. The median age was 49 years.

One patient died postoperatively of a cerebral hemorrhage. Nine patients had neurologic improvement for a median of 10 months. Four patients responded to systemic treatment, 1 completely, and 6 others had a stable course. The overall median survival was 6 months after craniotomy and 1 year after diagnosis. Five patients survived for 1 year to 26 months after craniotomy. For 4 patients relapse occurred only in the brain.

All patients with a solitary brain metastasis from lung cancer should be considered for systemic treatment. Neurosurgical resection should be considered more often in these cases. Long survival times have resulted with the use of conventional chemotherapy. Relapse in the brain, which is, however, not infrequent, may result from continuous intracranial spread from primary disease that is not well controlled by chemoradiotherapy.

▶ The results indicate that palliation is the only reasonable goal of resection of solitary metastases. In regard to this goal, the results were positive: 9 patients had neurologic improvement for a median of 10 months, and for selected patients, particularly younger individuals, aggressive resection of solitary metastases appears a reasonable approach. In elderly patients and those with multiple lesions, which may be detected with greater sensitivity by magnetic resonance imaging, surgical excision is less attractive.

Among 90 patients with carcinoma of the breast, brain metastases developed more commonly in patients with stage 3 disease at first diagnosis and in those who were premenopausal. Patients given whole brain irradiation for brain metastases lived longer (Snee et al.: *Clin. Radiol.* 36:365–367, 1985).—Robert M. Crowell, M.D.

Solitary Cerebellar Metastases: Clinical and Computed Tomographic Correlations
Leon A. Weisberg (Tulane Univ. and Charity Hosp. of New Orleans)
Arch. Neurol. 42:336–341, April 1985   21–10

Seventeen patients with solitary cerebellar neoplasms were diagnosed by computed tomography (CT). Fourteen of them underwent craniotomy and subsequent irradiation, while 3 were irradiated without surgical biopsy. Neurologic disorder preceded evidence of systemic cancer in 11 cases. The primary source of neoplasia was the lung in 15 cases and melanoma in 1 other case. The most frequent neurologic findings were gait instability, headache, and vomiting. Patients became symptomatic 5–28 days before diagnosis.

Computed tomography showed obstructive hydrocephalus in 17 cases, a homogeneously hypodense noncontrast density in 12 cases, and fourth ventricular effacement in 8 cases. A thick, irregular, complex ring was noted after contrast enhancement in 9 cases. The fourth ventricle consistently showed evidence of compression and distortion. Enhancement was apparent in all cases but 1 after contrast administration. Ten patients improved symptomatically after surgery or radiotherapy combined with steroid therapy. Only 1 patient lived long enough to exhibit CT evidence of recurrent cerebellar metastasis.

The CT finding of a solitary cerebellar lesion should prompt a careful search for primary systemic carcinoma. Surgical biopsy or autopsy may demonstrate a solitary cerebellar metastasis even if primary carcinoma is not identified. Bronchogenic carcinoma was the most frequent primary cancer in the present series. Indications for surgery may include a cystic lesion on CT, evidence of transtentorial herniation and obstructive hydrocephalus, papilledema, a radiation-resistant primary tumor, and CT evidence of a hemorrhagic neoplasm.

▶ In histologically proven solitary cerebellar metastases, CT consistently showed obstructive hydrocephalus and enhancement with fourth ventricular compression and distortion. Most cases showed hypodense lesions and often there was contrast enhancement.

Data from this report are insufficient to sustain indications for surgery. However, many surgeons believe that surgery is warranted for symptomatic solitary metastatic lesions (especially without known primary) in an effort to save life and prolong useful function, even when cure is deemed unlikely.—Robert M. Crowell, M.D.

Metastatic Melanoma in Brain: Rapid Treatment or Large Dose Fractions
Kwang N. Choi, H. Rodney Withers, and Marvin Rotman (State Univ. of New York, Downstate Med. Ctr., and Univ. of California at Los Angeles)
Cancer 56:10–15, July 1, 1985   21–11

The best dose fractionation for irradiation of melanoma remains to be determined. Various accelerated fractionation regimens were evaluated in 59 patients who received twice-daily irradiation for intracranial metastatic melanoma between 1972 and 1977. They had either brain metastasis as the only evidence of disease or complete resection of brain metastasis before irradiation. Seven different twice-daily fractionation schemes were utilized. Three involved an overall treatment time of 1 week and 4, a time of 2 weeks. Total dosage was increased gradually over the years from 3,000 to 4,800 rads.

Symptomatic improvement lasted longer in patients treated for 1 week. Patients with brain metastases only survived longer than those with disease elsewhere, especially if given 10 fractions within 1 week rather than 20 fractions in 2 weeks. The same was true for patients who had complete resection of an intracranial tumor before irradiation. Complete resection increased the likelihood of eliminating intracranial disease, but median survival was increased by less than 2 months. The advantage of 1-week irradiation was most evident in patients treated after resection of intracranial disease. About half the patients died primarily of intracranial metastasis.

A short overall radiotherapy time appears to be more important than large fractions in the management of metastatic intracranial melanoma. Local control is a more relevant end point than survival time, but it was difficult to assess in this study because of the terminal nature of the illness.

▶ Intracranial metastasis from melanoma remains a difficult challenge for treatment (Choi et al.: *Cancer* 56:1–9, 1985): 194 patients were treated at the M. D. Anderson Hospital (Houston) with a variety of techniques, including radiation of 3,000–4,800 rads for 2 weeks. Patients with complete surgical excision tended to do better. Of 43 patients for whom brain metastases were the only evidence of disease at the time of treatment, 32 subsequently developed extracranial disease. Of 32 patients who underwent complete resection before irradiation, the condition of only 8 were controlled by combined treatment.—Robert M. Crowell, M.D.

Pituitary Tumors

Long-Term Treatment of Acromegaly With the Somatostatin Analogue SMS 201–995

Steven W. J. Lamberts, Piet Uitterlinden, Louis Verschoor, Krijn J. van Dongen, and Emilio del Pozo (Erasmus Univ., Rotterdam, and Sandoz Ltd., Basel, Switzerland)

N. Engl. J. Med. 313:1576–1580, Dec. 19, 1985   21–12

The long-acting somatostatin analogue SMS 201–995 has a potent, prolonged inhibitory effect on growth hormone release and only a short-term effect on insulin. Long-term treatment with the analogue was undertaken in four acromegalic patients with classical clinical findings, three men and one woman aged 35–61 years. Three patients had not been treated previously but refused transsphenoidal surgery. One patient had a progressively extensive tumor despite three operations and radiotherapy. Long-term treatment began with 50 μg of SMS 201–995 twice or 3 times a day.

Plasma growth hormone was significantly inhibited by analogue therapy (Fig 21–4). Growth hormone levels were present for at least 2 hours after each 50-μg injection, and maximal inhibition was obtained with 100 μg twice or 3 times a day. Insulin profiles did not change markedly over the long range. Rapid clinical improvement, including a decrease in soft tissue swelling, occurred in all four patients, and resolution of hypertension occurred in two patients. Cranial nerve function returned in one case. Patients did well on self-administration of the analogue, and no side effects were observed.

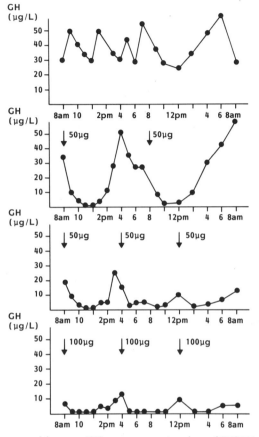

Fig 21–4.—Plasma growth hormone (GH) response to various doses of SMS 201–995 over 24 hours. Profiles are shown before treatment (**top graph**) and at 3 different treatment intervals. The mean (± SEM) daily levels of GH were 38.0 ± 2.5 µg/L before treatment, 20.7 ± 4.2 µg/L after 2 weeks of treatment with 50 µg twice a day, 7.5 ± 1.6 µg/L after 3 weeks of treatment with 50 µg 3 times a day, and 3.9 ± 0.9 µg/L after 6 weeks of additional treatment with 100 µg 3 times a day. (Courtesy of Lamberts, S.W.J., et al.: N. Engl. J. Med. 313:1576–1580, Dec. 19, 1985. Reprinted by permission of the New England Journal of Medicine.)

The somatostatin analogue 201–995 is suitable for long-term clinical use by subcutaneous administration, especially in patients who do not do well after surgery or radiotherapy, and in those who respond incompletely to dopaminergic drugs. Impaired carbohydrate tolerance and gastrointestinal dysfunction are theoretical side effects of this treatment.

▶ This preliminary report suggests that SMS 201–995 has useful long-term effects on acromegaly. Further studies will be needed to define side effects and administration schedules (possible only by injection today). The drug may take its place as adjunctive treatment along with surgery and radiotherapy, or even as primary treatment, depending on results of further studies.—Robert M. Crowell, M.D.

Visual Function in Prolactinoma Patients Treated With Bromocriptine

Mark L. Moster, Peter J. Savino, Norman J. Schatz, Peter J. Snyder, Robert C. Sergott, and Thomas M. Bosley (Univ. of Pennsylvania)
Ophthalmology 92:1332–1341, October 1985   21–13

Visual function was monitored in 10 patients with prolactinoma who were treated primarily with bromocriptine. All presented with visual dysfunction from prolactin-secreting pituitary macroadenomas. Therapy with bromocriptine was begun in a dose of 1.25 mg, with subsequent doses based on the response. The average follow-up on bromocriptine therapy was 15 months. The patients, all men, had an average age of 47 years.

The average serum level of prolactin fell from 6,630 to 85 ng/ml while patients were receiving an average daily bromocriptine dose of 13.5 mg. Seven patients had a dramatic visual response to treatment, and two with mild defects also improved. Visual acuity and fields eventually became normal in six patients, but 1 later had worsening of the visual fields. Improvement in vision paralleled the fall in serum prolactin and decreasing tumor size as revealed by computed tomography (CT). Two patients had complications; one became lightheaded while receiving 7.5 mg/day but became asymptomatic when the dose was reduced to 2.5 mg/day. The other patient, whose initial pretreatment CT scan revealed extension of the tumor into the sphenoid sinus with erosion of the floor of the sella turcica, developed a cerebrospinal fluid leak at 15 months.

The long-term effects of bromocriptine therapy for prolactinoma remain unknown, but early restoration of impaired vision can be expected unless visual loss has been present for years. Bromocriptine also may be given preoperatively to reduce tumor size and facilitate surgical removal. Bromocriptine is indicated for patients with residual tumor on CT scans or a persistently elevated level of serum prolactin after transsphenoidal hypophysectomy.

▶ These data indicate remarkable improvement in visual field defects after bromocriptine therapy for prolactinomas. Although the serum prolactin levels fell, normal levels were not achieved in many of the cases. Surely, bromocriptine is indicated for certain patients with residual tumor on CT scan, or persistently elevated prolactin levels following transsphenoidal hypophysectomy. For many patients with visual field defects associated with prolactinoma, transsphenoidal hypophysectomy offers prompt decompression of the optic apparatus and in some cases may be curative.—Robert M. Crowell, M.D.

The Effect of Dopamine Agonist Therapy on Large Functionless Pituitary Tumors

A. Grossman, R. Ross, M. Charlesworth, C. B. T. Adams, J. A. H. Wass, I. Doniach, and G. M. Besser (St. Bartholomew's Hosp., London, and Radcliffe Infirmary, Oxford, England)
Clin. Endocrinol. (Oxf.) 22:679–686, May 1985   21–14

Many pituitary tumors can be rapidly reduced in size with dopamine agonist therapy, but whether functionless tumors respond in this way is uncertain. Fifteen patients 22–59 years of age, 12 of whom were women, and who had large pituitary tumors but normal or minimally elevated prolactin levels, were studied prospectively during dopamine agonist therapy. The tumors were more than 1 cm in diameter and had greater than 1 cm of lateral and/or suprasellar extension. The serum prolactin concentrations were less than 1,000 mU/L. Nine patients were treated with bromocriptine, 5 with mesulergine, and 1 with pergolide. Dosage was increased until serum prolactin was undetectable.

Of 6 patients who had normal prolactin levels at the outset, 4 had total loss of residual anterior pituitary function; two of these 4 patients had diabetes insipidus. The mean follow-up of treatment was 9 months. All patients but 1 were eventualy operated on, usually because of a persistent visual field defect. Eleven tumors were chromophobe adenomas not staining for prolactin and growth hormone. One patient each had an eosinophilic adenoma, an epidermoid cyst, and a Rathke's pouch cyst. One patient had gradual shrinkage of a pituitary tumor, presumably because of a tumor infarction; regrowth did not follow the cessation of bromocriptine therapy.

Dopamine agonist therapy is unlikely to be helpful in patients with a large pituitary tumor and mild or no hyperprolactinemia. If there is no visual field response to a trial of treatment in a short time, surgical decompression of the visual pathways should be carried out.

► This report adds weight to the widely held opinion that dopamine agonist therapy is ineffective for functionless tumors of the pituitary gland. In such cases with visual disturbance, surgical decompression may be carried out without a preliminary trial of dopamine agonist treatment.

Bromocriptine treatment can lead to empty sella in cases of microprolactinoma (Demura et al.: *Acta Endocrinol.* [*Copenh*] 110:306–312, 1985).

Bromocriptine treatment for prolactinoma may lead to cerebral spinal fluid rhinnorhea requiring surgical correction (Kok et al.: *Neurology* 35:1193–1195, 1985).

In 12 cases where bromocriptine treatment was interrupted, hyperprolactinemia recurred, a finding which suggests that the medical treatment alone has no lasting curative effect (Kruhn et al.: *Presse Med.* 14:525–528, 1985).

Low doses of dopamine agonist are effective in the long-term treatment of macroprolactinomas (Liuzzi et al.: *N. Engl. J. Med.* 313:656–9, 1985). Of 38 patients treated, prolactin levels became normal in 30 and the tumor shrank in 29. After 2 years of treatment, in 21 patients doses were decreased to less than 10 mg per day without a change in prolactin level or tumor size. It was possible to withdraw the drug completely in only 1 patient.

Prolactin levels may remain low after drug withdrawal in the treatment of microprolactinomas with bromocriptine (Moriondo et al.: *J. Clin. Endocrinol. Metab.* 60:764–772, 1985). Effectiveness of the drug improves after prolonged administration. Dosage may be reduced in many patients and treatment may even be withdrawn in some, with no ill effects.

Bromocriptine treatment of large macroadenomas (macroprolactinomas) may not reduce tumor size (Boulanger, et al.: *Fertil. Steril.* 44:532–535, 1985).— Robert M. Crowell, M.D.

Stromal and Nuclear Markers for Rapid Identification of Pituitary Adenomas at Biopsy

Paul E. McKeever, Steve Laverson, Edward H. Oldfield, Barry H. Smith, Deborah Gadille, and William F. Chandler (Univ. of Michigan and Natl. Insts. of Health, Bethesda, Md.)
Arch. Pathol. Lab. Med. 109:509–514, June 1985   21–15

The intraoperative diagnosis of pituitary adenoma requires speed, simplicity, and accurate localization. Fluorescent and light microscopic markers were examined in an attempt to improve the recognition of these lesions at biopsy. The optimal staining procedure for direct visualization was found to include 3 μg of propidium iodide (PI) and 100 μg of fluorescein-conjugated *Ricinus communis* agglutinin 120 (RCA 120). Refrigerated solution was immediately available for use in the assessment of routine frozen sections. Sections were stained for 1 minute and viewed after saline rinse and coverslip application.

Fluorescein-labeled RCA 120, which binds galactose, localizes vascular stromata, whereas PI, which binds nucleic acids, stains nuclei. Visualization of the stromal configuration, nuclear morphologic features, and cell-to-stroma ratio can help distinguish between adenoma and adenohypophysis. The same features can be demonstrated by light microscopy with the use of peroxidase-conjugated RCA 120.

Pituitary adenomas can be rapidly and accurately distinguished from fragments of normal pituitary at biopsy by use of the combination of RCA 120 and PI. Fluoresceinated RCA 120 is a more reliable means of staining vessels and stromata than hematoxylin-eosin or labeled antibody to fibronectin and is more rapid than the fast method for reticulin. Slides must be read within a few days, and photographs must be taken if a permanent record is desired.

▶ The classification of pituitary neoplasms on the basis of staining by hematoxylin and eosin has been superseded by immunohistochemical diagnosis. Using these techniques, it is possible to identify the secretory products of the principal cellular elements and thus characterize the tumor in terms of its endocrine activity. Heretofore, these techniques have taken some time for accurate diagnosis such that same-day, "frozen section" diagnosis has not been feasible. McKeever and colleagues take the process one step further; the described methods provide histochemical diagnosis on a rapid basis, providing the surgeon with diagnostic information during the procedure. This method has now been used in many laboratories and appears to be reliable.

Although such data will not be crucial for intraoperative decision making in every case, one can imagine situations in which it could be of substantial importance.

Primary eosinophilic granuloma of the brain may be diagnosed by strongly positive S-100 immunoperoxidase stains from other conditions (Mosciniski and Kleinschmitt-Demantars: *Cancer* 56:284–288, 1985).

Glial fibulary acidic protein and S-100 markers are present in the foloicolo-stellate cell of the human pituitary, one of the six recognizable cell types within the gland (Hitchcock, M.: *J. Clin. Pathol.* 38:41–48, 1985).—Robert M. Crowell, M.D.

The Occurrence of Dural Invasion in Pituitary Adenomas
Warren R. Selman, Edward R. Laws, Jr., Bernd W. Scheithauer, and Sandra M. Carpenter (Case Western Reserve Univ. and Mayo Clinic)
J. Neurosurg. 64:402–407, March 1986   21–16

Dural invasion was investigated in a series of 60 patients with pituitary adenoma treated at the Mayo Clinic with transsphenoidal microsurgery between January 1983 and June 1984. Although the series was not consecutive, it did include almost every case in which the surgeon judged it safe to remove a separate dural specimen.

Microscopic dural invasion was evident in 51 (85%) of the cases, usually in the form of individual cells or cell clusters. In some cases, tongues of adenoma tissue dissected between the dural planes. Invasion was most frequent in larger tumors but could not be related to immunohistochemical characteristics of the tumors. Dural infiltration had to be distinguished from incorporation of normal pituitary cells within the sellar dura, arachnoidal cell clusters within the dura, and extensive hyalinization of the adenoma.

The incidence of surgical invasiveness (40%) was greater than that previously reported. More than 90% of tumors with suprasellar extension exhibited microscopic dural invasion. Prospective studies will be needed to determine whether frequent microscopic dural invasion warrants the use of such agents as alcohol or Zenker solution or routine postoperative radiotherapy to destroy residual tumor cells.

▶ This interesting report indicates a high frequency (85%) of microscopic dural invasion by pituitary adenomas. What does this mean? The frequency of symptomatic recurrence after transsphenoidal adenomectomy is far less in reported series. The frequency of "invasive pituitary adenoma," with aggressive basal extension, is quite low. Only long-term follow-up studies after radiologic grading and operative confirmation can disclose the implications of dural invasion as a prognostic factor. It may be that some constellation of features (e.g., suprasellar extension and dural invasion) may be identified with a prognosis grave enough to warrant routine postoperative x-ray (or even proton) irradiation.—Robert M. Crowell, M.D.

Cavernous Sinus Invasion by Pituitary Adenomas

Jamshid Ahmadi, Charles M. North, Hervey D. Segall, Chi-Shing Zee, and Martin H. Weiss (Univ. of Southern California)

AJR 146:257–262, February 1986   21–17

Cavernous sinus invasion by pituitary adenoma has been rarely diagnosed preoperatively. Review of 198 surgically explored adenomas revealed evidence of direct cavernous sinus invasion by high-resolution computed tomography (CT) in 19 patients, six of whom had had previous pituitary surgery. The study group included 14 male and 5 female subjects aged 16–85 years. Several patients were scanned in both the coronal and axial planes. Most studies were done with a rapid drip infusion of iodinated contrast material.

Computed tomography revealed unilateral involvement in 14 patients, with bilateral invasion in the other 5. Tumor size was variable, but a suprasellar component was present in all but 3 of the 19 patients. In 7, the tumor had grown outside the cavernous sinus into the middle or posterior fossa. In 5 patients, it was difficult to distinguish carotid artery engulfment from adjacent tumor. Intracavernous cranial nerves were displaced, compressed, or obliterated in 14 instances. Diffuse bone destruction was present in 7 patients, and invasion of the lateral wall of the cavernous sinus in the same number. Treatment included complete or partial tumor resection, bromocriptine, and radiotherapy. Two patients did well after total tumor resection. Two of 9 patients responded dramatically to radiotherapy alone.

Any type of pituitary tumor can invade the cavernous sinus, and such involvement makes complete tumor removal difficult. Computed tomography is the best means of evaluating patients with cavernous sinus involvement, of planning treatment, and of follow-up studies after treatment. It is especially useful in the absence of hormonal markers.

▶ Sir Geoffrey Jefferson described invasive pituitary adenomas and their extension into cavernous sinus (*Sherrington Lectures,* vol. 3, University of Liverpool, 1955). These lesions have generally been regarded as unresectable, and the results of all therapy have been discouraging.

The University of Southern California group details nicely the diagnosis of cavernous sinus invasion by computed tomography scanning. Their clinical results have also been impressive. In the two cases of "total" tumor resection, natural scepticism arises regarding the initial diagnosis of invasion or the brevity of follow-up, which could eventually disclose recurrence.

The very use of the term *invasion* needs to be carefully addressed regarding means of verification. Despite negative radiologic studies, Selman and colleagues have reported that 85% of patients undergoing adenomectomy have microscopic evidence of invasion of the dura of the sellar floor (*J. Neurosurg.* 64:402–407, 1986). Perhaps cavernous microscopic invasion is likewise more common than usually accepted.

Since these lesions have such a poor overall prognosis, special management may be needed, including radical surgery. The role of postoperative heavy particle (proton) therapy needs to be assessed.—Robert M. Crowell, M.D.

Absence of Intercavernous Venous Mixing: Evidence Supporting Lateralization of Pituitary Microadenomas by Venous Sampling
Edward H. Oldfield, Mary E. Girton, and John L. Doppman (Natl. Insts. of Health, Bethesda, Md.)
J. Clin. Endocrinol. Metab. 61:644–647, October 1985   21–18

A knowledge of the lateralization of a pituitary microadenoma may improve the outcome by allowing smaller tumors to be found or the tumor-containing tissue to be removed if no adenoma is observed. The superior orbital vein empties only into the ipsilateral cavernous sinus. The extent of mixing of blood flowing from this vein through the cavernous sinuses and inferior petrosal sinuses to the junction with the internal jugular vein was determined in adult rhesus monkeys. The superior orbital vein was infused with ^{99}Tc sulfur colloid with catheters present in the inferior petrosal sinuses.

Rapid injection of contrast into one superior orbital vein opacified both cavernous sinuses, but there was relatively little mixing of blood from the vein to the contralateral inferior petrosal sinus. There was no significant difference in variation of values from the contralateral inferior petrosal sinus or the peripheral blood compared with the ipsilateral inferior petrosal sinus. Isotope activity in the ipsilateral inferior petrosal sinus before recirculation from the periphery was at least 10-fold greater than that in the contralateral inferior petrosal sinus. Activity reaching the contralateral inferior petrosal sinus was not significantly different from that in the peripheral blood.

The finding that significant mixing of blood between the cavernous sinuses does not occur supports the ability to lateralize pituitary microadenomas by bilateral simultaneous inferior petrosal sinus sampling.

▶ Sampling of inferior petrosal sinus blood has been suggested as a method for lateralization of small lesions in functioning pituitary adenomas. Though unnecessary for the vast majority of cases, in selected instances the technique may have value. The present report from Oldfield and colleagues supports this approach by demonstrating absence of intercavernous venous mixing.

The basilar venous plexus of the posterior fossa is a potential source of error in petrosal sinus sampling (Doppman et al.: *Radiology* 155:375–378, 1985).—Robert M. Crowell, M.D.

Visual Recovery After Transsphenoidal Removal of Pituitary Adenomas
Alan R. Cohen, Paul R. Cooper, Mark J. Kupersmith, Eugene S. Flamm, and Joseph Ransohoff (New York Univ.)
Neurosurgery 17:446–452, September 1985   21–19

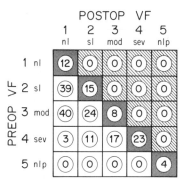

Fig 21–5.—Visual fields (VF) outcome for 100 patients (196 eyes). Scores along the shaded diagonal represent eyes with unchanged acuity. Scores below and to the left of the diagonal represent postoperative improvement. Scores above and to the right *(dashed lines)* represent deterioration. (Courtesy of Cohen, A.R., et al.: Neurosurgery 17:446–452, September 1985).

Visual outcome was assessed in 100 consecutively seen patients (median age, 52 years) with histologically documented pituitary adenoma who underwent transsphenoidal decompression of the optic paths between 1974 and 1984. Before surgery all patients had objective evidence of visual dysfunction. A simple scale was used to rank visual acuity and fields before and after surgery. Visual loss was the most frequent presenting symptom in this series, but 12 patients were unaware of visual problems. Bitemporal hemianopia was present in a majority of cases.

The mean follow-up was 26 months. Postoperative visual acuity was normal or improved in 79% of eyes and worse in 3% of eyes. Only two eyes had significantly worse acuity after surgery. The visual fields were normal or improved in 74% of eyes postoperatively and worse in none (Fig 21–5). The outcome in both respects was better in younger patients and in those with symptoms of shorter duration. Preoperative visual acuity was highly predictive of outcome, but the degree of preoperative deficit in visual fields was not related to outcome. Some patients with pronounced field deficits had considerable postoperative improvement. Two patients required repair for cerebrospinal fluid rhinorrhea. No patient had permanent diabetes insipidus. Only 1 patient required late surgery for recurrent tumor. There were no operative deaths.

These results compare favorably with those of other operative series, whether transsphenoidal or transcranial. Visual improvement was nearly always sustained during a follow-up averaging longer than 2 years. Inferior visual results were obtained in patients with previous surgery.

▶ This article nicely demonstrates that visual improvement is common after transsphenoidal surgery for pituitary adenoma. Significant worsening of acuity was rare (two cases), and no patient showed deterioration of visual fields. The data are presented in a dramatic fashion that is exemplary for presentation of the impact of surgery, as in Figure 21–5. The data are useful in advising patients for whom transsphenoidal surgery for pituitary tumor is considered.— Robert M. Crowell, M.D.

Treatment of Presumed Prolactinoma by Transsphenoidal Operation: Early and Late Results

J. A. Thomson, G. M. Teasdale, D. Gordon, D. C. McCruden, and D. L. Davies (Royal and Western Infirmaries and Southern Gen. Hosp., Glasgow, Scotland)

Br. Med. J. 291:1550–1553, Nov. 30, 1985　　　　　　　　　　21–20

The results of transsphenoidal surgery were reviewed in 77 patients with hyperprolactinoma who presented with amenorrhea, galactorrhea, and/or infertility and a persistently elevated level of serum prolactin, with impaired responses on dynamic testing with thyrotrophin-releasing hormone or metoclopramide. Sixty-one of the 69 patients with an identified tumor had a microprolactinoma 10 mm or less in diameter. The mean follow-up was 3½ years.

Changes in serum prolactin after surgery are shown in the table. Amenorrhea resolved after surgery in 39 (80%) of the 49 affected women with microadenomas, and galactorrhea in 32 of 40 patients. Infertility resolved in 82% of the cases. Four of 8 patients with macroadenomas had a satisfactory outcome. Four of 6 patients in whom tumor was not found at operation had a normal serum prolactin level after surgery. Three patients had recurrent hyperprolactinemia, including 2 of 22 patients with initially successful results who were followed up for longer than 5 years. The only serious complication of surgery was mild meningitis. One patient developed secondary hypothyroidism.

Transsphenoidal surgery is a reasonable approach in treating women with hyperprolactinemia thought to be due to a prolactinoma. The best results are obtained in cases with a small tumor where surgery is the primary treatment. Surgery is preferable to radiotherapy in patients who are intolerant of bromocriptine or who wish to avoid long-term drug therapy.

▶ The authors report excellent results for transsphenoidal surgery for 77 patients with prolactinoma. Operative morbidity was minor and symptoms resolved in about 80% of the patients. Only 3 patients had recurrence. The results support the contention that transsphenoidal surgery is a reasonable treatment approach in patients with small tumors and is preferable to radiotherapy in patients who are intolerant of bromocriptine or who wish to avoid long-term drug therapy.

Among 35 patients with prolactinomas treated by partial hypophysectomy, recurrence of hyperprolactinemia was rare even in large tumors, a finding which is more encouraging than other reports (Scanlon et al.: *Br. Med. J. [Clin. Res.]* 291:1547–1550, 1985).—Robert M. Crowell, M.D.

Long-Term Follow-Up of Large or Invasive Pituitary Adenomas

Nobuo Hashimoto, Hajime Handa, Junkoh Yamashita, and Tatsuhito Yamagami (Kyoto Univ., Japan)

Surg. Neurol. 25:49–54, January 1986　　　　　　　　　　21–21

CHANGES IN SERUM PROLACTIN CONCENTRATION AFTER TRANSSPHENOIDAL OPERATION IN 77 PATIENTS WITH SUSPECTED PROLACTINOMAS

Findings at operation	Range of preoperative serum prolactin (mU/l)	Early postoperative results		No of patients	Results after five years			
		No of patients	No (%) with prolactin <360 mU/l		No with prolactin <360 mU/l			No with sustained recurrence
					At initial follow up	After five years		
Microprolactinoma	560-11 700	61	46 (75·4)	28	21	19		2
Macroadenoma	2000-83 000	8	4 (50·0)	2	1	1		
Prolactinoma not found	1092-3880	8	3 (37·5)	2	1	1		
Total		77	53 (68·8)	32	23	21		2

(Courtesy of Thomson, J.A., et al.: Br. Med. J. [Clin. Res.] 291:1550–1553, Nov. 30, 1985.)

The long-term outcome of large and invasive pituitary adenomas was investigated in a series of 257 patients treated for pituitary tumor from 1965 to 1984. Transcranial removal of the adenoma followed by postoperative irradiation was the common therapy until the introduction of the computed tomography (CT) scan in 1976. In 1975, transsphenoidal microsurgery was introduced. Since 1979, radiotherapy was administered only in a few cases.

Sixty of 83 patients from the pre-CT era with mild or moderate suprasellar extension were still alive a mean of 13 years postoperatively. There were seven operative deaths in this group. All but 1 of 60 patients in the post-CT era were alive at a mean of 3½ years. Nineteen pre-CT and 32 later patients had huge and/or invasive adenomas. Four of the former patients died postoperatively; only 3 patients were still alive after a mean follow-up of 12 years. One of 32 post-CT patients died postoperatively; 29 of these patients were alive after a mean of 3 years. Three of 139 irradiated patients had radiation necrosis of the brain, 3 had cerebral ischemia ascribed to radiation angiopathy, and 1 patient had a postirradiation glioblastoma. Ten patients had cerebral ischemia during follow-up, including the 3 with radiation angiopathy. A majority of post-CT patients with large or invasive tumors were capable of normal activities.

Even large pituitary adenomas now can be removed transsphenoidally at low risk, with the aid of high-resolution CT. Large and/or invasive adenomas should be removed to the extent possible, primarily by the transsphenoidal route, and the patient then followed by CT. Drug therapy may be indicated in cases of functioning adenoma. Radiotherapy is recommended only for very large adenomas, biologically malignant neoplasms, and otherwise incurable functioning adenomas, and after reoperation for recurrent adenoma.

▶ Professor Handa and colleagues have carefully analyzed long-term follow-up data on a large group of patients with large or invasive pituitary adenomas. They conclude that the risk of regrowth of these lesions, in the era of CT and transsphenoidal surgery, is less than the risk of complications of irradiation, including radiation necrosis and angiopathy.

This report emphasizes complications of radiation therapy, but 9 of 12 deaths in the pre-CT patients were from undetermined causes, potentially unrelated to radiation. Also, the better results in the post-CT group could be related, at least in part, to the much shorter follow-up (mean, 3.2 years).

The Kyoto group presents an interesting point of view, but further data will be needed to overturn the conventional combination of subtotal resection and radiation therapy for large adenomas (Sheline, G. E., in Tindall, G. T., and Collins, W. F. [eds.], *Clinical Management of Pituitary Disorders.* New York: Raven Press, 1979, pp. 303–306).—Robert M. Crowell, M.D.

CT of the Sella Turcica After Transsphenoidal Resection of Pituitary Adenomas
Harvey C. Kaplan, Hillier L. Baker, Jr., O. Wayne Houser, Edward R. Laws, Jr., Charles F. Abboud, and Bernd W. Scheithauer (Mayo Clinic and Found.)
AJR 145:1131–1140, December 1985   21–22

The usefulness of computed tomography (CT) was assessed in 120 patients having transsphenoidal surgery for pituitary adenoma in 1979–1983.

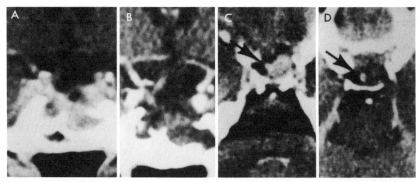

Fig 21–6.—ACTH macroadenoma at 9 (**A**) and 18 (**B**) months (5 and 15 months postirradiation, respectively). The typical decrease in contrast enhancement of residual tumor usually occurs 6–12 months after irradiation. Nonfunctioning adenoma at 6 (**C**) and 13(**D**) months (3 and 10 months postirradiation, respectively). Persistent enlargement and displacement of stalk (*arrows*), despite decreased enhancement and size of residual tumor after irradiation. (Courtesy of Kaplan, H.C., et al.: AJR 145:1131–1140, December 1985. Copyright 1985, by the American Roentgen Ray Society.)

High-resolution CT was performed before and after surgery. Functioning tumors were present in 95 patients, and nonfunctioning tumors in 25. All the latter tumors and 37 of the functioning tumors were macroadenomas more than 1 cm in size. Eight patients had had previous surgery.

CT Indicators of Success or Failure of Surgical
Treatment in 95 Cases of Functioning
Pituitary Tumors*

Finding	No. of Patients with Finding	No. of Patients "Cured" (Success) or with Residual Tumor (Failure) (%)
Success (*n* = 48):		
Pituitary stalk enlargement resolved	8	8 (100)
Pituitary stalk displacement resolved	11	10 (91)
No intrasellar abnormal enhancement	60	40 (66)
Empty or partly empty sella	47	22 (47)
Failure (*n* = 45):		
Pituitary stalk enlargement persisted or evolved	8	8 (100)
Pituitary stalk displacement persisted or evolved	28	20 (71)
Parasellar extension on preoperative CT	14	14 (100)
Intrasellar abnormal enhancement (inflammatory in 19%)	26	21 (81)

*This table summarizes the prevalence of various findings seen on preoperative and postoperative CT arranged in order of their relative value in predicting curative resection and residual tumor, as independently assessed by hormonal criteria. These trends were seen in both microadenoma and macroadenoma. Clinical status of "cure" is unknown in two cases pending follow-up hormonal and CT studies.

(Courtesy of Kaplan, H.C., et al.: AJR 145:1131–1140, December 1985. Copyright 1985, by the American Roentgen Ray Society).

Resolution of pituitary stalk enlargement was predictive of cure in all eight cases, and persistent enlargement predicted residual tumor in eight other patients. Resolution of stalk displacement predicted cure in 91% of the cases, but persistent displacement was a less reliable finding. Abnormal intrasellar enhancement predicted residual tumor in 81% of the cases. Tumor enhancement appeared in diffuse, mottled peripheral, focal, or nodular forms (Fig 21–6). None of 14 patients with functioning macroadenoma who had parasellar extension preoperatively were cured surgically. Seven of 11 patients with nonfunctioning macroadenomas and similar extension were not cured, while 4 had indeterminate outcomes pending follow-up CT. Radiotherapy and/or bromocriptine therapy frequently was associated with decreased tumor size and enhancement on follow-up CT.

Computed tomography indicators of outcome in cases of functioning pituitary tumor are shown in the table. Similar indicators should be applicable to nonfunctioning tumors, where hormonal methods are unrevealing.

▶ Detailed CT evaluation in coronal section is important to the postoperative management of patients with pituitary adenomas. Resolution of pituitary stalk enlargement is a highly reliable indicator of cure, as is resolution of pituitary stalk displacement. Intrasellar enhancement was a reliable finding with persistent tumor. These findings will be of importance in guiding further treatment, including radiotherapy and medical treatment.

Of additional interest in this study is the fact that despite enormous surgical experience, the Mayo group was unable to effect cures in 25 cases with parasellar extension. Total removal of pituitary macroadenomas with extrasellar extension is not a feasible goal.

After transsphenoidal hypophysectomy, fat is permanently recognizable on CT. Complications, including bleeding, compression by packing material, cerebrospinal fluid leaks, and pneumocephalus, can be identified. Residual enhancing intra- and parasellar lesions may still be identified (Dolinskas and Simeone: *AJR* 144:47–492, 1985).

Preoperative CT-surgical correlation in 113 cases of pituitary adenoma offered useful results (Davis et al.: *AJNR* 6:711–716, 1985). The 51 functioning and nonfunctioning macroadenomas had similar CT appearances. Only 34 of 97 secreting adenomas presented a discrete hypodense lesion; the rest were isodense. The location of normal pituitary tissue could not be determined by attenuation but only by infundibulum displacement or opposite to a focal hypodense lesion. Hemorrhage, infarction, and cyst formation were not distinguishable. Computed tomography abnormalities were uncommon in microadenomas of all types.—Robert M. Crowell, M.D.

Transsphenoidal Surgery Following Unsuccessful Prior Therapy: An Assessment of Benefits and Risks in 158 Patients
Edward R. Laws, Jr., Nicolee C. Fode, and Michael J. Redmond (Mayo Clinic)
J. Neurosurg. 63:823–829, December 1985   21–23

Transsphenoidal microsurgery is an effective primary treatment of sellar

---

Outcome After Secondary Transsphenoidal Surgery in
84 Patients With Pituitary Hyperfunction*

Patient Group	No. of Cases	Criterion for Success	Successful Patients	
			No.	Percent
pituitary hyperfunction				
acromegaly	12	GH ≤ 5 ng/ml	5	42
PRL adenoma	41	PRL ≤ 20 ng/ml	12	29
ACTH adenoma				
Cushing's disease	4	normal corticosteroids	1	25
Nelson's syndrome	24	ACTH ≤ 150 ng/ml	5	21
total cases	84		23	27
persistent hyperfunction†				
acromegaly	9		5	56
PRL adenoma	35		12	34
ACTH adenoma	19		5	26
total cases	63		22	35

*PRL, prolactin; ACTH, adrenocorticotropic hormone; GH, growth hormone.
†Patients whose only indication for surgery was persistent hyperfunction.
(Courtesy of Laws, E.R., Jr., et al.: J. Neurosurg. 63:823–829, December 1985.)

---

lesions such as pituitary tumors, but its value as follow-up treatment is uncertain. Data were reviewed on 158 patients who underwent transsphenoidal microsurgery after other treatment between 1974 and 1983. The mean follow-up was 37 months. Pituitary adenoma was present in 127 patients, craniopharyngioma in 20, and other lesions in 11. The patients were among a total of 1,210 who had transsphenoidal surgery in the 10-year review period. The current operation was performed for persistent hyperfunctioning endocrinopathy in 63 patients, visual loss in 72, and cerebrospinal fluid (CSF) rhinorrhea in 21.

Previous treatment had included surgery with and without adjunctive radiotherapy, radiotherapy alone, stereotactic radiofrequency thermocoagulation, and bromocriptine therapy for prolactinoma. The outcome after secondary surgery in cases of pituitary hyperfunction is shown in the table. Endocrinopathy was normalized in 35% of patients, and vision improved or stabilized in 59%. Repair for CSF rhinorrhea was successful in three fourths of the patients; rhinorrhea persisted in 2 cases despite subsequent measures. Mortality from disease including operative deaths was 5%.

Secondary transsphenoidal microsurgery carries a higher risk than exists in previously untreated patients, but impressive salvage can be obtained in difficult clinical situations, including endocrine hyperfunction, progressive visual loss, and CSF leakage.

▶ In this landmark article, Laws and colleagues document that in their experience, despite an increased complication rate, transsphenoidal surgery after unsuccessful prior therapy can lead to impressive salvage in a number of difficult clinical situations. It must be emphasized that these results were reported by a senior surgeon with an enormous experience that is unlikely to be duplicated in other centers. The individual surgeon should weigh this factor when considering reoperation. It is also worth keeping in mind that an experienced ear, nose, and throat surgeon may be quite helpful with the approach to the floor of the sella and reexploration of the transsphenoidal operation. It may be that proton beam therapy will play a role in the treatment of some of these failed cases.—Robert M. Crowell, M.D.

Notes on Pituitary Tumors

▶ Pituitary adenoma may present as isolated third nerve palsy (Saul and Hilliker: *J. Clin. Neuro. Ophthalmol.* 5:185–193, 1985).

Idiopathic hyperprolactinemia, without demonstrable pituitary or CNS disease, is a benign condition in which development of pituitary tumor is rare and improvement or resolution of amenorrhea and/or galactorrhea is common. Data for 41 patients who were studied for 11 years challenge the use of surgical therapy for idiopathic hyperprolactinemia (Martin et al.: *J. Clin. Endocrinol. Metab.* 60:855–858, 1985).

High-resolution computed tomography can detect unprotected parasphenoidal carotid artery in the preoperative evaluation (Johnson et al.: *Radiology* 155:137–141, 1985).

Giant cell granuloma of the pituitary may be associated with minimal pituitary enlargement and panhypopituitarism (Hassoun et al.: *Neurol. Neurosurg. Psychiat.* 48:949–951, 1985).

Rathke's pouch appears as an intra- or suprasellar, low-density mass with or without enhancement (Okamoto et al.: *AJNR* 6:515–519, 1985).

Pergolide and mesulergine may be effective drugs in the treatment of hyperprolactinaemia (Grossman et al.: *Clin. Endocrinol. (Oxf.)* 22:611–616, 1985).

Cyproheptadine, a serotonin receptor blocking agent used in treatment of pituitary tumors, inhibits prolactin release by blockade of calcium influx at the cell membrane (Lamberts et al.: *Life Sci.* 36:2257–2262, 1985).

Ishibashi et al. (*Acta Endocrinol. Copenh.* 109:474–480, 1985) report inhibition by cyproheptadine of growth hormone and prolactin from pituitary adenoma in culture.

Transsphenoidal removal of follicle-stimulating hormone (FSH) secreting pituitary adenomas can normalize levels of serum FSH and restore potency in men, according to Beckers et al. (*J. Clin. Endocrinol. Metab.* 61:525–528, 1985).

Bromocriptine normalized serum FSH levels and α-subunit levels to normal and improved visual field defects in a patient with a secretory pituitary adenoma (Vance et al.: *J. Clin. Endocrinol. Metab.* 61:580–584, 1985).

Ikuyama et al. (*J. Clin. Endocrinol. Metab.* 61:666–671, 1985) have demonstrated somatostatin receptors on pituitary adenoma cell membranes. The function of these tumors could thus be influenced by somatostatin.

Reports of radical resection of craniopharyngioma continue to appear (Al-Mefty et al.: *Neurosurgery* 17:585–595, 1985). Not all surgeons will be able to achieve good results by this approach. Intracystic radioisotope therapy has produced remarkable results for cystic tumors (Backlund: *Acta Chir. Scand.* 139:237–247, 1973). Proton beam therapy has relieved patients with solid craniopharyngiomas (Kjellberg: personal communication, 1985). The future probably holds advances in less invasive management of these formidable lesions.—Robert M. Crowell, M.D.

Other Benign Tumors

Colloid Cysts of the Third Ventricle: A Review of 36 Cases

M. Nitta and L. Symon (Inst. of Neurology, London)
Acta Neurochir. 76:99–104, 1985   21–24

Data were reviewed on operations for colloid cysts of the anterior third ventricle that were performed between 1949 and 1983 on 26 male and 10 female patients aged 12–65 years. Twenty-four patients presented more than 6 months after the onset of symptoms.

Thirty-three patients had headache, 14 had disordered mental function, 17 had visual disturbances such as blurred vision, and 7 reported episodes of unconsciousness. Six patients had leg weakness. Seven had an upper motor neuron palsy of the seventh nerve at presentation. Five had hyperreflexia with extensor plantar responses. Ventriculography has been supplanted by computed tomography (CT) as the major diagnostic procedure.

Resection has been done by transventricular exposure of the right foramen of Monro via a small postfrontal parasagittal burr hole flap. The operating microscope was used in 18 cases. Care is taken to avoid injury to the septal and thalamostriate veins. The craniotomy wound is left undrained.

Twenty-five (68%) of the 36 patients had an excellent operative result and 9 others had a good result with minimal morbidity. Two patients had a poor outcome. There were no operative deaths. Neither of two late deaths was ascribed to the colloid cyst or its treatment.

The diagnosis of colloid cysts of the third ventricle has been revolutionized by CT; ventriculography no longer is necessary. Excellent results have been obtained in most cases by resection with the use of the operating microscope. Colloid cysts can recur, but early diagnosis and excision should produce a permanent cure with minimal morbidity.

▶ This article shows that an experienced neurosurgeon can get excellent results by excising colloid cyst microsurgically through the lateral ventricle. To me, this classic surgical approach to the problem represents a record to be bested: so far the published results of the elegant but potentially more risky transcallosal approach have not been as good. Stereotaxic aspiration has been recommended to avoid craniotomy; however, many cysts cannot be aspirated and hemorrhage may be provoked in the effort. Professor Symon's results represent a standard of comparison.—Robert M. Crowell, M.D.

Management of Acoustic Neuromas, 1978–1983

Stephen G. Harner and Michael J. Ebersold (Mayo Clinic and Found.)
J. Neurosurg. 63:175–179, August 1985   21–25

Review was made of 162 consecutive operations for removal of acoustic

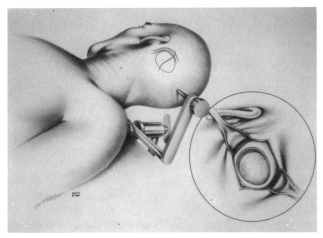

Fig 21–7.—Patient is supine with head fixed. The skin incision is 2 to 3 cm behind the ear. The craniectomy opening is approximately 4 cm in diameter. The transverse and sigmoid sinuses should be visible before the dura is opened. (Courtesy of Harner, S.G., and Ebersold, M.J.: J. Neurosurg. 63:175–179, August 1985. Printed by permission of the Mayo Foundation.)

neuroma performed on 160 patients (median age, 54 years) in a recent 6-year period. Two of 10 patients with neurofibromatosis had bilateral procedures. Nearly all operations were performed via a retrosigmoid suboccipital craniectomy (Fig 21–7), most of them with the cooperation of a neurosurgeon and an otologic surgeon. The bone defect averaged 3–4 cm in diameter. The tumor was exposed and removed from within the internal auditory canal and removed completely from the temporal bone. The final part of the dissection was individualized. Watertight dural closure is important; a dural graft substitute or pericranium should be used.

No intraoperative deaths occurred. One procedure was ended prematurely because of bleeding. The facial nerve was maintained intact in 81% of the cases and in all cases of a tumor 2 cm or less in size. Total tumor removal was achieved in all but 2% of the cases. The cochlear nerve was preserved in 55 patients, but only 14 had hearing. Cerebrospinal fluid otorhinorrhea occurred in 12% of patients and meningitis in 5%. Only 2 or 3 patients had a significant balance problem more than a year after operation. There have been 2 recurrences, 1 of them anticipated.

Acoustic neuromas can be removed totally with low mortality and morbidity. The posterior cranial fossa approach provides good exposure regardless of tumor size and facilitates control of bleeding. It has not been difficult to identify the facial nerve in the internal auditory canal. Spinal drainage and the use of the supine position and of mannitol or diuretics when indicated have minimized the need to retract or amputate the lateral part of the cerebellum. The CO_2 laser is now used to debulk some larger tumors. The facial nerve is monitored by electromyography with intermittent bipolar stimulation during surgery.

▶ This report demonstrates what experienced neurosurgeons can achieve with microsurgical suboccipital removal of acoustic neuromas. Technical points worthy of note include the use of the supine position, spinal drainage, and diuretics for reduction of brain bulk, identification of the facial nerve at the internal auditory canal, and use of the CO_2 laser with facial nerve monitoring. Total tumor removal was achieved in almost all cases without mortality or serious neurologic deficit. Preservation of the facial nerve was commonly possible in the entire group and routinely possible in tumors smaller than 2 cm. Preservation of hearing was only occasionally possible. In consideration of the approach for acoustic neuromas, these data should be compared with the results of other techniques.—Robert M. Crowell, M.D.

Cerebellopontine Angle Meningiomas: Clinical Manifestations and Diagnosis

Mark S. Granick, Robert L. Martuza, Stephen W. Parker, Robert G. Ojemann, and William W. Montgomery (Massachusetts Eye and Ear Infirmary and Massachusetts Gen. Hosp., Boston)

Ann. Otol. Rhinol. Laryngol. 94:34–38, Jan.–Feb. 1985   21–26

Meningioma is the second most frequent tumor at the cerebellopontine angle (CPA). Data on 32 patients seen between 1969 and 1979 with histologically confirmed CPA meningioma were reviewed. The 18 women and 14 men had a mean age of 55 years. No patient had bilateral tumors. The most frequent presenting symptoms were hearing loss, vertigo or imbalance, tinnitus, and altered facial sensation. Caloric responses were reduced or absent ipsilaterally in 19 of 20 patients, and sensorineural hearing loss was present in 17 of 23.

Computed tomography (CT) showed the tumor in all 27 patients examined, and in 19 it established the diagnosis. All but 15% of tumors were 3 cm or more in size on CT. Calcium was seen in one fourth of the studies and hydrocephalus in one third. All 6 brain stem auditory evoked response tests were abnormal. Ten of 21 temporal bone polytomograms yielded abnormal findings. Most patients underwent suboccipital craniectomy.

Cerebellopontine angle meningioma is often difficult to diagnose. The most useful measure is CT, and it should be performed whenever a CPA tumor is suspected. Angiography is helpful in preoperative planning. Cerebellopontine angle meningioma is a consideration in patients who have unilateral sensorineural hearing loss or symptoms of fifth nerve dysfunction.

▶ The diagnosis should be suspected in patients with hearing loss, dizziness, or altered facial sensation. Computed tomography is best in establishing the diagnosis, and the most reliable finding is a broad-based mass along the petrous ridge not centered over the porous acousticus. Angiography is a useful adjunct in planning surgery.—Robert M. Crowell, M.D.

Meningiomas of the Cerebellopontine Angle

Frank J. Laird, Stephen G. Harner, Edward R. Laws, Jr., and David F. Reese
(Mayo Clinic and Found.)

Otolaryngol. Head Neck Surg. 93:163–167, April 1985   21–27

About 10% of intracranial tumors arise in the cerebellopontine angle (CPA), and 10% to 15% of these are meningiomas. Records of 20 patients who had primary removal of a CPA meningioma between 1977 and 1982 were reviewed. None of the 14 female and 6 male patients (median age, 45 years) had neurofibromatosis.

Hearing loss was present in 60% of the patients and tinnitus in 50%; two thirds of the patients had dysequilibrium. Specific neurologic deficits were as frequent as in patients with acoustic neuroma. Three patients with meningioma had trigeminal neuralgia on the involved side. Abnormal ocular findings were the most frequent physical observation apart from hearing loss, followed by spontaneous nystagmus. Three patients had facial palsy. The median pure-tone hearing response was 18 dB, compared with 52 dB for patients with acoustic neuroma. The median speech discrimination scores were 76% and 8%, respectively. Vestibular testing gave abnormal responses in 9 of 10 patients with meningioma. Four of 17 patients had abnormal routine skull roentgenograms, and 2 of 12 had abnormal petrous apex tomograms. Seven of 13 angiograms showed a typical tumor blush and the vascular supply of a meningioma. Computed tomography (CT)

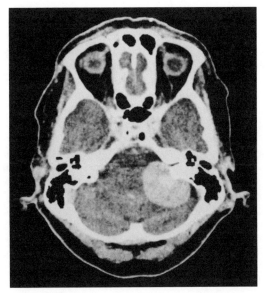

Fig 21–8.—Computed tomographic scan with contrast in a patient with 6.0-cm meningioma on left. The characteristic appearance of broad-based mass aligned with petrous ridge can be noted. The center of mass is posterolateral to the internal auditory canal. (Courtesy of Laird, F.J., et al.: Otolaryngol. Head Neck Surg. 93:163–167, April 1985.)

showed a hyperdense mass in all cases (Fig 21–8). In only two cases was the internal auditory canal involved by the meningioma. Meckel's cavity was invaded in six cases. Tumor removal was considered to be complete in 16 instances. Hearing was preserved in 6 of 18 patients.

The CT appearances of meningioma should prompt consideration of a retrosigmoid approach, rather than the suboccipital craniectomy used for acoustic neuroma. The most characteristic finding is a broad-based mass aligned with the petrous ridge and not centered over the internal auditory canal.

▶ Computed tomography, not magnetic resonance, is the diagnostic modality of choice in these cases. The posterolateral exposure including bone over the sigmoid sinus is recommended to obtain adequate exposure of these lesions. In some cases, particularly the smaller lesions less than 3 cm in diameter, translabyrinthine excision may be effective but will certainly eliminate hearing. Note that in the present series hearing could be saved in six of eighteen cases. This is a firm argument in favor of the suboccipital approach for these lesions.—Robert M. Crowell, M.D.

Operability of Intracranial Meningiomas: Personal Series of 353 Cases
B. Pertuiset, S. Farah, L. Clayes, J. Goutorbe, J. Metzger, and M. Kujas (Hôpital de la Pitié, Paris, and Antwerp, Belgium)
Acta Neurochir. (Wien) 76:2–11, 1985   21–28

Information was reviewed on 273 patients with intracranial meningioma who underwent surgery between 1958 and 1978 and 80 who underwent surgery between 1978 and 1984. In the later series, operability was assessed chiefly from the computed tomographic findings. The mean age for the 353 patients was 50 years (range, 21–74 years). Parasagittal and falx meningiomas were more prevalent in the later series. Only 9% of more recent patients had a neurologic deficit, compared with 30% in the earlier series. Intracranial hypertension was present in only 17% of the earlier group. No marked differences in seizures were apparent. Operability is questionable when a meningioma is closely related to a large artery of the skull base or to a smaller functional artery, when it is surrounded by cranial nerves, or when it is attached to the torcular. Radiotherapy is an alternative to surgery in some of these cases (Fig 21–9).

Mortality was 7% in the overall series. Fourteen patients were seen with recurrent disease. Of 53 later patients who were followed up, 90% returned to work or family life without sequelae. Operative mortality in the earlier series was highest among patients with sphenoidal ridge tumors. Most deaths were related to clipping or postoperative thrombosis of large arteries at the base of the brain.

Intracranial meningiomas are the most curable of brain tumors; surgery is advised for all patients for whom computed tomography has visualized a meningioma, although there are cases of questionable operability.

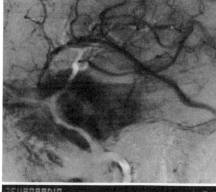

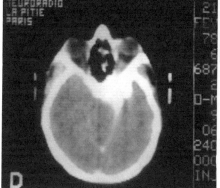

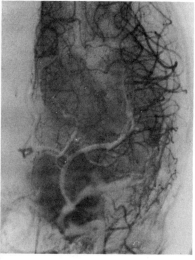

Fig 21–9.—Left-sided sphenocavernous meningioma. On the angiotomography, the internal carotid artery and its bifurcation were included in tumor. Patient refused open surgery and was given x-ray therapy, with good results during a 6-year follow-up. (Courtesy of Pertuiset, B., et al.: Acta Neurochir. [Wien] 76:2–11, 1985. Berlin-Heidelberg-New York: Springer.)

▶ Pertuiset is a master neurosurgeon with an enormous personal experience with intracranial meningiomas, including microsurgical experience. Ninety percent of patients in his more recent group returned to work or family life without sequelae. Operative disasters, particularly in the earlier group, seemed related to occlusion of large arteries at the base. Pertuiset's reflection on surgical indications will be helpful especially to the younger neurosurgeon: some meningiomas should be considered incurable, and an operation should be recommended only when there is a good chance that the patient will be better or at least no worse than prior to surgery.—Robert M. Crowell, M.D.

Schwannomas of the Jugular Foramen

Karl L. Horn, William F. House, and William E. Hitselberger (Otologic Medical Group, Inc., and House Ear Inst., Los Angeles)

Laryngoscope 95:761–765, July 1985   21–29

Schwann cell tumors arising from the cranial nerves of the jugular foramen frequently are misdiagnosed as glomus jugulare or acoustic neuroma. Experience with seven cases has shown that electronystagmography, cranial computed tomography (CT), carotid angiography, and auditory brain stem response recording all can be diagnostically useful. The site of origin of the schwannoma along the ninth and tenth cranial nerves in the pars nervosa of the jugular foramen determines its growth pattern. Proximal lesions enlarge in the posterior fossa and present with signs of a cerebellopontine angle lesion. There may be no palsy of cranial nerves IX, X, and XI, despite the presence of a large lesion. Retrocochlear hearing loss and/or vertigo may be the only presenting features. More distal lesions enlarge inferiorly through the skull base and produce palsies of the lower cranial nerves. The CT findings in one of the present cases are shown in Figure 21–10. All three patients having auditory brain stem response testing had findings consistent with the operative picture.

There is no consensus on the proper surgical management of schwannoma of the jugular foramen. A suboccipital, a transmastoid, and a combined otologic-neurosurgical approach all have been proposed. The au-

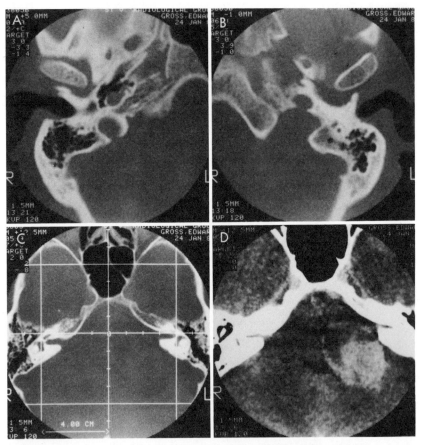

Fig 21–10.—Cranial computed tomography, case 4. **A,** normal right jugular foramen. **B,** smooth bony enlargement of the left jugular foramen. **C,** symmetric internal auditory canals. **D,** left intracranial extension of jugular foramen schwannoma. (Courtesy of Horn, K.L., et al.: Laryngoscope 95:761–765, July 1985.)

thors have used a single-stage procedure without increased morbidity. A translabyrinthine approach is useful when there is poor hearing and no cervical involvement, and a retrolabyrinthine approach if serviceable hearing is present. An infratemporal approach can be used when there is extracranial extension of disease into the neck. Complete tumor removal usually involves paralysis of cranial nerves IX, X, and XI. An attempt is made to preserve the auditory nerve in patients with serviceable hearing, but functional hearing is not always retained.

▶ The authors present results from seven cases of jugular foramen schwannoma. They point out that complete tumor removal usually involves paralysis of the lower cranial nerves. Efforts to save hearing have not usually been successful. An alternative approach is the suboccipital neurosurgical approach, which provides nice exposure of the lesion. When there is function of cranial nerves VII through XII in the presence of a large tumor, a radical debulking may be considered to preserve postoperative function. In this setting, postoperative radiation, possibly provided by proton beam, may be utilized to prevent substantial regrowth and symptoms. Loss of lower cranial nerve function is not a minor deficit, and we have seen bilateral vocal cord paralysis result from a unilateral tumor in this location.

Malignant epithelioid schwannoma can arise in a benign schwannoma (Yousem et al.: *Cancer* 55:2799–2803, 1985).—Robert M. Crowell, M.D.

Cranial Chordomas: Clinical Presentation and Results of Operative and Radiation Therapy in Twenty-six Patients
Corey Raffel, Donald C. Wright, Philip H. Gutin, and Charles B. Wilson (Univ. of California at San Francisco)
Neurosurgery 17:703–710, November 1985   21–30

Chordomas generally grow slowly, but their treatment is difficult because of local invasion and because of their proximity to critical structures. Twenty-six patients with intracranial chordoma were treated between 1940 and 1984. The 14 men and 12 women had a mean age at diagnosis of 40 years. Six of the patients had chondroid chordomas. Diplopia and headache were the most frequent symptoms. Computed tomography (CT) was highly useful in defining the extent of bony invasion and the exact relation of the tumor to adjacent neural structures (Fig 21–11). A total of 53 operations were performed. Two patients had significant postoperative complications. All but 3 patients received postoperative radiotherapy.

Eleven (42%) of the patients died during a mean follow-up of 5½ years. All 6 patients with chondroid chordoma were still alive. Six patients who received heavy charged particle irradiation were alive after a mean follow-up of 17 months. Fourteen patients had recurrent tumor after a mean of about 3 years. Two patients had metastases.

The outlook for patients with intracranial chordoma is not good at present, and it is unlikely that further surgical advances will prolong survival, since the tumor is pseudoencapsulated and locally invasive. Advances

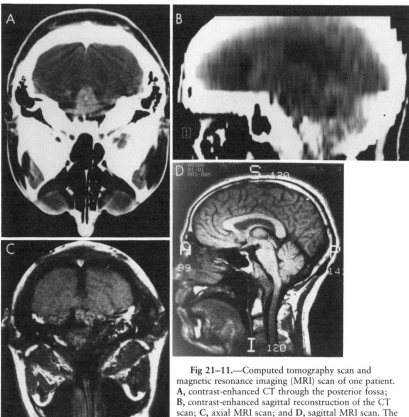

Fig 21–11.—Computed tomography scan and magnetic resonance imaging (MRI) scan of one patient. **A,** contrast-enhanced CT through the posterior fossa; **B,** contrast-enhanced sagittal reconstruction of the CT scan; **C,** axial MRI scan; and **D,** sagittal MRI scan. The precision with which the tumor is delineated on the MRI scans, especially in the sagittal views, can be noted. (Courtesy of Raffel, C., et al.: Neurosurgery 17:703–710, November 1985.)

in radiotherapy such as heavy charged particle irradiation, hyperfractionation, and brachytherapy may lead to longer survival and, perhaps, some cures. The optimal amount of postoperative radiotherapy is uncertain.

▶ Chordomas present as basisphenoid lesions with upper cranial nerve palsies or basioccipital lesions with lower cranial nerve palsies. Sagittal magnetic resonance imaging precisely depicts the pathologic conditions. Transoral needle biopsy can identify the occasional carcinoma for radiation or the soft, suckable chordoma for aggressive removal. The operative approach is dictated by the location of the lesion and the focus of symptoms. The authors emphasize anterior approaches, but approach to the clivus through the cerebellopontine angle may also be satisfactory, particularly when mass and symptoms are predominantly unilateral. Proton beam therapy has an impressive track record and should be offered.

In a related report on posterior fossa tumors, Gionnotta et al. (*Neurosurgery*

17:620–625, 1985) suggest that the translabyrinthine route may be used successfully for the removal of cerebellopontine angle meningiomas, even up to 5.5 cm in diameter. Careful cooperation of the neurosurgeon and the otologist is crucial to this approach, which we have also found valuable for such tumors. At first, the confined access hampers the neurosurgeon, but, with experience, even large lesions may be safely removed without brain retraction.— Robert M. Crowell, M.D.

Clinical and Pathologic Review of 48 Cases of Chordoma
Tyvin A. Rich, Alan Schiller, Herman D. Suit, and Henry J. Mankin (Harvard Med. School)
Cancer 56:182–187, July 1, 1985   21–31

Many chordomas are difficult to treat after a point because of their large size, but small lesions often can be controlled if treated to high radiation dose levels. Forty-eight chordomas seen between 1931 and 1981 were

SURVIVING PATIENTS AND TYPE OF TREATMENT

Site	Treatment	Status	Yr
Surgery			
Sacrum	R-hemipelvectomy	NED	8
Sacrum	Partial excision Radical excision segments S1-S2	NED	11
Sacrum	Radical excision segments S1-S2	NED	13
Sacrococcygeal	Partial excision Radical excision; coccyx and lower sacrum	NED	20
Radiation Therapy			
Base of skull	Biopsy 6100 cGy	NED	3.5
Base of skull	Biopsy 6970 cGy*	NED	3.0
Base of skull	Subtotal excision 6960 cGy*	NED	2.0
Base of skull	Subtotal excision 7660 cGy*	NED	2.0
Base of skull	Biopsy 7550 cGy*	NED	1.5
Base of skull	Biopsy 6490 cGy*	NED	1.0
Base of skull	Subtotal excision 6580 cGy*	NED	1.0
Base of skull	Biopsy 6580 cGy*	NED	1.0
L2 vertebra	Subtotal excision 6440 cGy; two more operations, specimen without tumor	AWD	8
C2 vertebra	Biopsy 7600 cGy*	NED	2.5
T6 vertebra	Subtotal excision for recurrent tumor 4000 cGy*	AWD	1.5
T4 vertebra	Subtotal excision 5040 cGy	AWD	1.5
Sacrum	Preoperative RT 5000 cGy; radical excision	NED	3.5
Sacrum	Preoperative RT 5000 cGy	AWD	2.5
Sacrum	Biopsy 6300 cGy	AWD	1.0
Sacrum	Biopsy 1200 cGy	AWD	0.5

R, right; RT, radiation therapy; AWD, alive with disease; NED, no evidence of disease progression.
*Mixed photons and 160 MeV protons.
(Courtesy of Rich, T.A., et al.: Cancer 56:182–187, July 1, 1985.)

reviewed. Pain was the most frequent symptom of vertebral column and sacral chordomas. Tumors at the skull base produced diplopia. Four skull base chordomas were of the chondroid type. Metastasis occurred in 18% of cases, always late in the disease.

Fourteen patients had surgery alone; the other 34 received radiotherapy as well. In 8 of the former group, distal sacral or coccygeal tumors were completely resected. One postoperative death occurred. Radiotherapy was given after partial tumor excision in 16 patients and after radical excision in 1. Radiation doses up to 6,000 centigrays were then used, and 3 patients received higher total doses. Palliative irradiation consistently relieved pain to some extent. Thirteen patients had local treatment failure only, and 9 others had both local and distant disease. Survival is related to management in the table. Patients who had partial or subtotal excision and radiotherapy did no better than those given radiotherapy only after biopsy, but follow-ups were short and tumor sizes were not comparable.

Patients with large chordomas occasionally do well after surgery, with or without radiotherapy. Small, unresectable lesions may respond to high-dose radiotherapy. Surgery is performed when feasible and is combined with radiotherapy whenever concern exists that the surgical margin will not be adequate. Surgical extirpation of vertebral and skull base tumors is unlikely unless they are extremely small.

▶ This report focuses on vertebral and sacral chordomas. Special note is made that patients with subtotal excision and radiotherapy fared no better than those with radiotherapy alone. Since cure by resection is possible only with very small lesions, substantial risk for loss of function should not be taken in the subtotal removal of larger lesions.—Robert M. Crowell, M.D.

Presentation of Central Nervous System Sarcoidosis as Intracranial Tumors

W. Craig Clark, James D. Acker, F. Curtis Dohan, Jr., and Jon H. Robertson (Univ. of Tennessee and Baptist Mem. Hosp., Memphis)
J. Neurosurg. 63:851–856, December 1985   21–32

Sarcoid involvement of the CNS has been described in an average of 3.5% of all sarcoid cases, but the presentation of sarcoid as an intracranial tumor mass is much rarer. Thirty such cases have been reported, 9 without systemic manifestations of disease. Five more patients with sarcoid presenting as an intracranial mass are described. Three had no signs of systemic sarcoid when first seen. The patients were seen between 1980 and 1984 at two hospitals in Memphis.

Woman, 42 years old, developed progressive hearing loss over 6 months, with occasional tinnitus, dizziness, and fasciculations of the left side of the face. Early morning headaches had also occurred for several months. A sensorineural hearing loss suggestive of acoustic neuroma was identified. Anosmia without abnormality of taste was later discovered. Computed tomographic (CT) cisternography showed a left cerebellopontine angle mass (Fig 21–12). The cerebrospinal fluid protein

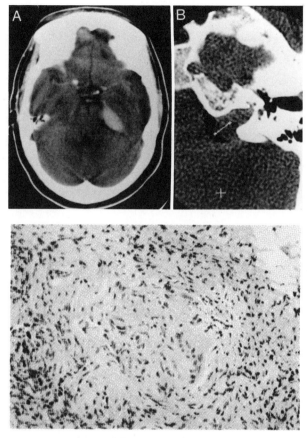

Fig 21–12.—**Top,** CT scan of the cerebellopontine angle mass (**A**). Enlargement of the scan (**B**) shows close apposition of mass along the edge of the posterior lip of the internal auditory canal suggestive of meningioma, **Bottom,** photomicrograph of biopsy material from the mass showing granulomatous inflammation. Hematoxylin-eosin; original magnification × 120. (Courtesy of Clark, W.C., et al.: J. Neurosurg. 63:851–856, December 1985.)

concentration was 119 mg/dl. At readmission for tumor removal, CT showed an enhancing anterior mass in the floor of the frontal fossa bilaterally and moderate associated parenchymal edema. Bifrontal craniotomy was performed, and necrotizing granulomatous inflammation with multinucleated giant cells was found (Fig 21–12). The cerebellopontine angle mass was also consistent with sarcoidosis, and permanent sections confirmed the diagnosis.

Computed tomography is helpful in the diagnosis and follow-up of patients with CNS sarcoidosis. The granulomatous nature of these tumor masses can be confirmed only by tissue sampling. Surgery may be useful for debulking the mass if intracranial pressure is increased. Many of these lesions respond to high-dose corticosteroid therapy, and a trial is probably advisable if specific contraindications are lacking.

▶ Neurosurgeons should be aware that sarcoidosis can occasionally present as a primary tumor of the CNS in the absence of systemic manifestations. In this circumstance, open biopsy is needed to direct further therapy, often with long-term systemic steroids.—Robert M. Crowell, M.D.

Notes on Other Benign Tumors

▶ The infralabyrinthine approach to skull base lesions involves mastoidectomy, anterior transposition of facial nerve, neck dissection, removal of the lateral tympanic bone, exposure of the jugular foramen, and exposure of the infratemporal carotid artery (Lambert et al.: *Otolaryngol. Head Neck Surg.* 93:250–258, 1985). This approach markedly enhances surgery of skull base lesions, including large glomus jugulare tumors.

Through a transsylvian microsurgical exposure, the rostral half of the tentorial hiatus may be exposed (Vorkapič et al.: *Zentralbl. Neurochir.* 46:2–10, 1985).

Meningioma cysts are probably more common than is usually realized (Worthington et al.: *Neurology* 35:1720–1724, 1985).

In tumors near the skull base, dynamic CT using arterial bolus may offer improved delineation of tumor or vascular pathology (Gointo et al.: *Radiology* 157:529–530, 1985).

After tumor removal from one side, contralateral intracerebral bleeding can occur (Shulz et al.: *Zentralbl. Neurochir.* 46:156–158, 1985).

Lithium carbonate may cause pseudotumors cerebri (Saul et al.: *JAMA* 253:2869–2870, 1985).—Robert M. Crowell, M.D.

22 Ischemia

Introduction

Bad news for cerebrovascular surgery: The extracranial-intracranial bypass study shows no benefit in protection against stroke by superficial temporal-middle cerebral artery bypass grafting (Digest 22–23). The study has appeared methodologically exemplary, but Sundt has pointed out that many patients in study centers underwent surgery outside the study, which thus raises the question as to whether the "best cases" were actually removed from the study, tipping the balance against surgery (American Association of Neurological Surgeons Meeting, Denver, April, 1986). A blue ribbon panel is investigating the implications of the exclusion of these cases from the study. It seems likely, however, that one result of this study is that the acceptable indications for this operation will diminish dramatically. Neurosurgeons in several states are fighting efforts by third party payers to refuse payment for the procedure. These efforts should be supported in that there are still indications, for example, as in cases of giant aneurysms, for which the operation remains warranted.

More bad news for neurovascular surgery: Large population studies of carotid endarterectomy indicate poor results that cannot substantiate an advantage over natural history (*JAMA*, 1986). With morbidity and mortality around 10%, the operation cannot be justified in patients with asymptomatic disease (Digest 22–1). To nail down the indications for surgery in symptomatic patients, a multicenter study is being formed with randomization as a key feature. Though such a study will be difficult to perform, the results will be worth it, because endarterectomy is under scrutiny and attack.

Studies of natural history appeared in 1986 regarding several ischemic conditions. In 32 patients with internal carotid artery occlusion, follow-up indicated that these cases do not necessarily have a worse outlook than those of patients with similar presentation and patent carotid arteries (Digest 22–2). True migrainous infarct is extremely rare and migraine may coexist in a patient with cerebral infarction from another cause (Digest 22–3). Spontaneous dissection of the extracranial vertebral artery is more common than generally recognized (Digest 22–4). Forty-three percent of patients deteriorate after hospitalization for stroke, and 25% regress markedly (Digest 22–5).

Laboratory studies have expanded knowledge about cerebral ischemia. A useful model of temporary middle cerebral artery occlusion in rats has provided information on the pathophysiology of cerebral infarction (Digest 22–6). Immunohistochemical investigation of cerebral ischemia in gerbils indicates permanent injury within an hour (Digest 22–7). Canine studies disclose a threshold of regional cerebral blood flow (CBF) for producing hemorrhagic infarction at about 50% of the preocclusion level (Digest 22–8).

Evaluation of diagnostic techniques continues. Swiebel et al. compared ultrasound and intravenous digital subtraction angiography for carotid evaluation and found similar results (Digest 22–10). Transcranial doppler sonography of the carotid and middle cerebral arteries can be used to diagnose stenosis and occlusions (Digest 22–11). Dissection of the internal carotid artery can be visualized by magnetic resonance (Digest 22–12). In experimental studies, iodine [123]IMP scintigraphy demonstrated reversible ischemia, while magnetic resonance imaging demonstrated structural damage (Digest 22–9).

Medical treatment is focused on expansion of vascular volume and induced hypertension. Keller and colleagues demonstrate improved CBF in focal cerebral ischemia induced by augmentation of cardiac output (Digest 22–13). Dopamine can improve CBF and somatosensory evoked responses in focal cerebral ischemia (Digest 22–14). Cerebral blood flow is regulated by changes in blood pressure and blood viscosity alike (Digest 22–15). Induced hypertension produces improvement in CBF in patients with cerebral ischemia after subarachnoid hemorrhage (Digest 22–16). Studies of cardiogenic brain embolism indicate that anticoagulant therapy is helpful for the prevention of brain embolus, but large infarcts and hemorrhage cases should not receive a potentially dangerous drug in the early phase (Digest 22–17).

Surgical therapy was evaluated by several studies. Emergency carotid endarterectomy for patients with acute carotid occlusion and severe deficit can produce helpful improvement (Digest 22–18). Laser endarterectomy is superior to standard endarterectomy in a rabbit model (Digest 22–19). Sundt and colleagues describe excellent results from excision and grafting of distal extracranial internal carotid artery aneurysms (Digest 22–20). Reimplantation of a tortuous internal carotid artery may be a useful technique during carotid endarterectomy (Digest 22–22). The Cleveland Clinic group describes improvement in the retinal circulation after superficial temporal to middle cerebral artery bypass (Digest 22–24). Studies with positron emission tomography show improved flow and metabolism after superficial temporal-middle cerebral artery bypass grafting in patients with stroke (Digest 22–25). Superficial temporal-middle cerebral artery bypass grafting is associated with good results in cases of moyamoya disease (Digest 22–26). In this disease, an onlay graft of the superficial temporary artery (STA) over the surface of the brain may be helpful (Digest 22–27). Emergency embolectomy for acute occlusion of the middle cerebral artery is sometimes helpful to the patient (Digest 22–28).

Robert M. Crowell, M.D.

Natural History

Natural History of Asymptomatic Extracranial Arterial Disease

M. Hennerici, D. Neuerburg-Heusler, and H. Steinfort (Univ. of Düsseldorf and Aggertalklinic Engelskirchen, Federal Republic of Germany)
Q. J. Med. New Series 55:109–118, May 1985   22–1

The proper management of asymptomatic carotid artery disease is uncertain, because it is unclear whether the risk of stroke exceeds the morbidity and mortality associated with angiography and endarterectomy. Seventy-six patients with extracranial arterial disease on angiography but no neurologic symptoms were followed up without treatment. The 65 men and 11 women had a mean age of 57 years. Risk factors included smoking in 71 patients, hypertension in 44, and diabetes in 21. All but 8 patients had a history and/or signs of peripheral artery disease and 28 of coronary artery disease. Twenty-five patients had obstructive disease in only one vessel.

Forty-six patients died during 10 years of observation, 25 of coronary artery disease. Six patients had fatal stroke, and 5 had a stroke before dying of other causes. One surviving patient had sudden stroke. Five others had transient ischemic attacks, followed by stroke in 2. The overall cumulative rate of stroke was 18%, but only two strokes involved the same territory as the original extracranial carotid lesion. Progressive arterial disease was more evident in patients who became symptomatic, but 2 asymptomatic patients had marked deterioration.

These findings suggest no obvious benefit from prophylactic carotid surgery in patients with asymptomatic extracranial disease. Severe multivessel disease may be an exception. The authors presently reexamined patients at quarterly intervals and educate them in recognizing symptoms of cerebral ischemia. The occurrence of cerebrovascular symptoms calls for immediate reevaluation.

▶ Although there are problems with this study (no controls, extent of disease poorly delineated), nonetheless the main point is clear: in patients with asymptomatic extracranial arterial occlusive disease the stroke rate was quite low, averaging 1.8% per year, with only two of the infarctions involving the same territory as the original lesion. These data add to the growing conception that there is no benefit to be obtained from prophylactic endarterectomy in these cases. The authors conceive that multivessel disease may be an exception, and, certainly, patients should be alert to the development of symptoms that would trigger surgical intervention.

Asymptomatic carotid stenosis appears to carry a risk so low that prophylactic endarterectomy is probably not justified (Colgan et al.: *Br. J. Surg.* 72:313–314, 1985). Among 209 cases of asymptomatic stenosis followed for 4 years with Doppler ultrasound and spectral analysis, stroke-free survival of 97% at 3 years was reported. Four strokes were reported: 13.5% of the arteries showed disease progression, only three in association with symptoms. Eight arteries became occluded, all asymptomatically. Of the four cases with stroke, one had less than 50%, two greater than 50%, and one greater than 75% stenosis of the internal carotid artery, which suggests a lack of correlation between the degree of stenosis and the risk of stroke.—Robert M. Crowell, M.D.

Internal Carotid Artery Occlusion: Clinical and Therapeutic Implications
Vivian U. Fritz, Chris L. Voll, and Lewis J. Levien (Johannesburg Hosp. and Univ. of Witwatersrand, Johannesburg, South Africa)
Stroke 16:940–944, Nov.–Dec. 1985   22–2

Residual symptoms and significant stroke following internal carotid occlusion are less frequent than previously thought. Among 500 patients studied at a cerebrovascular clinic, 32 were found to have 34 internal carotid occlusions. The patients were followed up for a mean of 18 months and compared with age- and sex-matched patients with similar presenting symptoms but patent internal carotid arteries on angiography. The 21 men and 11 women in the study had a mean age of 59 years (range, 44–69 years). Three patients were totally asymptomatic, while 17 presented with transient ischemic episodes, 7 had fixed initial neurologic deficit, and 5 had transient carotid events that were ignored and subsequent stroke.

Nineteen patients (59%) had no further symptoms on follow-up. Nine patients required surgery; 4 had external carotid endarterectomy; 4, internal carotid endarterectomy; and 1, extracranial-to-intracranial bypass. Twenty-nine patients (91%) of the 32 patients were well and without symptoms at follow-up. Two patients were lost to follow-up, and 1 died of contralateral stroke. Three control patients without occlusion died, 3 had late strokes, and 2 had myocardial infarction.

Patients with total internal carotid artery occlusion do not necessarily have a worse prognosis than those with similar presenting features but patent arteries. Surgery is helpful in patients with severe contralateral internal and ipsilateral external disease. Higher stroke rates in patients without occlusion may be explained in part by the lack of a common etiology of symptoms.

▶ With small numbers of patients managed in various ways and with various presentations, it is difficult to reach conclusions regarding the value of intervention. Previous long-term follow-up studies of patients with internal carotid artery occlusion has suggested a low rate of subsequent cerebral infarction from relevant ipsilateral carotid occlusion, probably in the range of 1%–2% per year. In the absence of subsequent symptomatology, long-term therapy for patients with carotid occlusion cannot be recommended. Other studies have suggested a moderate rate of progression of symptoms within the first month or so after carotid occlusion, thus giving rise to the practice of short-term anticoagulant therapy. In the absence of subsequent symptomatology, it is difficult to recommend long-term medical therapy or specific surgical intervention.—Robert M. Crowell, M.D.

Ischemic Strokes and Migraine
M. G. Bousser, J. C. Baron, and J. Chiras (Hôpital de la Salpêtrière, Paris)
Neuroradiology 27:583–587, November 1985   22–3

Lasting neurologic deficits have been documented in patients with migraine, but the precise role of migraine in the pathogenesis of ischemic stroke is uncertain. Motor or sensory deficits, speech disturbance, and visual field defects can persist after migraine attacks. Computed tomography has shown anomalies suggestive of cerebral infarcts in such patients (Fig 22–1). Areas of decreased density are seen, with or without contrast enhancement and sometimes with a moderate mass effect. The angiographic findings are diverse and often conflicting. When a major artery is occluded, angiography should be repeated after a few months, since recanalization, confirming dissection (Fig 22–2), or an arterial aneurysm (Fig 22–3) may be discovered. Few hemodynamic studies have been performed on patients with migrainous sequelae, and pathologic studies are uncommon.

Recent evidence suggests that focal symptoms of classic migraine may be secondary to a neuronal phenomenon rather than to ischemia. Computed tomography and some pathologic studies, however, suggest that the oligemic wave that follows the aura is severe enough to cause ischemia and infarction. Vasospasm has been implicated when symptoms of the aura persist after a severe attack, but spasm has only exceptionally been visualized in classic migraine. In most instances, there is no close relation between migraine and stroke. "True" migrainous infarcts are extremely rare in view of the prevalence of migraine.

▶ Cerebral infarction can occur in patients with classic migraine (Fig 22–1). In most published case reports of long-lasting migraine deficits, cerebral angio-

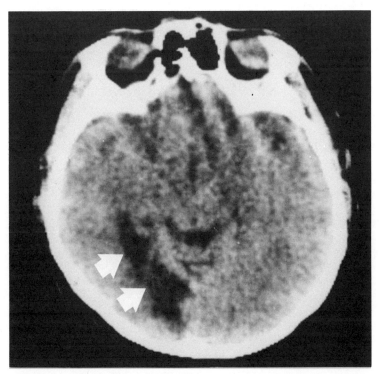

Fig 22–1.—Computed tomographic scan of a patient who had had ophthalmic migraine since childhood. After severe attack, he was left with permanent upper left homonymous quadrantanopia. The scan shows a focal hypodensity suggestive of an infarct in the right occipital lobe. (Courtesy of Bousser, M.G., et al.: Neuroradiology 27:383–387, November 1985. Berlin-Heidelberg-New York: Springer.)

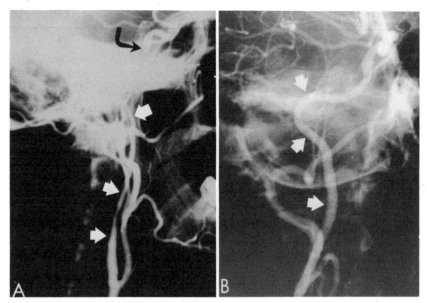

Fig 22–2.—Left carotid angiogram of a 48-year-old woman, with a long-lasting deficit in the middle cerebral artery territory after attack of classic migraine. **A,** irregular stenosis of the left internal carotid artery typical of dissection. **B,** three months later, the internal carotid artery is normal. (Courtesy of Bousser, M.G., et al.: Neuroradiology 27:583–587, November 1985. Berlin-Heidelberg-New York: Springer.)

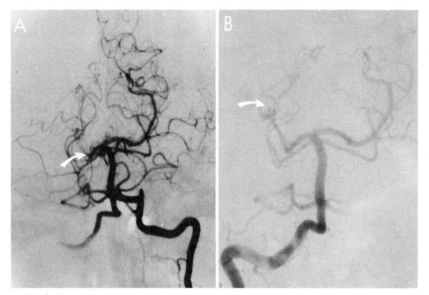

Fig 22–3.—Vertebral angiography in the patient represented in Figure 22–1. **A,** occlusion of left posterior cerebral artery. **B,** 1 year later, a small aneurysm of the left posterior cerebral artery is visible. (Courtesy of Bousser, M.G., et al.: Neuroradiology 27:583–587, November 1985. Berlin-Heidelberg-New York: Springer.)

graphs are normal. Occasionally, studies have indicated occlusion of the posterior cerebral, the middle cerebral, or the anterior cerebral arteries, and, exceptionally, the internal carotid arteries. Occlusions have been attributed to a variety of causes, such as intraluminal thrombus, kinking, fibromuscular dysplasia, and dissections. Pathologic studies on 3 patients have confirmed infarction without identification of arterial pathology.

Until recently, it has been thought that the neurologic symptoms of a migrainous aura were due to focal ischemia secondary to vasospasm. Recent cerebral blood flow (CBF) studies have indicated that the decrease in CBF appears after the aura and that oligemia progressed over the hemisphere like spreading depression. This suggests that symptoms might be due to a primary neural phenomenon. Recent positron emission tomography studies showing increased CBF with decreased oxygen extraction support this concept.—Robert M. Crowell, M.D.

Spontaneous Dissecting Aneurysm of the Extracranial Vertebral Artery (20 Cases)
J. Chiras, S. Marciano, J. Vega Molina, J. Touboul, B. Poirier, and J. Bories (Hôpital de la Salpetrière, Paris)
Neuroradiology 27:327–333, July 1985   22–4

Only 14 cases of spontaneous dissecting aneurysm of the vertebral artery have been reported as a cause of vertebrobasilar ischemic stroke. Twelve

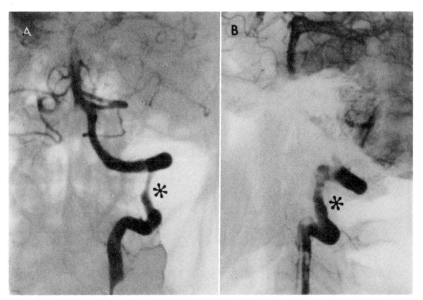

Fig 22–4.—A (front view) and **B,** (lateral view) left vertebral angiography showing localized stenosis of the third segment of the left vertebral artery (* as in figure set) due to a dissecting aneurysm. The patient also had fibromuscular dysplasia of the renal arteries. (Courtesy of Chiras, J., et al.: Neuroradiology 27:327–333, July 1985. Berlin-Heidelberg-New York: Springer.)

female and 3 male patients, aged 26 to 64 years, presented with a dissecting aneurysm of the extracranial part of the vertebral artery not due to trauma or iatrogenic factors. All patients had conventional arteriography and 10 had preliminary computed tomography (CT). Two lesions were surgically confirmed.

Predisposing factors included hypertension in eight cases, fibromuscular hyperplasia in five, oral contraception in four, and migraine in one. Eight patients had preliminary lateral cervical pain, and five had vertebrobasilar transient ischemic attacks. Two cases were discovered during exploration of bilateral dissecting internal carotid aneurysms. The angiographic appearances are shown in Figure 22–4. Stenosis was present in 17 instances, and occlusion in 3. Most stenoses were irregular, eccentric, and long. Good clinical improvement was the rule; only 2 of 15 patients had slight neurologic sequelae. Three of seven vessels evaluated 3 months after the onset had normal angiographic appearances, and two had only slight or moderate stenosis.

Dissecting aneurysm of the extracranial part of the vertebral artery is a cause of vertebrobasilar stroke, especially in younger patients. Bilateral involvement is frequent, and bilateral vertebral angiography is necessary. The frequent occurrence of acute hypertension and fibromuscular dysplasia justifies angiographic evaluation of the carotid or renal arteries.

▶ Traumatic dissection of the vertebral artery, particularly following neck manipulation, has been recognized as a cause of brain infarction for some years. More recently, Caplan has drawn attention to similar vertebral dissections without antecedent trauma. Angiography makes the diagnosis. Clinical improvement with conservative therapy is the rule, but we have seen patients devastated by these cases of cerebral infarction, particularly when it is in relation to a contralateral occlusion. The clinician should be aware that with reperfusion, especially in the setting of hypertension, infarction may develop into cerebral hemorrhage. Thus, CT scan and lumbar puncture are essential prior to institution of any coagulants in these patients. No role for surgery has been established, although it has been recommended for dissections of the proximal vertebral artery.

Digital subtraction angiography disclosed posttraumatic occlusion of both vertebral arteries in a 24-year-old patient (Laugareil et al.: *J. Radiol.* 66:605–608, 1985).—Robert M. Crowell, M.D.

Progression of Stroke After Arrival at Hospital
Mona Britton and Åsa Rödén (Karolinska Inst., Stockholm, and Danderyd Hosp., Sweden)
Stroke 16:629–632, July–August 1985   22–5

The progression of paresis and speech disorder following admission to hospital was examined in 402 consecutive stroke patients seen in a nonintensive stroke unit between 1976 and 1979. The unit had about half of all stroke cases admitted to the hospital, and the cases were representative of those of patients with stroke in population studies.

The condition of 43% of the patients deteriorated to some extent after hospitalization; that of 25% showed marked deterioration. Deterioration occurred in about one third of 39 patients for whom all symptoms had resolved at admission. Progression occurred mostly in the first 24 hours in hospital. Limb paresis characterized progression in 82% of the cases. The degree of dysfunction at arrival could not be related to the subsequent course, but progression was associated with a poorer outcome. Mortality, however, was comparable in patients with and those without progression. No clinical characteristics were found that distinguished patients who deteriorated after admission from those who did not. Patients with hemorrhage and ischemia deteriorated comparably often.

Progression of stroke after admission to hospital is a major problem. Careful supervision will detect changes in performance without delay. Nurses might usefully record a limited, standardized function test at regular intervals. The administration of heparin is preferred when progression is confirmed and hemorrhage is ruled out. Aspirin might be tried in patients with ischemic lesions, whereas in cases of hemorrhage the long-range solution is chiefly surgical. If brain edema, arterial spasm, synaptic crisis in the edge zones of an infarction, or hypotension are implicated in progression, other preventive measures such as oxygen therapy and hemodilution might be appropriate.

▶ Since fully a quarter of stroke victims deteriorate after admission to the hospital, frequent close monitoring often in a setting is reasonable to detect this untoward development. Appropriate treatment with heparin when hemorrhage is ruled out and with hypervolemic hemodilution may salvage some of these cases.

Computed tomography scanning provides useful information in a minority (28%) of patients with first stroke, who may be selected on the basis of uncertain diagnosis, cerebellar pathology, need to exclude hemorrhage, or deterioration atypical for stroke (Sandercock et al.: *Br. Med. J. [Clin. Res.]* 290:193–197, 1985).—Robert M. Crowell, M.D.

Laboratory Studies

Recirculation Model Following MCA Occlusion in Rats: Cerebral Blood Flow, Cerebrovascular Permeability, and Brain Edema

Taku Shigeno, Graham M. Teasdale, James McCulloch, and David I. Graham (Wellcome Surgical Inst. and Univ. of Glasgow, Scotland)
J. Neurosurg. 63:272–277, August 1985   22–6

Middle cerebral artery (MCA) occlusion in the rat appears to be a good model of human stroke. Previous studies have revealed a disorder of the blood-brain barrier after transient halothane-induced hypotension in this model. The development of brain edema was studied by measuring tissue-specific gravity in a model in which a snare ligature is introduced at the stem of the MCA just distal to the lenticulostriate branches (Fig 22–5) and occlusion and recirculation performed by pulling on and release the thread. This method is preferable to use of a clip, which damages the artery

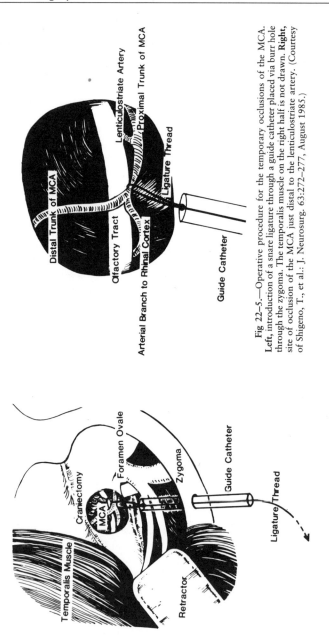

Fig 22–5.—Operative procedure for the temporary occlusions of the MCA. **Left**, introduction of a snare ligature through a guide catheter placed via burr hole through the zygoma. The temporalis muscle on the right half is not drawn. **Right**, site of occlusion of the MCA just distal to the lenticulostriate artery. (Courtesy of Shigeno, T., et al.: J. Neurosurg. 63:272–277, August 1985.)

without good recirculation. Local cerebral blood flow was measured by use of ^{14}C-labeled iodoantipyrine, and cerebrovascular permeability with ^{14}C-labeled amino isobutyric acid. Brain water was quantified by the microgravimetric technique.

Cortical blood flow was reduced about 75% during MCA occlusion, and flow in the caudate nucleus was reduced by about 65%. Reactive hyperemia was noted in the periphery of the ischemic area adjacent to the cingulate cortex on recirculation, after 30 minutes or 2 hours of ischemia. Postocclusion flow subsequently tended to become subnormal in the core region. Cerebrovascular permeability was not altered by recirculation. A significant reduction in specific gravity was evident in the entire MCA territory 4 hours after permanent occlusion. Recirculation produced no significant changes in brain specific gravity.

This model of reperfusion following focal cerebral ischemia is especially useful in autoradiographic studies. Thresholds for reperfusion cell injury can be established by varying the duration and depth of ischemia.

▶ The study of pathophysiology as therapy for focal cerebral ischemia has been hampered by difficulty with experimental models. In particular, there has not been a suitable inexpensive small animal model that permitted temporary MCA occlusion. In the past few years, a rat model for permanent MCA occlusion has been introduced. The present report contributes a modification of a snare ligature for temporary middle cerebral occlusion. The authors are to be congratulated for accomplishing this surgical tour de force. The model should be useful in the study of substantial numbers of animals for generation of statistical validity in a situation known to be highly variable.

Indomethacin caused marked enhancement of reactive hyperemia following temporary MCA occlusion in cats (Shigeno et al.: *Stroke* 16:235–240, 1985).— Robert M. Crowell, M.D.

Immunohistochemical Investigation of Cerebral Ischemia During Recirculation

Toshiki Yoshimine, Kazuyoshi Morimoto, Joan M. Brengman, Henry A. Homburger, Heitaro Mogami, and Takehiko Yanagihara (Mayo Clinic)
J. Neurosurg. 63:922–928, December 1985   22–7

Rapid disappearance of immunohistochemical reactivities for tubulin and creatine kinase BB isoenzyme (CK-BB) from the vulnerable area of gerbil brain has been seen within 5 minutes of common carotid occlusion, but it is unknown whether this phenomenon is reversible after reestablishment of the cerebral circulation. Recovery from ischemia was examined by estimating levels of tubulin, CK-BB, and astroprotein-glial fibrillary acidic protein. Animals were followed from 15 minutes to 1 month after a 30-minute ischemic insult or were examined 7 days after a 5 to 30-minute ischemic period.

The postischemic lesion, characterized by loss of reactivity for tubulin and CK-BB, developed within 60 minutes of reperfusion in the hippocampus (Fig 22–6) and cerebral cortex and within 3 hours in the caudoputamen and thalamus. The preexisting ischemic lesion resolved only after an ischemic period of less than 10 minutes in the cerebral cortex and caudoputamen and one of less than 15 minutes in the thalamus. Ischemia developed after 5 minutes in the CA1-CA2 region of the hippocampus and was largely irreversible at this site.

The immunohistochemical technique is useful in delineating recovery

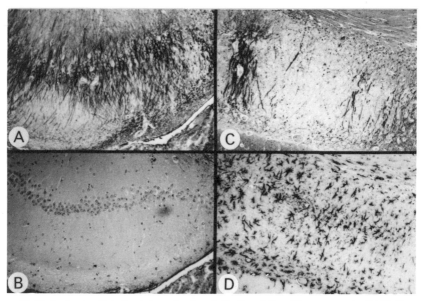

Fig 22–6.—Immunohistochemical reaction for tubulin (**A** and **C**) and for astroprotein-glial fibrillary acid protein (**B** and **D**) in CA1 region of the hippocampus after an ischemic period of 30 minutes without reperfusion (**A** and **B**) and after reperfusion for 2 weeks following an ischemic period of 30 minutes (**C** and **D**). Cell nuclei were visualized with Harris' hematoxylin, × 100. The patchy loss of the reaction for tubulin after ischemia for 30 minutes (**A**) and widespread loss of the same reaction after reperfusion for 2 weeks but with dark surviving neurons (**C**) are evident. No abnormality was found with the reaction for astroprotein-glial fibrillary acidic protein after ischemia for 30 minutes (**B**), but there were many reactive astrocytes, particularly along the stratum pyramidale after reperfusion for 2 weeks (**D**). (Courtesy of Yoshimine, T., et al.: J. Neurosurg. 63:922–928, December 1985.)

from or progression of ischemic lesions in the postischemic period. In conjunction with biochemical markers for various cellular and subcellular components, the method may help elucidate various pathophysiologic conditions of the nervous system.

▶ The authors present striking evidence of cellular injury after 5 minutes of focal ischemia in gerbils subjected to carotid occlusion. These immunohistochemical changes appear before histologic damage is evident.

Immunohistochemistry can be expected to help elucidate the pathoanatomy and treatment of focal cerebral ischemia. Application to a more clinically relevant model, such as a monkey, will doubtless provide useful data.—Robert M. Crowell, M.D.

Hemodynamics in Hemorrhagic Infarction: An Experimental Study
Hirobumi Seki, Takashi Yoshimoto, Akira Ogawa, and Jiro Suzuki (Tohoku Univ., Sendai, Japan)
Stroke 16:647–651, July–Aug. 1985   22–8

Little is known of the pathophysiology of hemorrhagic infarction. A canine model of thalamic infarction was used to examine hemodynamics, CO_2 responses, and thalamic EEG alterations after 6 hours of vascular occlusion and recirculation. Four of the 7 dogs that were studied exhibited hemorrhagic infarction. None of the 3 dogs without hemorrhagic infarction had signs of anemic infarction at autopsy.

The threshold of regional cerebral blood flow (CBF) for producing hemorrhagic infarction was about 50% of the preocclusion level. Hyperperfusion due to recirculation was observed initially in dogs with hemorrhagic infarction and was followed by a flow rate below baseline after a relatively short time. Disordered CO_2 responses were observed both during occlusion and after release of occlusion. The thalamic EEG was nearly flat during occlusion, and no recovery was evident on recirculation. In dogs without hemorrhagic infarction, regional CBF rapidly recovered to baseline on recirculation, and the CO_2 response recovered. The thalamic EEG was well preserved during occlusion and after release of occlusion in these dogs.

A prolonged decrease in regional CBF due to vascular occlusion, to below half the preocclusion level, leads to disordered cerebral hemodynamics. Dehiscence of tight capillary junctions has been described. A sudden increase in perfusion pressure on recirculation is followed by leakage of blood components at weak points and hemorrhagic infarction. A rise in tissue pressure, a decrease in regional blood flow, and damage to surrounding brain tissue result.

▶ The canine model for hemorrhagic infarction in the thalamus has been used with modern techniques for the determination of CBF. The suggestion of a threshold at 50% of preocclusion CBF accords with other measures of infarction thresholds. The results again emphasize the importance of blood pressure control, for both the upper level as well as the lower level in the care of patients with cerebral vascular ischemic disease.—Robert M. Crowell, M.D.

Comparison of I-123 IMP Cerebral Uptake and MR Spectroscopy Following Experimental Carotid Occlusion
B. Leonard Holman, Ferenc A. Jolesz, Joseph F. Polak, James F. Kronauge, and Douglass F. Adams (Harvard Univ. and Brigham and Women's Hosp., Boston)
Invest. Radiol. 20:370–373, July 1985   22–9

Both N-isopropyl I-123 p-iodamphetamine (^{123}I-IMP) cerebral perfusion imaging and magnetic resonance (MR) imaging have been used to evaluate patients with cerebrovascular disease. Uptake of ^{123}I-IMP was compared with alterations in T_1 and T_2 relaxation times in the gerbil brain following internal carotid artery ligation. Total brain tissue water was quantified as an index of cerebral edema. A dose of 100 μCi of ^{123}I-IMP was injected about 3 hours after carotid ligation.

About half the experimental animals developed severe hemiparesis. Radionuclide uptake was decreased on the side of ligation (Fig 22–7), regardless of whether or not severe hemiparesis was present. Only symp-

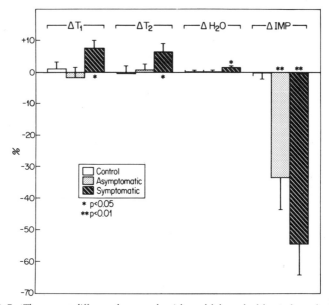

Fig 22–7.—The percent difference between the right and left cerebral hemispheres for T_1 and T_2 relaxation times, tissue water, and I-123 IMP concentration in the control, asymptomatic, and symptomatic gerbils. (Courtesy of Holman, B.L., et al.: Invest. Radiol. 20:370–373, July 1985.)

tomatic animals had a significant interhemispheric difference in T_1 or T_2 relaxation times. Relaxation times were longer on the ligated side in all instances. The only significant difference in total tissue brain water content was in symptomatic animals, with an increase of 1.4% on the side of carotid ligation.

These findings suggest that structural brain damage and edema are necessary for a change in T_1 or T_2 relaxation times after carotid occlusion. Markedly altered perfusion is observed even in the absence of symptoms. Imaging with ^{123}I-IMP may demonstrate reversible ischemia or, in a patient without MR abnormality, the presence of transient ischemia or a prestroke syndrome. Magnetic resonance imaging can demonstrate structural damage and edema.

▶ These experimental studies suggest that single photon emission, computed tomography, or magnetic resonance spectroscopy may help distinguish ischemia from infarction. As such, these studies may be helpful in the acute treatment of ischemic stroke.—Robert M. Crowell, M.D.

Diagnostics

Comparison of Ultrasound and IV-DSA for Carotid Evaluation
William J. Zwiebel, Charles M. Strother, Charles W. Austin, and Joseph F. Sackett (Univ. of Wisconsin)
Stroke 16:633–642, July/August 1985   22–10

STATISTICAL SUMMARY, PLAQUE DETECTION—HRS AND IV-DSA

	HRS			IV-DSA		
	All (n = 180)	CC & IC (n = 120)	Exclude grades 3 & 4* (n = 138)	All (n = 180)	CC & IC (n = 120)	Exclude grades 3 & 4* (n = 145)
Sensitivity	84%	95%	84%	81%	86%	82%
Specificity	77%	100%	76%	77%	100%	76%
Positive predictive value	96%	100%	96%	96%	100%	97%
Negative predictive value	46%	33%	50%	36%	16%	38%
False (−)	19	minimum plaque thickness		27	minimum plaque thickness	
	3	moderate plaque thickness		3	moderate plaque thickness	
	3	severe plaque thickness				

Severity of the plaque: most of the false-negatives were in the minimum thickness range. Minimum thickness <% diameter.

*Poor or inadequate examinations excluded.

(Courtesy of Zwiebel, W. J., et al.: Stroke 16:633—642, July/Aug. 1985. By permission of the American Heart Association, Inc.)

A total of 60 carotid bifurcations in 34 symptomatic patients were examined prospectively by both intravenous digital subtraction angiography (IV-DSA) and duplex ultrasonography, which includes high-resolution B-mode ultrasonography and a Doppler flow assessment (HRS). The average patient age was 65 years. Twelve studies were done for asymptomatic bruits, 12 for ipsilateral carotid transient ischemic attacks or transient unilateral visual symptoms, and 11 for other neurologic complaints.

The overall quality of examination was better with DSA than with the ultrasound study. Imaging of the external carotid artery was especially difficult with sonography. Both methods were more than 80% sensitive in the detection of atherosclerotic plaque (table). All internal carotid occlusions were detected by ultrasonography, and IV-DSA correctly identified five of the six occlusions. Both methods detected 95% of lesions producing 70% or greater stenosis. Specificity was good at all levels of obstruction.

Both ultrasonography and IV-DSA are potentially effective in the detection of cervical carotid artery disease. The range-gated Doppler technique can sensitively detect common and internal carotid plaque, whereas IV-DSA may overlook minimal plaque involvement. Either study can be used to select potential surgical candidates when at least 70% luminal stenosis is present. It is preferable to use IV-DSA if the chance of surgery is high and the surgeon favors operating solely on the basis of the angiographic findings.

► This study demonstrates once again that DSA and duplex ultrasonography are roughly equivalent in detection of stenosis and occlusion of the internal carotid artery. In this setting, since the ultrasonographic examination carries no risk and DSA has a small risk, it is rational to choose duplex Doppler examination for screening of certain cases, including questionable cases, high-risk cases, and follow-up examinations. Patients with cerebral infarction and typical TIAs continue to require standard angiographic evaluation, in my opinion. This is the only technique that can accurately depict intracranial stenosis and sensitively detect ulceration of the carotid artery.

Neufang and Friedmann (*Eur. J. Radiol.* 5:139–146, 1985) discussed indications for various techniques in the diagnosis of cerebrobasilar insufficiency. They suggest that duplex scanning (B-mode imaging plus Doppler flow analysis) is the first choice because it is really noninvasive and gives the same results as intravenous DSA. For precise planning of surgery, intraarterial DSA provides the safest high-quality images. Postoperative examinations of the carotid bifurcation can be done with ultrasound and IV-DSA. Extracranial bypasses are demonstrated with IV-DSA. Extracranial and intracranial bypasses require intraarterial DSA.

For patients with symptoms of cerebral vascular disease, digital intravenous angiography may be helpful, but additional testing is required in as many as 56% of the patients (Roederer et al.: *J. Vasc. Surg.* 2:327–331, 1985).—Robert M. Crowell, M.D.

Transcranial Doppler Sonography of the Cerebral Supply Arteries: Noninvasive Diagnosis of Stenoses and Occlusions of the Carotid Syphon and Medial Cerebral Artery
E. B. Ringelstein, H. Zeumer, G. Korbmacher and F. Wulfinghoff (Neuklinikum RWTH, Aachen, Federal Republic of Germany)
Nervenarzt 56:296–306, June 1985   22–11

The recently developed transcranially recorded Doppler system, TC2–64, has been successfully used for evaluation of vascular spasms after subarachnoid hemorrhage. Intracranial stenoses of the internal carotid and medial cerebral artery were diagnosed by way of transtemporal and transorbital ultrasonic recording, with angiographic control. In 16 patients with clinical or computer-tomographic evidence of an embolizing or hemodynamically active lesion, the usual Doppler sonography was used at the extracranial segments, with regular findings in 13 instances on extracranial examination. Of 9 patients with pathologic Doppler results, 3 had been admitted with severe neurologic deficits a few hours after the acute insult. In the latter, Doppler sonography of the extracranial carotid arteries had suggested intracranial "occlusion" of the internal carotid artery, a diagnosis which, on further analysis by way of transcranial Doppler sonography, proved to be high-grade stenoses (Fig 22–8). Moreover, transcranial Doppler sonography proved a reliable means of monitoring patients under anticoagulation treatment for intracranial stenoses, thus avoiding unnecessary control angiographies.

Although this small number of patients does not allow definitive conclusions regarding the sensitivity and specificity of the method, it is evident that transcranial Doppler sonography is a valuable tool in clinical neuroangiology.

▶ Further experience with transcranial Doppler ultrasonography is presented. It is suggested that this method is a reliable means of monitoring patients with

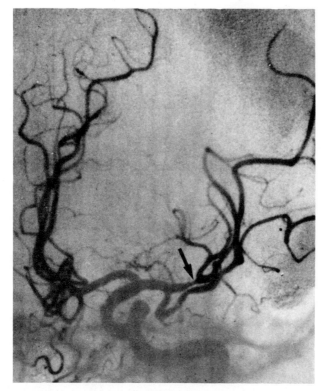

Fig 22–8.—Angiographic and Doppler-sonographic findings in a patient with stenosis of a main branch of the medial cerebral artery. **A,** the moderate degree stenosis is marked by *arrow.* The poststenotic dilatation of the adjoining vascular segment is striking. (Courtesy of Ringelstein, E.B., et al.: Nervenarzt 56:296–306, June 1985. Berlin-Heidelberg-New York: Springer.)

intracranial stenosis. To clearly establish the utility of this method for demonstration of hemodynamically significant intracranial stenotic lesions, reference to a commonly accepted standard will be needed; it is difficult to escape the need for correlation of transcranial Doppler studies with cerebral angiography.—Robert M. Crowell, M.D.

Cervical Internal Carotid Artery Dissecting Hemorrhage: Diagnosis Using MR

Herbert I. Goldberg, Robert L. Grossman, John M. Gomori, Arthur K. Asbury, Larissa T. Bilaniuk, and Robert A. Zimmerman (Univ. of Pennsylvania)
Radiology 158:157–161, January 1986   22–12

Prompt diagnosis of carotid dissecting hemorrhage (CDH) of the cervical internal carotid artery can prevent complicating embolic stroke. The "string" sign is a highly characteristic but not completely specific angiographic sign. A false lumen is rarely seen in CDH. Magnetic resonance

(MR) imaging was carried out in 2 men with spontaneous dissection of the internal carotid artery, after intervals of 12 and 16 days, respectively. T_1-weighted images were obtained in both patients, T_2-weighted images in 1.

Man, 49 years old, had difficulty swallowing and speaking 2 weeks before admission, followed by hoarseness and progressive dysphagia, severe headache over the left side of the face and head, and drooping of the left upper eyelid. The symptoms began 5 days after a severe upper respiratory infection with marked coughing. Examination showed paralysis in the area of the left ninth through twelfth cranial nerves. Carotid angiography showed irregular narrowing of the left internal carotid artery (Fig 22–9). Magnetic resonance imaging (Fig 22–10) showed crescentic thickening of the arterial wall that spiraled distally around the artery, involving the medial, then the posterior, and finally the posterolateral portions. Computed tomography (CT) showed no relevant abnormality. Repeat MR imaging 7 weeks later showed normal appearances on both T_1- and T_2-weighted images.

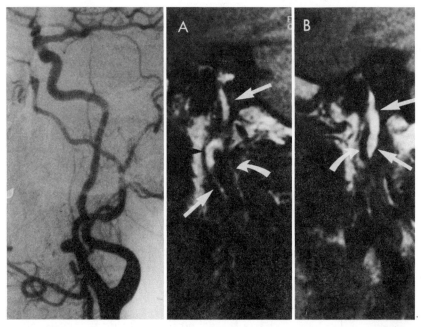

Fig 22–9 (left).—Case 1. Anterior oblique projection, left common carotid angiogram demonstrates a rippled irregularity along both walls of the internal carotid artery beginning about 4 cm distal to the bifurcation and extending into the horizontal portion of the petrous canal segment. There is only minimal narrowing of the artery just below the petrous bone.

Fig 22–10(A,B).—Case 1. Adjacent sagittal T_1-weighted 3-mm-thick sections through the middle and distal cervical and proximal petrous segments of the left ICA. A sharply marginated hyperintense mass *(straight arrows)* appears first in the anterior wall in A and spirals around the lumen *(curved arrows)* to be mainly within the posterior wall in the distal cervical and petrous segments of the ICA (**B**). Because of tortuosity, only a portion of the ICA is seen in any one section. In A, the section does not pass through the ICA lumen in the upper cervical region but does show the hyperintensity of the mural hematoma *(upper straight arrow)*, which could be confused with an interstitial fat plane.

(Courtesy of Goldberg, H.I., et al.: Radiology 158:157–161, January 1986. Reproduced with permission of the Radiological Society of North America.)

Magnetic resonance imaging can demonstrate the arterial wall and vascular lumen noninvasively without the need for contrast material. The MR findings in the present cases corresponded exactly to the luminal changes seen at angiography. This modality appears useful for the demonstration of CDH through visualization of the intramural clot and luminal stenosis. If specific vessel wall changes are detected in the first days, more cases might be diagnosed before the occurrence of embolic infarction, which may be prevented by the institution of antithrombotic or antiplatelet therapy.

▶ The clinical presentation of internal carotid dissection is distinctive. Cranial pain, abrupt hemispheric deficit, and ipsilateral Horner's syndrome often belie the diagnosis. But, on occasion, the diagnosis may be obscure (the cranial nerve signs in the reported case histories are not characteristic). In such cases, angiography is the key diagnostic study. Usually, a "string sign" or distal aneurysmal pouch will clinch the diagnosis (Fisher, et al.: *Can. J. Neurol. Sci.* 5:9–19, 1978). Often the artery will recanalize, and the best treatment is usually anticoagulation.

The advent of noninvasive diagnosis for cervical (and perhaps intracranial) dissections is welcome. The present report shows nicely that cervical carotid dissection can be detected by MR imaging. Hodge and co-workers in Syracuse have presented transverse CT images that also demonstrate dissections. Further investigations will be needed to clarify the roles of these promising approaches.—Robert M. Crowell, M.D.

Medical Treatment

Modification of Focal Cerebral Ischemia by Cardiac Output Augmentation
Ted S. Keller, John E. McGillicuddy, Virginia A. LaBond, and Glenn W. Kindt (Univ. of Michigan)
J. Surg. Res. 39:420–432, November 1985   22–13

Intravascular volume expansion is effective as an adjunct to the treatment of ischemia from cerebral vasospasm after subarachnoid bleeding from ruptured aneurysm, but the physiologic mechanisms involved are not understood. The effects of cardiac output and hemodilution were examined in a primate model of focal cerebral ischemia. Local cerebral blood flow (CBF) estimates in anesthetized adult rhesus monkeys were made by the hydrogen clearance technique after unilateral middle cerebral artery occlusion and blood volume expansion with Dextran 40 or isovolumic hemodilution with the cardiac output kept constant. In the former group, 20–50-ml boluses of warmed 10% Dextran 40 were given until the cardiac output plateaued at its peak level.

A significant increase in local CBF occurred in ischemic regions only and only in response to augmentation of cardiac output. Isovolumic hemodilution produced no significant changes in local CBF. Gross pathologic findings were minimal, as expected from ischemia lasting only 3 to 6 hours.

Ischemic regions of the brain are selectively vulnerable to changes in cardiac output, apart from blood pressure alterations. Changes in blood viscosity may be only a minor factor. Intravascular volume expansion and cardiac output augmentation seem to have an important role in the management of acute ischemic stroke. Collateral circulation to an area of brain normally supplied by an occluded vessel presumably is augmented by increased systemic circulatory activity. Intravascular volume expansion has been useful in the treatment of patients with carotid occlusive disease and ischemic stroke, especially those in whom clinical dehydration or hypovolemia is present.

▶ The authors present experimental data indicating that augmentation of cardiac output (but not isovolemic hemodilution) improves local CBF in experimental focal cerebral ischemia. This implies that volume expansion is important, whereas rheologic improvement of viscosity may be less so. Wood and colleagues (*J. Neurosurg.* 56:80–91, 1982) emphasized that hemodilution was a critical mechanism in improved CBF after volume expansion. In their experiments, however, cardiac output was also improved (+58%–114%, depending on the infusion).

Regardless of the precise mechanism, the present report and others tend to support the concept that intravascular volume expansion may provide a useful edge in the treatment of cerebrovascular insufficiency. Clinical studies likewise support this concept, especially if clinical dehydration or hypovolemia is present.

Grotta et al. (*Stroke* 16:790–795, 1985) report safe and successful monitoring of pulmonary wedge pressure in nine patients undergoing hemodilution therapy for acute cerebral ischemia.—Robert M. Crowell, M.D.

Effects of Dopamine on Cortical Blood Flow and Somatosensory Evoked Potentials in the Acute Stages of Cerebral Ischemia
Yoku Nakagawa, Hitoshi Kinomoto, and Hiroshi Abe (Hokkaido Univ., Japan)
Stroke 17:25–30, Jan.–Feb. 1986   22–14

Maintenance of blood flow is critical in the management of acute cerebral ischemia. The efficacy of infused dopamine was examined in a canine model of cerebral ischemia produced by middle cerebral artery occlusion. Cortical blood flow (CBF) was monitored by the H_2 clearance technique, and somatosensory evoked potentials (SSEPs) were recorded. The P_1-to-N_1 peak-to-peak amplitude was obtained by stimulating the contralateral sciatic nerve. Dopamine was infused in doses of 25–65 γ. The study lasted 2½ hours.

Cortical blood flow and the SSEP recovered at doses of 5–10 γ dopamine, with little rise in systemic arterial pressure. Both parameters were restored at doses of 20 and 30 γ, with a rise in mean systemic arterial pressure of 5–15 mm Hg. Recovery of the SSEP was slight at the 65-γ dose of dopamine, despite definite increases in arterial pressure and CBF.

Dopamine has a vasodilatory effect at low doses and a blood pressure-enhancing effect at high doses. Enhanced cerebral blood flow can be expected at high dose levels, but brain edema may become worse. Careful control of dopamine infusion is necessary when used to maintain cortical blood flow in acute cerebral ischemia.

▶ Dopamine infusion can increase CBF in normal and ischemic brain tissue (von Essen et al.: *Surg. Neurol.* 13:181–188, 1980). The report by Nakagawa and colleagues emphasizes that low-dose dopamine (β-action) can improve CBF without elevation of arterial pressure and without cerebral edema. These deleterious effects are common with high-dose dopamine (α-action). Direct CBF measurements are helpful in guiding dopamine therapy for cerebral ischemia.—Robert M. Crowell, M.D.

Cerebral Blood Flow Is Regulated by Changes in Blood Pressure and in Blood Viscosity Alike
J. Paul Muizelaar, Enoch P. Wei, Hermes A. Kontos, and Donald P. Becker (Med. College of Virginia)
Stroke 17:44–48, Jan.–Feb. 1986   22–15

The influence of blood viscosity on cerebral blood flow (CBF) remains uncertain, but a previous study in cats showed good correlation between mannitol-induced change in blood viscosity and changes in pial arteriolar diameter. Cerebral blood flow was estimated with use of microspheres in 23 cats in which autoregulation was disturbed in the left caudate nucleus by microsurgical occlusion of the middle cerebral artery. Hypotension was induced with adenosine triphosphate (ATP) and hypertension with angiotensin. Mannitol was given as a 25% solution in water at 37 C in a dose of 1 gm/kg of body weight in 1 minute.

In all cats, blood viscosity decreased an average of 16% at 15 minutes and increased 10% in 16 cats at 75 minutes after administration of mannitol. Changes in CBF were minimal in areas of normal autoregulation, but, with impaired autoregulation, CBF decreased 21% with hypotension and 18% with increased viscosity. Cerebral blood flow increased 56% in the left caudate with hypertension, and 47% with lower viscosity. Comparable observations were made in the ectosylvian cortex, which is nearly exclusively supplied by the middle cerebral artery in cats.

Lower blood viscosity leads to vasoconstriction when autoregulation is intact, thus maintaining CBF constant but decreasing cerebral blood volume with an ensuing decrease in intracranial pressure, whereas with a defective autoregulation the lower viscosity from mannitol leads to an increase in CBF without an effect on vessel diameter, cerebral blood volume, or intracranial pressure.

▶ Mannitol causes a decrease in blood viscosity and an increase in CBF in ischemic brain tissue. Muizelaar and colleagues provide persuasive evidence that the effects on local CBF caused by mannitol do not require a change in blood pressure, cerebral blood volume, or intracranial pressure. The results are encouraging for use of mannitol in cases of focal cerebral ischemia. Dr.

Jafar of our department has collected a series of clinical case histories that bear out these expectations: mannitol infusion in patients with ischemia due to vasospasm has resulted in improved CBF and neurologic status, without evidence of increases in blood pressure or intracranial pressure (Jafar et al.: *J. Neurosurg.* 64:754–759, 1986).—Robert M. Crowell, M.D.

Induced Hypertension for the Treatment of Cerebral Ischemia After Subarachnoid Hemorrhage: Direct Effect on Cerebral Blood Flow

J. Paul Muizelaar and Donald P. Becker (Med. College of Virginia)
Surg. Neurol. 25:317–325, April 1986   22–16

Cerebral infarction from vasospasm remains one of the leading causes of morbidity and mortality in patients with aneurysmal subarachnoid hemorrhage. Five of 43 patients operated on for ruptured aneurysms of the anterior circulation postoperatively developed clinical cerebral ischemia. For 4 of these patients, vasospasm was diagnosed by cerebral blood flow (CBF) measurement. Arterial hypertension was induced with phenylephrine in these 5 patients and, in 1 patient, hemodilution was also instituted.

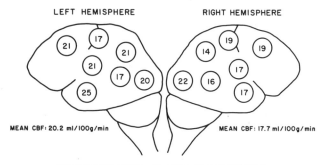

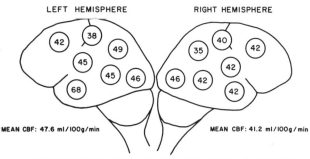

Fig. 22–11.—Effect of induced hypertension on regional CBF. (Courtesy of Muizelaar, J.P., and Becker, D.P.: Surg. Neurol. 25:317–325, April 1986. Reprinted by permission of the publisher. Copyright 1986, Elsevier Science Publishing Co., Inc.)

Hemispheric blood flow increased in both the operated on and contralateral sides, and a positive clinical effect was noted in all instances.

Woman, 39 years old, had a sudden severe headache 5 days before admission, for which she visited an emergency room. She presented with a loss of consciousness that had preceded a motor vehicle accident. She was conscious and neurologically intact an hour later, when cranial computed tomography (CT) showed much blood in the basal cisterns. Deep coma ensued, with decerebrate posturing to painful stimuli. Computed tomography showed more subarachnoid blood and moderate hydrocephalus. An intraventricular catheter was inserted. Angiography showed right posterior communicating and middle cerebral aneurysms and moderate basilar artery spasm. Both aneurysms were clipped, and a third one on the anterior choroidal artery was reinforced with muslin. Left hemiplegia developed 6 days after surgery. Phenylephrine reversed the deficit and increased the CBF on the right side from very low values (Fig 22–11). Treatment continued for a week. The patient had recovered completely 3 weeks after the subarachnoid hemorrhage and returned to work shortly after.

Measurements of CBF are preferable to cerebral angiography, especially in comatose patients with subarachnoid hemorrhage, in whom it is difficult to recognize focal signs.

▶ Induced hypertension caused an increase in CBF and clinical improvement in all 5 patients with vasospasm after subarachnoid hemorrhage. This report bolsters previous claims for the effectiveness of induced hypertension (Kassell et al.: *Neurosurgery* 11:337–343, 1982), particularly by showing enhanced CBF in previously ischemic zones.

A novel feature of the report is the contention that CBF measurement is an adequate study for diagnosis of vasospasm. However, it has always been difficult to diagnose vasospasm with certainty, unless angiography has been performed. The variability of test-retest values with CBF determination is considerable. Before we can rely on CBF determinations to diagnose spasm, we need data correlating CBF levels and angiographic evidence of arterial narrowing.—Robert M. Crowell, M.D.

Cardiogenic Brain Embolism
Cerebral Embolism Task Force
Arch. Neurol. 43:71–84, January 1986   22–17

One of every six ischemic strokes is caused by cardiogenic embolism. Embolic stroke is often extensive and functionally devastating and is usually preceded by warning transient ischemic attacks. Many patients with ischemic stroke have both a potential cardiac source of emboli and cerebral vascular disease, so that it is often difficult to determine which accounts for the stroke in an individual patient. Nonrheumatic atrial fibrillation is the most frequent underlying disorder; patients with this dysrhythmia have a fivefold increase in the risk of stroke. The other major sources of cardioembolic strokes are ischemic heart disease (25%), rheumatic mitral stenosis (10%), and a prosthetic cardiac valve (10%). Mitral valve prolapse is associated with cerebral ischemia, but the risk of stroke in affected young adults is low. Less frequent causes of embolic stroke are mitral annulus calcification, calcific aortic stenosis, nonbacterial thrombotic endocarditis, atrial myxoma, and bacterial endocarditis. Paradoxical embolism is seen in congenital heart disease.

A program for the management of anticoagulant therapy in embolic stroke was developed. The optimal range of anticoagulation for preventing and treating brain embolism is uncertain, and properly designed clinical studies are unavailable. Platelet antiaggregation agents have been evaluated in patients with prosthetic heart valves, but their use in other types of cardiogenic brain embolism remains empirical. The best time to begin anticoagulation after aseptic cardiogenic brain embolism is also unknown, but immediate heparinization probably reduces the risk of early recurrent embolism. The risk of symptomatic brain hemorrhage with immediate anticoagulation is difficult to determine. Immediate anticoagulation of small- to moderate-sized embolic strokes may, however, be beneficial if a computed tomographic scan, performed 24–48 hours after stroke, shows no bleeding. Delayed hemorrhagic transformation may be more likely with a large embolic infarct, and it may be wise to postpone anticoagulation for 5–7 days in these cases.

▶ Heparin clearly reduces the risk of recurrent cerebral embolism. But pale infarcts may become hemorrhagic after heparinization. This leaves the clinician in a quandary: should the patient with an embolic stroke be anticoagulated?

This report provides data upon which to base a treatment plan. The algorithm in Figure 7 in the original article represents a rational approach to the patient with cardiogenic brain embolism, and I recommend it be sought out.

It is important to remember that the carotid bifurcation is another common source of emboli to the brain.—Robert M. Crowell, M.D.

Surgical Treatment

Emergency Carotid Endarterectomy for Patients With Acute Carotid Occlusion and Profound Neurological Deficits

Fredric B. Meyer, David G. Piepgras, Burton A. Sandok, Thoralf M. Sundt, Jr., and Glenn Forbes (Mayo Clinic and Mayo Graduate School of Medicine)
Ann. Surg. 203:82–89, January 1986   22–18

Emergency carotid endarterectomy generally has been considered contraindicated in patients with acute occlusion and profound ischemic deficit; however, the natural course of such patients is grave. From January 1973 to November 1984, 2,036 carotid endarterectomies were performed at the Mayo Clinic. Of these, 34 emergency endarterectomies were done for acute occlusion with profound neurologic deficits. Three patients had a progressing deficit. There were 20 male and 14 female patients with an average age of 68 years. Twenty patients had occlusion of a known high-grade internal carotid stenosis; for 10 of these, administration of heparin was discontinued in anticipation of elective endarterectomy. In 9 patients, occlusion occurred within 1 hour of cerebral angiography, 8 of these being performed by direct carotid puncture. The average follow-up was 5.4 years.

A shunt was used in 33 patients. A Fogarty catheter (no. 3 or no. 4) was used to assist thrombus removal in 10 cases. Nine patients returned to normal after endarterectomy, and 4 others made a good recovery. Ten patients made a fair recovery, 4 had a poor outcome, and 7 (21%) died. The operation was technically successful in 32 (94%) of the patients. Two deaths were due to hemorrhagic infarction. The outcome was not closely related to the time of oligemia, but patients with middle cerebral artery embolism had a poor prognosis. Collateral flow was a factor in the outcome.

Emergency carotid endarterectomy may be indicated in selected cases of acute internal carotid occlusion with profound neurologic deficit. Full preoperative angiography may identify those patients who would benefit from surgical intervention and reduce the surgical mortality. Surgery is not recommended after a long delay. The most favorable prognostic factors in the present series were good collateral flow and the absence of middle cerebral artery embolism.

▶ Emergency carotid endarterectomy can sometimes reverse severe deficits from acute carotid occlusion. The present report supports this conclusion, reported some years ago by Fisher and Ojemann (*Clin. Neurosurg.* 22:214–263, 1975). Several preoperative findings indicate little chance for recovery; these include dense hemiplegia with drowsiness, large hypodense lesion on computed tomography, and middle cerebral artery embolism with poor collateral. Favorable findings indicating a good chance for recovery include stuttering or partial deficit and good collateral on angiography.

Emergency endarterectomy should be reserved for the neurosurgeon who has established a good track record with elective endarterectomy. Be sure that the family is aware of the patient's preoperative condition to confirm the deficit.—Robert M. Crowell, M.D.

Experimental Arteriosclerosis Treated by Conventional and Laser Endarterectomy
John Eugene, Stephen J. McColgan, Marc E. Pollock, Marie Hammer-Wilson, Earl W. Moore-Jeffries, and Michael W. Berns (VA Med. Ctr., Long Beach; Univ. of California at Irvine; and Beckman Laser Inst. and Med. Clinic, Irvine)
J. Surg. Res. 39:31–38, July 1985   22–19

Laser vaporization of atheromatous plaques by catheter methods is feasible, but target localization and uneven depth of plaque penetration are problems. The open laser and conventional methods of endarterectomy were compared in a rabbit model of arteriosclerosis. The aorta was exposed thoracoabdominally, and either conventional endarterectomy or a laser procedure was performed, the latter with an argon ion laser at a power of 1.0 W. Exposures of 1–5 joules were used to create a line of craters

0.4–0.5 mm in diameter at the ends of the atheroma. The craters were connected by exposures of 10–20 joules, which developed a cleavage plane within the media. The plaque finally was removed and the end points fused by continuous radiation at 10–20 joules.

The end points of laser endarterectomies were more even and better defined than those of conventional surgery. In conventional cases the cleavage plane was just beneath the internal elastic lamina. There was no damage to other layers of the vessel wall. Carbonization of remaining tissues was minimal in the laser specimens. A majority of distal end points showed a smooth transition, in contrast to the rough transitions seen in most conventional surgery specimens.

Argon ion laser endarterectomy is superior to standard endarterectomy in the rabbit model. There is no good animal model for severe calcified human arteriosclerosis, but open laser endarterectomy provides a uniform technique for studying the effects of laser radiation on arteriosclerotic arteries in initial clinical trials.

▶ This interesting report suggests that laser endarterectomy performed in an open fashion may produce a superior anatomical result in rabbits. Whether this could produce a superior endarterectomy in humans remains to be demonstrated. I can imagine that in circumstances in which a limited removal of plaque is desired—for example, the redo-endarterectomy for recurrence stenosis for which a cleavage plane may be extremely difficult to identify—such a technique might offer some clinical advantage. Another circumstance might be that of the extremely pitted wall of certain invasive plaques, in which superficial laser lesions might produce a smoother luminal lining.

A different application of laser in this field has been suggested with regard to coronary arteriosclerosis: a transvascularly placed fibrooptic laser probe has been introduced into the coronary arteries to vaporize coronary plaque. A similar technique might be utilized to vaporize carotid plaque; it would be important to devise a method for egress of vapor and debris without cerebral embolization. Much investigation remains to be done before this space-age partnership can be tested clinically.—Robert M. Crowell, M.D.

Surgical Management of Aneurysms of the Distal Extracranial Internal Carotid Artery
Thoralf M. Sundt, Jr., Bruce W. Pearson, David G. Piepgras, O. Wayne Houser, and Bahram Mokri (Mayo Clinic)
J. Neurosurg. 64:169–182, February 1986   22–20

Nineteen patients had surgery for unilateral aneurysmal lesions of the extracranial internal carotid artery (ICA) from 1978 through 1985, and 1 had two procedures for bilateral aneurysms of this vessel. Dissection of the ICA was the most common underlying cause; there were seven traumatic dissections and six spontaneous dissections. Fourteen patients presented with ischemic symptoms.

Treatment was individualized according to the site and size of the aneu-

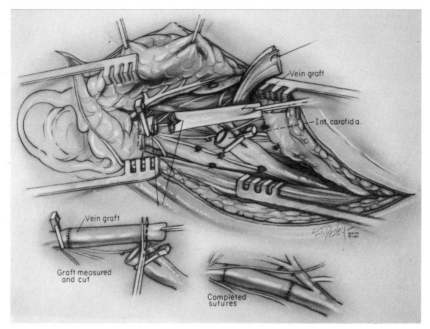

Fig 22–12.—The proximal and distal ICAs are temporarily occluded with soft low-pressure intracranial vascular clips. Proximal and distal ends of ICA are prepared in fishmouth fashion as is the sphenous vein, which is sewn into place distally with the aid of the operating microscope, with interrupted 7–0 or 8–0 monofilament nylon sutures and microvascular instruments. The proximal end of the anastomosis is constructed with 6–0 interrupted Prolene sutures. Although proximal and distal self-retaining retractors are illustrated in this diagram, less traumatic retraction is provided by the use of spring or elastic activated fishhook restraints. (Courtesy of Sundt, T.M., Jr., et al.: J. Neurosurg. 64:169–182, February 1986.)

rysm, symptoms, and the hemodynamic findings from radioxenon clearance studies. Seven patients had resection of the aneurysm with placement of an interposition saphenous vein graft (Fig 22–12). Five others had resection with end-to-end anastomosis of the ICA. Internal carotid artery ligations were performed in 3, aneurysmal clipping was carried out in 1, and extracranial-to-intracranial bypass in 4. One patient had mild permanent impairment of hand function from cerebral ischemia. Four patients had transient dysphagia. The long-term outcome has been excellent, except in 1 patient with severe preoperative dysphagia. Postoperative angiograms confirmed the patency of all interposition grafts and bypass pedicles.

Intraoperative cerebral blood flow estimates and EEG monitoring can help prevent cerebral ischemic complications during surgery for aneurysm of the distal extracranial internal carotid artery. The operating microscope is used when suturing an interposition vein graft. Resection of the stylomandibular ligament allows the mandible to be displaced anteriorly. It is not necessary to resect the mandible or dislocate the jaw or to resort to any other potentially disfiguring approaches to gain access to the distal ICA.

▶ The authors present a spectacular series of cases with anatomical reconstructions and good results in nearly all patients. It is important to remember that (1) most carotid dissections are best treated conservatively, and that (2) Dr. Sundt and colleagues have enormous experience with carotid endarterectomy. These cases are not for the occasional endarterectomy surgeon.—Robert M. Crowell, M.D.

Extracranial Carotid Aneurysms: Report of Six Cases and Review of the Literature
Thomas A. Painter, Norman R. Hertzer, Edwin G. Beven, and Patrick J. O'-Hara (Cleveland Clinic)
J. Vasc. Surg. 2:312–318, March 1985   22–21

Direct reconstruction of cervical carotid artery aneurysms can be performed by use of modern methods of cerebral protection and revascularization, with risks nearly comparable with those of carotid endarterectomy for occlusive disease. Six patients have had such reconstructions since 1977, among more than 1,500 patients requiring carotid artery surgery at The Cleveland Clinic.

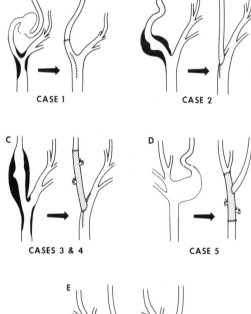

Fig 22–13.—Surgical management of extracranial carotid aneurysms at The Cleveland Clinic. (Courtesy of Painter, T.A., et al.: J. Vasc. Surg. 2:312–318, March 1985.)

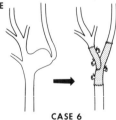

Woman, 60 years old (Case 1), was found during evaluation of angina to have bilateral carotid bruits. A saccular aneurysm of the right internal carotid artery was found, with advanced, ulcerated stenosis of the carotid bifurcation. Severe multivessel coronary disease was also present. Right carotid endarterectomy was performed, with segmental resection of the aneurysm and axial reanastomosis of the internal carotid artery (Fig 22–13). There were no neurologic sequelae, and a satisfactory technical result was found on angiography. An atherosclerotic aneurysm was diagnosed. A coronary bypass was performed uneventfully 6 weeks later, and the patient was asymptomatic 4 years thereafter.

A short, straight shunt usually has been employed in the patients for whom graft replacement is necessary. Direct reconstruction of extracranial carotid aneurysms can give satisfactory late results with few complications if appropriate precautions are taken. Saphenous vein interposition grafts were used in 4 of these 6 patients; the other 2 had aneurysm resection in conjunction with reanastomosis of the internal carotid artery. One vein graft had to be revised, but there were no surgical deaths or permanent strokes. Patients have been asymptomatic during follow-up for as long as 6 years after surgery.

Management of the Tortuous Internal Carotid Artery
Dipankar Mukherjee and Toshio Inahara (Oregon Health Sciences Univ., Portland)
Am. J. Surg. 149:651–655, May 1985 22–22

Opinions differ on the clinical significance of coiling or kinking of the internal carotid artery (ICA), but most investigators agree that it is a significant finding at endarterectomy. Twenty-six tortuous ICAs were found in a 22-year period, representing 3% of carotid endarterectomies done in this period. All 14 patients with transient ischemic attacks had endarterectomy, and 5 were found to have hemodynamically significant stenoses at the carotid bifurcation. Ten patients had symptoms of embolism of the retinal circulation. Ten patients had findings of an abdominal aortic aneurysm.

Seventeen reconstructions were done in 15 patients by the reimplantation technique. Two early patients had neurologic deficits after endarterectomy without correction of kinking. None of 17 patients having reimplantation of the ICA lower on the common carotid artery had neurologic dysfunction. One of 5 patients having other reconstructive procedures had a permanent deficit related to the operation.

Reimplantation of a tortuous ICA in its lower half is illustrated in Figure 22–14.

Angulation occlusion is likely to occur after standard endarterectomy in these cases. In addition, a tortuous proximal carotid artery contributes to intimal ulceration. In cases of tortuosity high in the internal carotid, completion angiography is recommended after endarterectomy of the bifurcation lesion.

▶ Tortuous ICA rarely, if ever, occurs because of intracranial ischemia. How-

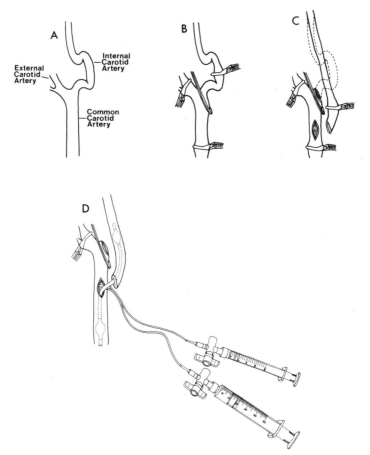

Fig 22–14.—Reimplantation of a tortuous and redundant ICA by use of an indwelling Inahara-Pruitt shunt. (Courtesy of Mukherjee, D. and Inahara, T.: Am. J. Surg. 149:651–655, May 1985.)

ever, this anatomy distal to carotid stenosis may prove a technical challenge to the neurosurgeon. When faced with this problem, I have initially attempted to leave the tortuosity firmly embedded by adventitia in place if possible. In some instances, carotid endarterectomy can be performed without disturbing the loop. Distal control may sometimes be obtained above the loop without disturbing its course. In one rare instance in which distal atheroma required entry into the loop, I resected the loop and performed end-to-end anastomosis of the two ends of the internal carotid artery with an onlay patch graft. The described reimplantation technique appears logical and feasible, and the results in this report were satisfactory. However, the surgeon should be aware that these techniques are not simple and require great care, particularly with the tailoring and suturing.—Robert M. Crowell, M.D.

Failure of Extracranial-Intracranial Arterial Bypass to Reduce the Risk of Ischemic Stroke: Results of an International Randomized Trial

The EC/IC Bypass Study Group
N. Engl. J. Med. 313:1191–1200, Nov. 7, 1985   22–23

A randomized trial of the value of an anastomosis of the superficial temporal artery to the MCA was carried out on a multicenter prospective basis in 1,377 patients with recent hemispheric stroke, retinal infarction, or transient ischemic attacks who had atherosclerotic involvement of the internal carotid artery (ICA) or middle cerebral artery (MCA). All were entered in the trial within 3 months of the presenting event. Bypass surgery was added to medical management in 663 cases, while the remaining 714 patients (52%) received medical treatment alone. The average follow-up was 56 months.

During surgery and the subsequent 30 days, 20 major strokes occurred: 16 nonfatal (2.5%) and 4 fatal (0.6%). The bypass patency rate was 96% after surgery. Both fatal and nonfatal strokes occurred more often and earlier in the group that had surgery. Secondary survival analyses of the two groups demonstrated a similar lack of benefit from surgery (Fig 22–15).

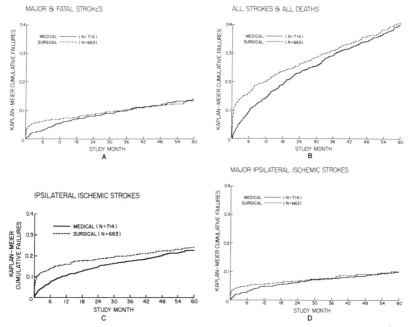

Fig 22–15.—Results of secondary analyses showing the failure of bypass in the total surgical cohort, as compared with total medical cohort, to reduce occurrence of major stroke and stroke death (**A**), all strokes and all deaths (**B**), all ischemic strokes ipsilateral to the side of symptoms for which randomization was carried out (**C**), and major ischemic strokes ipsilateral to the side of such symptoms (**D**). (Courtesy of EC-IC Bypass Study Group: N. Engl. J. Med. 313:1191–1200, Nov. 7, 1985. Reprinted by permission of The New England Journal of Medicine.)

Fatal and Nonfatal Stroke Among Clinically Interesting Subgroups*

PATIENTS†	MEDICAL GROUP			SURGICAL GROUP			MANTEL–HAENSZEL CHI-SQUARE
	NO.	OBSERVED	EXPECTED	NO.	OBSERVED	EXPECTED	
				number of patients			
All patients	714	205	218.3	663	205	191.7	1.72
Excluding those with ICA occlusion, no symptoms‡	438	133	148.0	418	148	133.0	3.23
Including only those with							
ICA occlusion, no symptoms‡	276	72	69.9	245	57	59.1	0.13
ICA occlusion, symptoms§	147	51	61.7	140	64	53.3	4.04
Including only severe¶							
ICA stenosis	72	26	27.1	77	29	27.9	0.10
MCA stenosis	59	14	20.5	50	22	15.5	4.74
Including only							
Bilateral carotid occlusion	43	17	17.4	31	14	13.6	0.02
MCA occlusion	79	18	16.9	80	16	17.1	0.15
1st TIA within 3 mo. of entry and total TIAs >3	87	27	31.5	109	41	36.5	1.32
Center size							
Smaller (<25 patients)	350	98	112.1	337	113	98.9	3.81
Larger (≥25 patients)	364	107	105.9	326	92	93.1	0.02
Geographical region							
North America	352	115	126.8	327	120	108.2	2.37
Europe	247	60	64.9	230	63	58.1	0.77
Asia	115	30	26.8	106	22	25.2	0.78

*Values listed under "Observed" indicate the observed number of patients in each treatment group who had a stroke. Those listed under "Expected" indicate the number of patients in each treatment group who would be expected to have stroke if surgery had no effect, taking into account differences in sample size and duration of follow-up;
†TIA, transient ischemic attack.
‡No symptoms were experienced between angiographic demonstration of the occlusion and randomization.
§Symptoms were experienced between angiographic demonstration of occlusion and randomization.
¶Severe stenosis is stenosis of 70% or more of the luminal diameter.
(Courtesy of EC-IC Bypass Study Group: N. Engl. J. Med. 313:1191–1200, Nov. 7, 1985. Reprinted by permission of The New England Journal of Medicine.)

Separate analyses in patients with different angiographic lesions did not identify a subgroup with any benefit from surgery (table). Patients with severe stenosis of the MCA and those with persistent symptoms after occlusion of the ICA fared worse if operated on.

These findings failed to confirm the value of extracranial-intracranial bypass surgery in preventing cerebral ischemia in patients with atherosclerotic disease in the carotid or MCA system. No substantial difference in functional outcome was found between patients with surgery and medically managed patients with mild or moderate stroke in this large series, which suggests that bypass surgery does not hasten or improve neurologic recovery.

▶ The EC-IC Bypass Study is outstanding in many respects: it provides a randomized controlled trial of a commonly performed neurosurgical procedure.

Surgical performance was excellent, with 96% overall patency. Surgical and medical groups were comparable in all important respects analyzed. Follow-up was maintained for each one of the 1,377 patients entered. Cross-overs were minimal. Statistical surveillance and analysis were of the highest quality.

Thus, it is difficult to find fault with the results and conclusions as published. Both fatal and nonfatal strokes occurred more frequently in the surgical group. No benefit was demonstrated for subgroups, including MCA stenosis, ICA occlusion with subsequent symptoms, and ICA occlusion without further symptoms. There has been some concern expressed that 10 of the strokes ascribed to surgery occurred after randomization, but before the surgical procedure; however, the results are not different, even with deletion of these cases, which are appropriately tagged to surgery, according to accepted statistical protocol.

The EC-IC Bypass Study does not provide data relevant to several types of cases. These include patients with transient ischemic attacks despite anticoagulation, patients with acute ischemia, and those with such adverse physiologic findings as altered regional cerebral blood flow and O_2 metabolism. It may yet be that a small group of patients could benefit from EC-IC bypass. Such patients might be identified by physiologic testing, such as positron emission tomography, as suggested by Donnan et al. (*Aust. NZ J. Med.* 15:386–391, 1985).

At present, it seems appropriate that EC-IC bypass not be used routinely for the prevention of ischemic stroke. However, further investigation of the operation seems warranted regarding potential benefit in subgroups not specifically examined by the EC-IC Bypass Study. The operation remains a valuable adjunct in treatment of certain aneurysms when additional collateral is needed for protection during therapeutic arterial occlusion.—Robert M. Crowell, M.D.

Improvement in the Retinal Circulation After Superficial Temporal to Middle Cerebral Artery Bypass
Michael Standefer, John R. Little, Robert Tomsak, Anthony J. Furlan, Hernando Zegarra, and George Williams (Cleveland Clinic Found.)
Neurosurgery 16:525–529, April 1985   22–24

Ophthalmodynamometry and fundus fluorescein angiography were used to evaluate the retinal circulation prospectively before and after superficial temporal artery-middle cerebral artery (STA-MCA) bypass in 35 patients. Twenty-two patients had symptomatic internal carotid occlusion, and 13 had severe, inaccessible carotid stenosis. The 27 men and 8 women had a median age of 60 years. All but 6 patients had visual symptoms, most often amaurosis fugax and blurred vision. Twenty-one patients had had at least one transient ischemic attack.

The most frequent baseline abnormalities were venous stasis retinopathy and visual field deficit. Venous stasis retinopathy resolved in 4 of 11 patients within 2 months after the operation. Ophthalmologic abnormality was worse in only 1 patient after the operation. Ophthalmodynamometric values improved in 71% of the patients after surgery. Fluorescein angiographic values improved significantly in 88% of the patients with abnormal preoperative values. The postoperative status was better in patients with normal fundus findings before surgery than in those with venous stasis retinopathy.

These findings show the value of STA-MCA anastomosis in patients who have retinal ischemia secondary to severe ipsilateral, inaccessible carotid stenosis, or occlusion. Clinical findings of ocular ischemia improve after bypass, and the retinal circulation time and retinal artery pressure improve. The diastolic retinal artery pressure improves less than after carotid endarterectomy, but improvement continues to occur over time after bypass.

▶ The data suggest that several parameters relative to retinal circulation improve following STA-MCA bypass grafting. The key clinical parameter, namely improved clinical results, has not yet been demonstrated by appropriate controlled studies.—Robert M. Crowell, M.D.

Effects of Extra-Intracranial Arterial Bypass on Cerebral Blood Flow and Oxygen Metabolism in Humans

Y. Samson, J. C. Baron, M. G. Bousser, A. Rey, J. M. Derlon, P. David, and J. Comoy (Service Hospitalier Frederic Joliot, Hôpital de la Salpetriere, and Hôpital Lariboisiere, Paris; Centre Hospitalier Universitaire Cote de Nacre, Caen; and Hôpital de Bicetre, Kremlin-Becetre, France)
Stroke 16:609–616, July–Aug. 1985   22–25

Positron emission tomography (PET) with $C^{15}O_2$ was used to measure regional cerebral blood flow, oxygen extraction fraction, and cerebral metabolic rate of oxygen ($CMRO_2$) in 12 patients (mean age, 56 years) who had successful extracranial-intracranial arterial bypass (EIAB), 11 for internal carotid obstruction and 1 for middle cerebral artery occlusion.

Both cerebral blood flow and $CMRO_2$ increased significantly in both hemispheres after EIAB, approaching values found in age-matched controls. Mean oxygen extraction fraction was not, however, altered by EIAB. A bilateral effect of EIAB on blood flow and $CMRO_2$ was confirmed by studying relative regional variations. Increases in cerebral blood flow and $CMRO_2$ were observed only in patients in whom angiographic reperfusion was provided by a proximal artery that itself had an obstructing lesion, not in those in whom spontaneous reperfusion came from the contralateral, disease-free carotid artery.

Extracranial-intracranial arterial bypass can relieve long-standing unilateral "misery perfusion" and produce increases in cerebral blood flow and $CMRO_2$ in both cerebral hemispheres. The findings suggest that long-standing hemodynamic failure can lead to cerebral metabolic depression that is potentially reversible through surgical revascularization. Further studies are needed to determine how long the increase in $CMRO_2$ lasts after bypass, and what effects the procedure has on neuropsychologic function and the occurrence of further cerebral ischemic events.

▶ These results suggest that bypass can reverse the cerebral blood flow and metabolic changes attendant with certain forms of occlusive cerebral vascular disease. The results compare with data obtained with positron emission tomography. However, these parameters must be correlated with critical measures of clinical outcome, such as those provided by the Extracranial-Intracranial Bypass Study. The results suggest, however, that physiologic measures might be used to identify particularly favorable candidates for bypass with regard to clinical outcome. It is to be hoped that a marriage of physiologic techniques for patient selection and careful statistical means for assessment of clinical outcome can be utilized to study this important subgroup of patients with cerebral vascular disease.

Whisnant et al. describe long-term follow-up after superficial temporal artery-middle cerebral artery bypass (*Mayo Clin. Proc.* 60:241–246, 1985). Among 239 patients, there were no deaths during surgery or for 30 days thereafter; mortality was then 3% per year. The survival rate at 5 years was 84%, compared with an expected survival rate of 89%. Of 25 deaths during follow-up, 2 were due to stroke and 16 to cardiac causes. Of 28 strokes, 5 occurred during the day of surgery and 3 others within 30 days after surgery. Thereafter, strokes occurred at the rate of 2.5% per year, with one third of the strokes contralateral to the side of surgery. In regard to the probability of stroke, the condition of patients with bypass compared favorably with that of patients having transient ischemic attacks of undetermined cause. However, compared with 139 surgical patients with ischemic symptoms related to proven internal carotid artery occlusion, patients with bypass had stroke at a comparable frequency. Superficial temporal artery-middle cerebral artery bypass should be reserved for patients with progression of neurologic symptoms after established internal carotid artery occlusion.—Robert M. Crowell, M.D.

Basal Arterial Occlusive Disease
Donald O. Quest and James W. Correll (Columbia Univ.)
Neurosurg. 17:937–941, December 1985   22–26

Basal arterial occlusive disease refers to progressive stenosis of arteries at the base of the brain or moyamoya disease. The internal carotids are affected distal to the carotid siphon and usually distal to the ophthalmic artery, along with the proximal parts of the anterior and middle cerebral arteries. Deep perforating vessels in the basal ganglia proliferate to provide collateral supply.

Seventeen patients with radiographic findings of basal arterial occlusive disease were seen in the past 4 years. Nine patients had bilateral involvement. Six patients were children; all but 2 were female. The presentation was either ischemic or hemorrhagic. Eight of the 9 patients with bilateral disease had ischemic episodes. Four of 5 hemorrhages were intracerebral or intraventricular, while one was subarachnoid. Of 8 patients with bilateral disease who underwent superficial temporal-middle cerebral artery bypass procedures, the condition of 6 improved. One patient died with bilateral carotid occlusion, and another had a stroke. For the five patients with unilateral disease who had bypass procedures, all improved. Another patient was treated for a basilar artery aneurysm.

Superficial temporal-middle cerebral artery bypass has been an effective approach to the treatment of basal arterial occlusive disease. An aggressive policy is warranted by the significant morbidity and mortality that can occur with this disease and the impressive surgical results obtained in many cases. An alternative method is encephaloduroarteriosynangiosis, in which the superficial temporal artery with its pedicle is joined to the dura via a strip craniectomy.

▶ These results suggest that superficial temporal artery-middle cerebral artery bypass may be helpful in the treatment of patients with moyamoya disease. The results compare with previous published results from Japan, including the reports of Kikuchi. It is important to note that the generally negative results of the Extracranial-Intracranial Bypass Study did not include patients with moyamoya disease and therefore do not refute the conclusions of this report.— Robert M. Crowell, M.D.

The Specificity of the Collaterals to the Brain Through the Study and Surgical Treatment of Moyamoya Disease
Yoshiharu Matsushima and Yutaka Inaba (Tokyo Med. and Dental Univ.)
Stroke 17:117–122, February 1986   22–27

Moyamoya disease, which involves chronic progressive stenosis or occlusion that starts in the periphery of both internal carotid arteries, is a clinical model of chronic brain ischemia. All of the collateral networks are not available in the early stages of ischemia because of the watery layer of subarachnoid fluid between the cortical and dural vessels and the bony enclosure that intervenes between the arterial networks of the dura and scalp. These barriers serve to isolate the brain from the abundant supply of the external carotid system. Irreversible ischemic changes may occur before adequate transdural anastomoses are formed.

A surgical procedure termed *encephaloduroarteriosynangiosis* (EDAS) has been developed to place the scalp artery directly on the surface of the brain through fixation to the incised dural edge via a narrow craniotomy (Fig 22–16). The goal is to promote formation of spontaneous transdural anastomoses. The scalp vessel is used with a narrow strip of galea attached, for fixation to the dura.

Seventy operations have been done on 38 pediatric patients with moyamoya disease, and no deterioration has ensued. The dural arteries are markedly dilated 1 to 3 months after operation, and the donor artery gradually enlarges. The brain is revascularized 6 months after surgery in almost all cases. The moyamoya vessels have disappeared in some cases. Ischemic episodes ceased in all cases an average of 11½ months after surgery. Improvement in findings on EEGs was consistently noted. Some existing motor deficits improved, but intellectual function did not improve substantially.

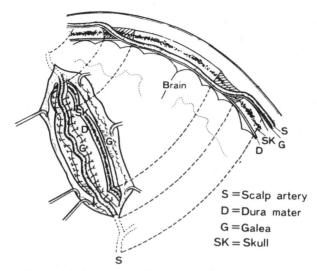

Fig 22–16.—The EDAS: bird's eye view and vertical cut surface. (Courtesy of Matsushima, Y., and Inaba, Y.: Stroke 17:117–122, February 1986. By permission of the American Heart Association, Inc.)

The external carotid system with its good collateral capacity can be used to revascularize the brain in cases of moyamoya disease through the EDAS procedure. Revascularization has been consistently obtained, and varying degrees of symptomatic improvement have resulted.

▶ Matsushima and colleagues provide an interesting overview of brain collateral circulation at various levels and the important, increasingly recognized problem of moyamoya disease. A new operation, an onlay graft of superficial temporal artery and its pedicle, is suggested. The group confirms that such grafts can sprout many tiny collaterals to the brain tissue, without the need for direct anastomosis. The resulting increase in collateral is reminiscent of the implant grafts directly inserted into the brain that are described by Khodadad and the onlay momental grafts described by Yasargil and Goldsmith. Goldsmith has evidence that omental grafts contain angiogenesis factor, and it seems likely that the superficial temporal artery onlay graft does too.

Overall, this particular approach of synangiosis (an onlying arterial graft without interruption of scalp or cortical vasculature) has several advantages: a very low risk, ease of performance, speed of operation, and high patency rate in a setting without vascular occlusions. However, the proof of the pudding is still in the eating: clinical studies will be required to demonstrate improvement in clinical outcome following this type of procedure. At the moment it is unknown whether this procedure or standard superficial temporal artery-middle cerebral artery bypass grafting can improve the course of moyamoya disease.

The prognosis of 27 patients with moyamoya was studied by Kuokawa et al. (*Pediatric Neurology* 1:274–276, 1985). Intellectual deterioration and neurologic deficits increased over time; 19% of the patients were normal, 33% had occasional transient ischemic attacks, 26% had mild impairment, 11% had special needs, 7% required 24-hour care, and one patient (3%) died. Poor prognosis was correlated with early agent onset and hypertension.—Robert M. Crowell, M.D.

Emergency Embolectomy for Acute Occlusion of the Middle Cerebral Artery

Fredric B. Meyer, David G. Piepgras, Thoralf M. Sundt, Jr., and Takehiko Yanagihara (Mayo Clinic and Mayo Graduate School of Medicine)
J. Neurosurg. 62:639–647, May 1985   22–28

The data on 20 patients who underwent an emergency embolectomy for acute middle cerebral artery (MCA) occlusion in 1970–1983 were reviewed. The 10 male and 10 female patients had an average age of 55 years. The embolus arose in the heart in seven cases, in the carotid artery in seven, and in the aorta in three. The left MCA was involved in all but three cases. Surgery was done via a pterional craniotomy. Nontraumatic aneurysm clips were placed on the main divisions of the MCA distal to the embolus before the arteriotomy was made and the embolus was milked out.

Before surgery all patients had a severe neurologic deficit and impaired consciousness. Seven patients had an excellent or good outcome, with no more than minimal residual neurologic deficit. Seven others had a fair outcome, 4 patients had a poor result, and 2 (10%) died. Two hemorrhagic infarctions occurred, and 1 patient had a cerebrospinal fluid leak. Of 3 patients in whom flow could not be restored, 2 had aortic emboli. Patients with MCA occlusion associated with carotid occlusion did poorly. Good collateral flow to ischemic tissue was associated with a better outlook.

Embolectomy can provide a good outcome in a significant number of patients with acute, profound deficits from MCA occlusion. The outlook is not good in cases of aortic embolism or when a prolonged delay precedes embolectomy. Good collateral flow to the MCA complex is a favorable prognostic indicator.

▶ Meyer and colleagues indicate that good results can be obtained in some cases in emergency embolectomy. There are, however, some patients who have poor results, even a fatal outcome. This procedure should be reserved for patients who develop the embolus in the hospital—in a setting in which an experienced and prepared neurovascular team is ready to undertake this surgery at a moment's notice.

Controlled studies in rabbits do not indicate definite benefit of streptokinase clot lysis in acute occlusion of the rabbit cranial circulation (Centeno et al.: *AJNR* 6:589–594, 1985).—Robert M. Crowell, M.D.

Notes on Ischemia

Carotid Endarterectomy

▶ Among 181 patients who underwent computerized tomography (CT) prior to endarterectomy, findings on CT were not helpful in patients undergoing elective surgery but were very helpful in patients undergoing urgent carotid endarterectomy (Ricotta et al.: *Ann. Surg.* 202:783–787, 1985).

Neurosurgeons will be interested to learn that a controlled study of symptomatic carotid stenosis treated by endarterectomy is being organized. This study is likely to be supported by the National Institutes of Health, multicentered, and influential in its results. Stay tuned!

Hennerici et al. (*Q. J. Med.* 55:109–118, 1985) present a 10-year follow-up study of 76 patients with angiographic carotid stenosis. There were 46 deaths (often due to coronary disease) and 17 strokes, but only 2 in the area of the diseased carotid, and only 1 without premonitory transient ischemic attacks. Prophylactic endarterectomy seems inadvisable.

Mukherjee and Inahara (*Am. J. Surg.* 149:651–655, 1985) describe repair of tortuous internal carotid artery by anastomosis of the internal carotid artery take-off to a more proximal site on common carotid artery. [Tortuous carotids are rarely symptomatic.—Robert M. Crowell]

Findlay et al. (*J. Neurosurg.* 63:693–698, 1985) report on the effects of platelet inhibition on postcarotid endarterectomy mural thrombus formation. Studies with radiolabeled platelets showed a significant reduction in platelet accumulation at the operative site in patients treated with antiplatelet drugs. Use of aspirin/dipyridamole in the perioperative period may reduce the risk of operative stroke and recurrent carotid stenosis.

Pribil and Powers (*J. Neurosurg.* 63:771–775, 1985) joined rat carotid artery end-to-end with the Argon laser. Over time, stenosis and pseudoaneurysm were noted at the anastomotic site. Further studies are needed.

External carotid artery endarterectomy in four patients with ipsilateral internal carotid artery occlusion and cerebral symptoms led to cessation of symptoms (Takolander et al.: *Acta Chir. Scand.* 151:647–650, 1985).

External carotid artery reconstruction may be helpful in the management of cerebral ischemia. Twenty-one patients undergoing 22 external carotid artery endarterectomies all had ipsilateral internal carotid artery occlusion and external carotid artery stenosis or cul de sac of the internal carotid artery. The internal carotid artery was divided at its origin and external carotid endarterectomy carried out. Of 19 symptomatic patients, all became asymptomatic during a follow-up of 32 months.

In a controlled study of antiplatelet drugs in carotid endarterectomy, thrombotic complications were less frequent in the treated group (Edwards et al.: *Ann. Surg.* 765–770, 1985).

Local anesthesia was carried out for carotid endarterectomy in 41 cases, with good results (Shifrin et al.: *Isr. J. Med. Sci.* 21:511–513, 1985).

A marked drop in ocular systolic pressure following carotid endarterectomy identifies early occlusion and may be used to select patients for reoperation (Ricotta et al.: *J. Vasc. Surg.* 2:415–418, 1985).

Intraoperative angiography through a butterfly needle is recommended for assessment of arterial patency (McCready et al.: *Gynecology and Obstetrics* 160:367–368, 1985).

External carotid artery endarterectomy in four patients with ipsilateral internal carotid artery occlusion and cerebral symptoms led to cessation of symptoms (Takolander et al.: *Acta Chir. Scand.* 151:647–650, 1985).

New Procedures for Ischemia

The occipital artery may be joined end-to-side to the vertebral artery above C1 when vertebral occlusion is needed for vertebral aneurysm (Hadley et al.: *J. Neurosurg.* 63:622–625, 1985). An alternative is balloon catheter occlusion of the vertebral artery with the patient awake.

The transverse cervical artery may be joined to the vertebral artery (Donaldson et al.: *J. Vasc. Surg.* 2:917–920, 1985). Indications for this procedure have not been established.

Grotta et al. (*Stroke* 16:790 795, 1985) report safe and successful monitoring of pulmonary wedge pressure in nine patients undergoing hemodilution therapy for acute cerebral ischemia.

Among 30 patients with vertebral artery revascularization, occlusion developed in five, with one bad result, while 19 were cured and 7 improved (Habozig and Rambaud: *Lyon Chirurgie* 82:110–113, 1985).

Arterial Ectasia

Taptas et al. (*Neurochirurgie* 31:237–249, 1985) review 169 cases in the literature and add the case reports of six of their own patients with dolichoectasia of the intracranial arteries. They present pathologic material indicating a defect in the elastic lamina without atherosclerosis.

Hegedüs (*Surg. Neurol.* 24:463–469, 1985) describes defects in the elastic lamina in basilar ectasia. Similar less severe changes are present in berry aneurysms but not in atherosclerotic arteries.

Serial contrast computed tomography scans can demonstrate progression of cerebral arterial dolichoectasia, according to van Tassel and Gammal (*Neuroradiology* 27:440–442, 1985).

When dopamine is withdrawn during treatment of cerebral ischemia, a decrease in cerebrospinal fluid of 25% or more indicates need for further hypertensive therapy (Mandelon et al.: *J. Neurol. Neurosurg. Psychiatry* 49:35–38, 1986).

In controlled feline studies, three opiate antagonists did not reduce infarct size (Baskin et al.: *J. Neurosurg.* 64:99–103, 1986).

Norris and Hachinski report a double-blind randomized controlled study of high-dose steroid treatment for cerebral infarction (*Br. Med. J.* [*Clin. Res.*] 292:21–23, 1986).

Freitag et al. report on 11 patients with percutaneous carotid angiography for symptomatic atherosclerosis (*Neuroradiology* 28:126–127, 1986). In 8 patients, good angiographic and clinical results were obtained. In 3, angioplasty was unsuccessful, with transient symptoms in 1.

Among 1,930 patients undergoing carotid endarterectomies, 8 suffered postoperative intracerebral hemorrhage (Solomon et al.: *J. Neurosurg.* 64:29–34, 1986). Seven of the 8 had high-grade stenosis, and defective autoregulation with postoperative hyperperfusion probably played a role in pathogenesis.

Biller and colleagues review literature on intraluminal clot in the carotid artery and add nine new cases (*Surg. Neurol.* 25:467–477, 1986). They conclude that optimal treatment is not known and that surgical and medical treatments need further evaluation.

Courbier and colleagues recommend intraoperative carotid angiography to correct defects (*J. Vasc. Surg.* 3:343–350, 1986).

Among 79 carotid endarterectomies studied after 2 years with digital subtraction angiography, one asymptomatic occlusion and one symptomatic restenosis with three external carotid artery occlusions were noted. Vein patch grafting appears to protect the internal carotid artery but not the common carotid artery from restenosis (Sundt et al.: *Ann. Surg.* 90–100, 1986).

Basilar artery stenosis progressed to occlusion after superficial temporary artery superior cerebellar artery anastomosis (Minakason et al.: *Surg. Neurol.* 25:39–42, 1986).

Recovery from the locked-in syndrome is possible after bilateral vertebral occlusions (Cabezudo et al.: *Surg. Neurol.* 25:185–190, 1986).—Robert M. Crowell, M.D.

23 Hemorrhage

Introduction

For cerebral aneurysms, delay in referring to neurosurgical attention often results in worse outcome (Digest 23–1). Percutaneous obliteration of basilar aneurysms has been attained with detachable balloon catheters (Digest 23–2).

Regarding arteriovenous malformations, posterior fossa lesions remain formidable with 13% mortality and 14% serious morbidity in the most experienced surgeons (Digest 23–3). Angiographically occult angiomas are more common than is generally recognized and may occasionally warrant operative excision (Digest 23–4). Polyvinyl alcohol enhances embolization of cranial and spinal arteriovenous malformations (Digests 23–5, 23–6).

Intracranial hematomas may be imaged by high-resolution magnetic resonance, but lesions within the first 72 hours are difficult to detect (Digest 23–7). Evacuation of large-volume cerebral hematomas is warranted for deteriorating patients (Digest 23–8).

Robert M. Crowell, M.D.

Aneurysms

Delay in Referral of Patients With Ruptured Aneurysms to Neurosurgical Attention

N. F. Kassell, G. L. Kongable, James C. Torner, H. P. Adams, Jr., and Haia Mazuz (Univ. of Iowa)
Stroke 16:587–590, July–Aug. 1985   23–1

Deaths from rebleeding and vasospasm following subarachnoid bleeding have prompted a renewed interest in earlier surgery, but this requires early referral to specialized facilities. Reasons for delayed referral were analyzed in a series of 150 patients with proved aneurysmal bleeding, all admitted consecutively between 1977 and 1983. Subarachnoid hemorrhage was confirmed in all cases by lumbar puncture, computed tomography (CT), surgery, or autopsy, and an aneurysm was demonstrated by CT, angiography, or autopsy.

The median delay from the first clear symptoms and signs of subarachnoid bleeding to the patient's arrival at the stroke unit was 3½ days (Fig 23–1). Delay exceeded two days in 64% of cases and three days in 59%. Multiple bleeding before admission was suspected in one third of the cases. Delay correlated closely with the severity of initial bleeding. Delay exceeded two days in all cases in which the initial event was focal and in 72% of cases where it was minor. Physicians' diagnostic problems caused the delay in 37% of cases, and a delayed referral policy was responsible in 23%. Logistical reasons for delay were identified in 12% of the cases.

Excessive delay in the referral of patients with aneurysmal rupture ap-

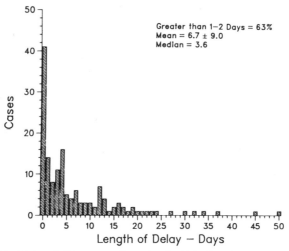

Fig 23–1.—Distribution of 150 cases according to length of delay from first sign or symptom to arrival at the Acute-Care Stroke Unit. (Courtesy of Kassell, N.F., et al.: Stroke 16:587–590, July–August 1985. By permission of the American Heart Association, Inc.)

pears to be universal. Most of the delay is avoidable. Physician education in the clinical features of subarachnoid hemorrhage will help, along with a policy of prompt referral of patients to neurosurgical attention. It is likely that more lives will be saved in this way for the rest of the decade than with further advances in treatment.

► This important report documents that delay of referral of aneurysm cases is common, lethal, and avoidable. Physician education and policies of early referral provide the best chance for diminishing the devastating effects of subarachnoid hemorrhage.

Synowitz et al. (*Zentralbl. Neurochir.* 46:11–30, 1985) reported on giant aneurysms. Of 11 patients, they were able to clip 8; 4 patients had superior temporal artery-middle cerebral artery bypass grafts. One patient had carotid ligation. Five did well, 2 had severe complications, and 1 died.

Preoperative treatment with nimodipine does not have deleterious effects on anesthesia for cerebral aneurysm clipping (Stullken et al.: *Anesthesiology* 62:346–348, 1985).

Scanning and transmission electron microscopy failed to reveal structural changes in cerebral arteries taken from dogs up to 9 days after injection of autologous blood into the basal cistern (Pickard et al.: *J. Neurol. Neurosurg. Psychiatry* 48:256–262, 1985).—Robert M. Crowell, M.D.

Balloon Embolization in the Treatment of Basilar Aneurysms
H. Zeumer, H. Brückmann, D. Adelt, W. Hacke, and E. B. Ringelstein (Aachen, Federal Republic of Germany)
Acta Neurochir. 78:136–141, 1985

23–2

Transvascular obliteration by modern neuroradiologic methods is an alternative to surgical treatment when a vertebrobasilar aneurysm is not amenable to direct clipping at reasonable risk.

Woman, 61 years old, with severe headache a few months previously, presented in a comatose and tetraparetic state after a second attack of severe headache. There

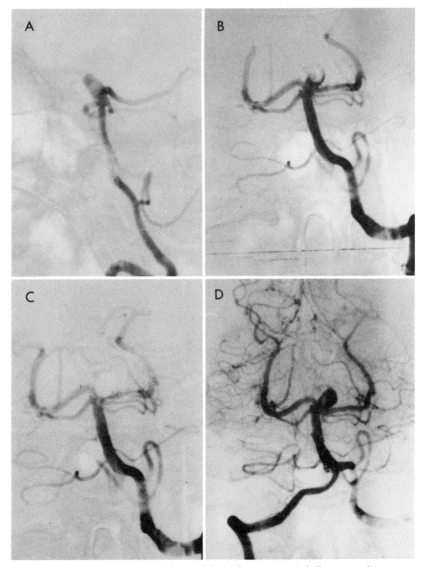

Fig 23–2.—**A,** oblique projection of the top of the basilar aneurysm. **B,** balloon enters the aneurysm. **C,** balloon occluding the aneurysm. **D,** reappearance of the aneurysm after deflation of the balloon 3 weeks later. (Courtesy of Zeumer, H., et al.: Acta Neurochir. 78:136–141, 1985. Berlin-Heidelberg-New York: Springer.)

was a history of hypertension and mild cardiac insufficiency. Computed tomography showed subarachnoid bleeding and minor clots within the third and lateral ventricles. Some improvement occurred, and angiography showed the top of a basilar aneurysm with a diameter of 8 mm. A latex balloon on a teflon catheter was advanced via a right axillary artery approach (Fig 23–2), and a transfemoral catheter was inserted into the vertebral artery for contrast injection. The balloon was filled with dye under somatosensory evoked potential monitoring, and the catheter was tied off and left buried under the puncture site. Almost complete obliteration of the aneurysm was seen. The balloon deflated over the next 3 weeks, and significant clinical improvement occurred. Angiographic study after 6 weeks showed the nearly completely deflated balloon within the aneurysm, which remained largely thrombosed. The patient has done well for 10 months.

Aneurysmal rupture and occlusion of perforating arteries are major risks of direct embolic occlusion; however, it is sometimes possible to induce a spontaneous thrombosis of a basilar aneurysm by altering blood flow within the basilar artery. The risk of surgery in older patients is very high. Close cooperation among neurosurgeons, neuroradiologists, and neurologists will help in the planning of the best treatment in individual cases of vertebrobasilar aneurysm.

▶ Transvascular obliteration of intracranial aneurysms remains an attractive goal. The present report documents that the general approach can be used for posterior circulation aneurysms.

The usual application of detachable balloons involves proximal occlusion of parent artery (or arteries) at a distance from the lesion ("Hunterian" ligation). In the case of the vertebral artery, one must position the balloon above C1, and thus distal to deep muscular collateral circulation, which can foil a more proximal occlusion. To avert the risk of recanalization with eventual balloon deflation, we have used one or two gianturco coils proximal to the balloon to promote solid thrombosis of the cervical vertebral artery. Unilateral vertebral occlusion can result in thrombosis of a vertebral posterior inferior cerebral artery (PICA) aneurysm with preservation of PICA.

The placement of detachable balloons *within* aneurysms has been less successful. Positioning is difficult, and aneurysmal rupture has occurred. Moreover, if the aneurysm is not completely thrombosed (as in the case reported here), there is still risk of a subarachnoid hemorrhage (SAH). Direct surgical clipping is recommended for many basilar apex lesions such as seen in Figure 23–2.

Notes on Subarachnoid Hemorrhage (SAH)

Among multiple aneurysms, the site of rupture can be identified with a high degree of confidence (Nehls et al.: *J. Neurosurg.* 63:342–348, 1985). Focal spasms of mass or serial change were highly reliable but infrequent signs. Irregular shape and nipple were very reliable, and larger size rather reliable.

Acute hydrocephalus after a SAH is ominous, according to van Gijn et al. (*J. Neurosurg.* 63:355–362, 1985). Thirty-four of 174 consecutive patients exhibited acute hydrocephalus. Of these, 20 were dead within 1 month, 6 from rebleeding, and 11 from infarction, which was often related to hyponatremia.

Rodriguez y Baena et al. (*Surg. Neurol.* 24:428–432, 1985) suggest that arachidonate metabolism may play a role in the genesis of vasospasm following SAH.

In experimental animals, disturbance of arterial wall permeability after SAH probably accounts for postcontrast enhancement and probably is involved in the pathogenesis of vasospasm (Sasaki et al.: *J. Neurosurg.* 63:433–440, 1985).

Shaw et al. (*J. Neurosurg.* 63:699–703, 1985) found no difference in postoperative ischemic deficits between patients with aneurysmal SAH and comparable groups treated with dipyridamole and placebo.

Isobutyl-2-cyanoacrylate embolization incites foreign-body giant cell reaction in cerebral arteriovenous malformations, according to Klara et al. (*J. Neurosurg.* 63:421–425, 1985).

Auer et al. describe removal of intracerebral hemorrhage via an endoscopic method (*Eur. Neurol.* 24:254–261, 1985).

Dujovny et al. have reported an important study of aneurysm clip motion during magnetic resonance imaging (*Neurosurgery* 17:543–548, 1985). Yasargil, Sugita, Heifetz Elgiloy, and Vari-Angle McFadden clips do not deflect. Mayfield, Heifetz, Vari-Angle, Pivot, and Sundt-Kees Multi-Angle clips deflect or slip off aneurysms. Thus, this latter group should be avoided if magnetic resonance imaging is to be used. (See also Digest 20–11.)

Ausman et al. (*Surg. Neurol.* 24:625–635, 1985) comment on myths and facts in current management of cerebral aneurysms. They favor early surgery and temporary clips.

Guegan et al. (*Surg. Neurol.* 24:441–448, 1985) present four case histories of patients with difficult intracranial aneurysm treated with deep hypothermia and circulatory arrest with extracorporeal circulation. The use of other methods, including temporary clips with cerebral protection, may produce good results without the use of the extreme step of total circulatory arrest.

Symon advocates use of somatosensory evoked potential monitoring and temporary clips in the treatment of internal carotid artery and middle cerebral artery aneurysms (*Acta Neurochir.* 77:1–7, 1985).—Robert M. Crowell, M.D.

Arteriovenous Malformations

Posterior Fossa Arteriovenous Malformations
Charles G. Drake, Allan H. Friedman, and Sydney J. Peerless (Univ. of Western Ontario)
J. Neurosurg. 64:1–10, January 1986

23–3

Sixty-six cases of infratentorial arteriovenous malformation (AVM) in patients aged 5–69 years were reviewed. All but 5 patients had presenting symptoms related to subarachnoid or intraparenchymal bleeding. The physical findings localized disease to the posterior fossa in all 27 patients with known intraparenchymal hematoma and in 24 of 34 with only subarachnoid bleeding. Nine of 12 concomitant aneurysms had ruptured. Fifteen patients did not have excision of the AVM, and 5 had exploration only. Four patients had intraoperative embolization. Complete excision

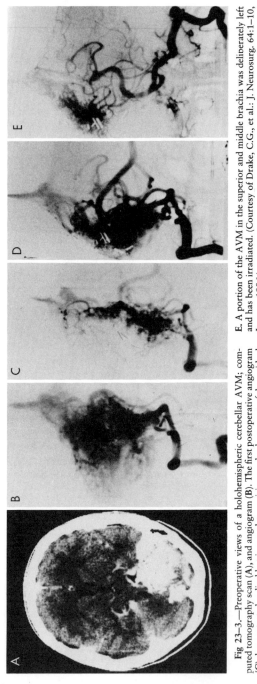

Fig 23-3.—Preoperative views of a holohemispheric cerebellar AVM; computed tomography scan (A), and angiogram (B). The first postoperative angiogram (C) demonstrated radical but incomplete excision, and enlargement of the residual medial AVM was seen 9 months later (D). The extent of final excision is seen in E. A portion of the AVM in the superior and middle brachia was deliberately left and has been irradiated. (Courtesy of Drake, C.G., et al.: J. Neurosurg. 64:1–10, January 1986.)

was attempted in 51 cases and was achieved in 47 of them. Twelve of 14 malformations confined to a single hemisphere were excised via suboccipital craniectomy. One of two holohemispheric lesions appeared to be completely resected (Fig 23–3). Twenty-one vermian and vermian-paramedial AVMs were excised. Only 2 of 15 lesions involving the brain stem were excised.

The best results were obtained when no significant clot was present in the cerebellum or brain stem. Nineteen patients had excellent results after excision of the AVM, and 2 others after exploration only. Twenty-six patients had a good outcome, 18 after excision of the AVM. Five of 9 poor results were due solely to preoperative hematoma. Six of 10 deaths were due to postresection clots.

Seventy-one percent of patients in this series had an excellent or good outcome, while 15% died. Most surgical morbidity was due to massive postoperative hemorrhage, presumably related to inadequate hemostasis. Better means are needed of obliterating small, fragile feeding arteries during surgery for posterior fossa AVM.

▶ Drake and colleagues, leaders in the field, present their results for posterior fossa AVMs. Complete excision was possible in 47 of 66 cases. Only 2 of 15 lesions involving the brain stem were excised. Five of 9 poor results were due to preoperative hematoma; 71% of the patients had an excellent or good outcome, but 15% died. Most of the surgical morbidity was due to postoperative hemorrhage.

Judging from this experience, the optimum treatment for these lesions has not been established. In instances in which the most experienced neurosurgeons encounter substantial morbidity and mortality, less experienced surgeons will do well to decline operative intervention. Proton beam therapy may have a role for some of these lesions.

Cerebellar venous angiomas can bleed with serious neurologic sequelae (Biller et al.: *Arch. Neurol.* 42:367–370, 1985).

Stenosis of afferent vessels to intracranial AVMs may lead to thrombosis (Omojola et al.: *AJNR* 6:791–793, 1985).

Latex balloons in high-flow fistuli are encased by fibrosis but remain nonadherent up to 12 weeks, and close of the fistula requires the balloon to remain inflated for at least 7 days (Quisling et al.: *AJNR* 6:583–587, 1985).—Robert M. Crowell, M.D.

Angiographically Occult Angiomas: A Report of Thirteen Cases With Analysis of the Cases Documented in the Literature
Susumu Wakai, Yasuichi Ueda, Satoshi Inoh, and Masakatsu Nagai (Dokkyo Univ., Tochigi, Japan)
Neurosurgery 17:549–556, October 1985   23–4

Angiographically occult angioma (AOA) can cause epilepsy or intracerebral hemorrhage. Fifteen patients with lobar hematoma and 2 with intracerebellar hematoma without abnormal vessels on angiography were operated on in the past 8 years. Angioma was confirmed pathologically in 9 patients and hemangioblastoma in 5. Four other patients with AOA without hemorrhage were operated on in the same period. Symptoms developed suddenly in the 9 patients with hematoma. Calcifications were present in 3 of those without hemorrhage. No patient had abnormal vessels, early veins, or a vascular blush on angiography. The angiomas were less than 2 cm in 9 patients and more than 6 cm in only 1. Nine patients had a good surgical outcome, 3 were left with a moderate deficit, and 1 was disabled. Twelve lesions were diagnosed as arteriovenous malformation (AVM) and 1 as cavernous angioma.

A total of 159 pathologically verified cases of AOA have been reported. Most cases were accompanied by hemorrhage. One third of the patients with bleeding did not have typical hemorrhagic symptoms. Ten patients who bled had definite hypertension. The usual computed tomographic (CT) finding was a round to oval intraparenchymatous hematoma. Diffuse or nodular enhancement was seen in about half the cases. A large majority of angiomas were supratentorial. Nearly 80% of the lesions that bled were less than 2 cm, whereas about half the nonbleeding lesions were 2 to 6 cm. Surgery was followed by a good outcome in 99 patients, a fair outcome in 15, and disablement in 2. Seven patients died. In another 46 patients the outcome was unknown.

Surgery seems to be indicated for any suspected AOA with suggestive CT features in an accessible location, whether or not recent hemorrhage has occurred. High-risk elderly patients may be an exception. The lesion should be completely removed. The therapeutic options for lobar hematoma are uncertain.

▶ This report emphasizes an important point—AVM may exist in the brain despite normal angiographic results. The authors, by collecting 13 personal cases and reviewing 159 from the literature, document that this phenomenon is more frequent than usually believed. However, a single normal angiogram early after subarachnoid hemorrhage (SAH) does not exclude AVM. Not infrequently, 2–3 months after SAH, when hematoma has diminished to permit AVM filling, repeat angiography will disclose the AVM. In some instances, contrast enhancement on CT may be seen, suggesting AVM (6 of the reported patients did not undergo CT with infusion). Magnetic resonance imaging may show some of these lesions that are not seen angiographically. Totally occult AVM remains distinctly rare.

The risk of recurrent SAH from such occult lesions is not precisely known. Therefore, the need for excision is difficult to gauge. The tendency to operate in the face of persistently normal angiographic findings seems greater in the younger nonhypertensive patients with hemorrhage in an accessible zone. Surely it is necessary to evacuate hematoma in deteriorating patients with accessible lesions, even if angiographically silent. However, careful follow-up may be the best course for elderly patients or those with inaccessible lesions. Proton beam therapy might also be considered for younger patients with lesions in eloquent zones.

In related work, Brismar and Sundbärg (*J. Neurosurg.* 63:349–354, 1985) report that prognosis after SAH of unknown origin is good: only 0.6% per year suffer recurrent SAH and 88% return to full work.—Robert M. Crowell, M.D.

Small Particle Polyvinyl Alcohol Embolization of Cranial Lesions With Minimal Arteriolar-Capillary Barriers
R. G. Quisling, J. P. Mickle, and W. Ballinger (Univ. of Florida)
Surg. Neurol. 25:243–252, March 1986   23–5

Experience with six patients has shown that very small particle polyvinyl alcohol (PVA) foam can embolize arteries in lesions with minimal arteriolar-capillary barriers. Particles less than 150 μm in diameter were used. Feeding vessels are subselectively catheterized with a benzalkonium-heparin-coated catheter, and particles injected under fluoroscopic monitoring with contrast medium. Preliminary subtraction angiography is performed.

Five dural arteriovenous fistulas and a vascular hemangioma were treated. There were areas of fistulization within a more complex matrix, or only a scant capillary matrix, implying minimal arteriolar-capillary barriers. In five patients, there were other complicating factors, such as venous aneurysms (Fig 23–4) or direct venous communication with major dural sinuses of intracerebral veins. Decreased arterial circulation after embolization greatly facilitated surgical removal of the lesions. In nonsurgical patients, follow-up angiography showed persistent obliteration of the primarily embolized vessels in 4 instances. Vessels lacking PVA foam particles remained patent. Three patients received additional embolizations. Symptoms improved or resolved in all patients, and subarachnoid hemorrhage did not recur.

Microparticle-sized PVA foam can be used to embolize cranial lesions associated with either fistulization or only minimal complexity in the matrix of the vascular malformation. Symptomatic improvement can be obtained and blood flow controlled, even if the malformation is not completely eradicated.

▶ Such new materials as small particle PVA are likely to extend the applicability of embolization for treatment of intracranial AVMs and tumors.—Robert M. Crowell, M.D.

Spinal Arteriovenous Malformations: Advances in Therapeutic Embolization
Jacques Théron, Rees Cosgrove, Denis Melanson, and Romeo Ethier (Montreal Neurological Inst. and McGill Univ.)
Radiology 158:163–169, January 1986   23–6

Embolization of intramedullary spinal arteriovenous malformations (AVMs) has been considered dangerous because of the risk of occlusion of the anterior spinal artery, but newer techniques permit safer endovas-

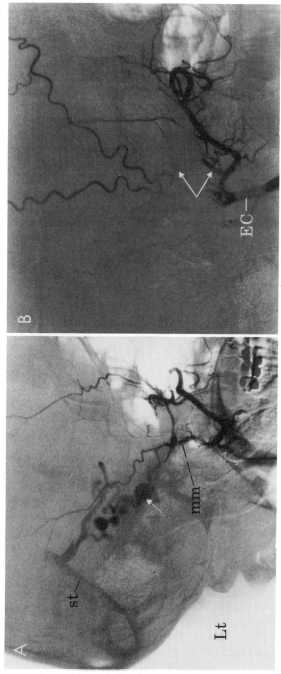

Fig 23-4.—A, oblique-lateral projection, left internal maxillary angiography demonstrates filling of a dural arteriovenous malformation (*white arrow*) having multiple venous aneurysms. Feeding vessels arise primarily from small branches of the left middle meningeal artery (mm) and to a lesser extent from dural branches of the meningohypophyseal trunk of the left internal carotid artery. The capillary matrix is minimal. Venous drainage is via the petrosal vein, lateral anastomotic mesencephalic vein, and subsequently into the vein of Galen and straight sinus (st). In this oblique view, the proximal segments of the middle meningeal and superficial temporal arteries are superimposed. **B,** lateral projection, left carotid (EC) angiograph obtained after subselective middle meningeal, small particle PVA foam embolization. No persistent filling of the arteriovenous fistula was evident by either route or from contralateral dural vessels at the time. (Courtesy of Quisling, R.G., et al.: Surg. Neurol. 25:243–252, March 1986. Reprinted by permission of the publisher, Copyright 1986, Elsevier Science Publishing Co., Inc.)

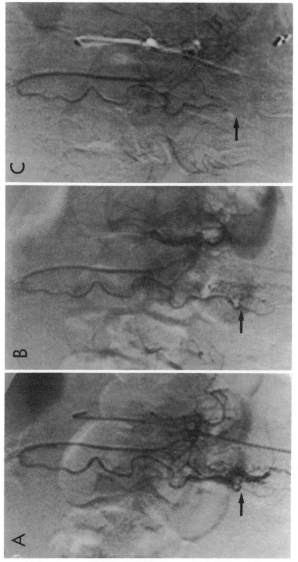

Fig 23–5.—Extramedullary lumbar AVM supplied by a slightly dilated Adamkiewicz artery. There is progressive occlusion of malformation (*arrow*) with preservation of the anterior spinal artery. **A,** preembolization image. **B,** image obtained during embolization. There is modification of AVM, with slight decrease in caliber of anterior spinal artery, as compared with **A. C,** postembolization image shows occlusion of AVM. (Courtesy of Théron, J., et al.: Radiology 158:163–169, January 1986. Reproduced with permission of the Radiological Society of North America.)

cular treatment of such lesions. These methods include the use of polyvinyl alcohol (PVA) in calibrated particles and temporary balloon occlusion of the vertebral artery in cervical AVMs that are supplied by a pedicle that arises from the vertebral artery. Serial digital subtraction angiography also has been helpful.

Five patients with spinal AVMs that were supplied at least in part by the anterior spinal artery were treated with embolization in the past year. Included were two cervical and two dorsolumbar intramedullary malformations and one extramedullary lumbar lesion. Two patients had Klippel-Trénaunay-Weber syndrome. All procedures were done under local anesthesia with the use of calibrated PVA particles 150 to 250 μ in size in normal saline.

Total occlusion of the AVM was obtained in all cases. Motor deficits improved markedly in three patients, but the other two had no change in neurologic status. No complications occurred. The angiographic findings in 1 case are shown in Figure 23–5. Both follow-up angiograms showed persistent occlusion of the AVM.

Spinal intramedullary AVMs now may be embolized more safely than in the past. The use of small, calibrated PVA particles permits occlusion of the nidus of the malformation with preservation of the anterior spinal artery and of the normal central spinal arteries. Serial digital subtraction angiography allows more precise control over the rate of occlusion of the nidus.

▶ Polyvinyl alcohol particles can be used to obliterate spinal AVMs with preservation of the anterior spinal artery and good clinical results. Obviously, such difficult embolizations should be attempted only by those with substantial experience with percutaneous embolization methods.

In a small number of cases, the group from the Montreal Neurological Institute reports excellent results. Technical advances include the use of PVA particles and serial digital subtraction angiography. If these results can be duplicated, embolization may become the treatment of choice for many of these lesions.—Robert M. Crowell, M.D.

Spontaneous Hemorrhage

Intracranial Hematomas: Imaging by High-Field MR

John M. Gomori, Robert I. Grossman, Herbert I. Goldberg, Robert A. Zimmerman, and Larissa T. Bilaniuk (Univ. of Pennsylvania)
Radiology 157:87–93, October 1985   23–7

Low-field magnetic resonance (MR) images of acute hematomas are isointense to parenchyma, whereas subacute and chronic hematomas are hyperintense at all pulse sequences. The high-field MR findings were examined in 20 intracranial hematomas ranging in age from 1 day to more than 1 year. Imaging was performed with a 1.5-T unit and spin-echo pulse sequences. Three patients had two separate hematomas. Fifteen intracerebral and four subdural hematomas and one chronic epidural hematoma were evaluated.

Acute hematomas less than 1 week old were characterized by central hypointensity on T2-weighted images. Subacute hematomas aged 1 week to 1 month exhibited peripheral hyperintensity on T1-weighted images and then on (T2-WI). Hyperintensity filled in the hematoma in the chronic stage. Both subacute and chronic lesions showed hypointensity on T2-weighted images in the immediately adjacent brain tissue. White matter near acute and subacute hematomas appeared hyperintense on T2-weighted images, which is consistent with edema.

The preferential T2 proton relaxation enhancement seen in the center of acute hematomas and in the parenchyma adjacent to subacute and chronic hematomas is attributed to deoxyhemoglobin in intact red blood cells. Hemosiderin in macrophage lysosomes in adjacent brain is probably the cause of a peripheral hypointensity pattern. These relaxation effects are proportional to the square of the magnitude of the main magnetic field. The peripheral hyperintensity extending inward in subacute hematomas at all field strengths is probably due to methemoglobin proton-electron dipolar-dipolar proton relaxation enhancement. Iron is to high-field MR imaging what calcium is to computed tomography.

▶ Magnetic resonance imaging does not image intracranial hematomas well in the first 72 hours. Thereafter, MR imaging may provide helpful diagnostic information not available from CT, particularly when lesions are isodense on CT. Clinicians will need to become familiar with the heterogenous appearance of hematomas on MR imaging in order to use this newly gleaned data for patient care.—Robert M. Crowell, M.D.

Lobar Intracerebral Hemorrhage: Etiology and a Long-Term Follow-Up Study of 32 Patients
Yasufumi Tanaka, Makoto Furuse, Hideaki Iwasa, Toshio Masuzawa, Ken Saito, Fumiaki Sato, and Yoshikuni Mizuno (Jichi Med. School, Tochigi, Japan)
Stroke 17:51–57, Jan.–Feb. 1986   23–8

Thirty-two patients (23 men and 9 women, with a mean age of 47 years) were admitted in a 6½-year period with lobar intracerebral hemorrhage. Patients with hemorrhages in the basal ganglia and thalamic regions or with obvious cerebral trauma or hemorrhagic infarction had been excluded. Computed tomography (CT) was done with intravenous contrast, and 28 patients had cerebral angiography as well. Hypertension was a known factor in 13 patients, and arteriovenous malformation (AVM) in 5. The temporal or temporoparietal region was involved in half the cases. Three patients had multiple hemorrhages.

The onset was sudden in 31 cases. One patient was initially diagnosed as having a brain tumor by CT scan, but only a hematoma was found at operation (Fig 23–6). Three patients, 2 of them comatose when admitted, died in hospital. Thirteen patients had surgical evacuation. Two of the 5 patients noted to have ventricular extension died. Four patients died during

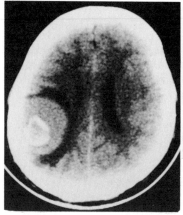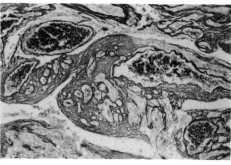

Fig 23–6.—Left, CT scan for a 15-year-old with a cavernous angioma in the left temporoparietal region; a round high-density area with central calcification and perifocal edema was seen. **Right,** histologic examination revealed sinusoidal, thin-walled vessels without intervening neural tissue; reticulin staining; × 40. (Courtesy of Tanaka, Y., et al.: Stroke 17:51–57, Jan.-Feb. 1986. By permission of the American Heart Association, Inc.)

a mean follow-up of 42 months, 1 of transtentorial herniation at recurrence. Thirteen patients recovered completely, whereas 12 were left with mild to moderate disability. No patient was confined to a wheelchair or bedridden at follow-up.

This limited experience suggests that surgery may be advisable in young, normotensive patients with lobar intracerebral hemorrhage and an accessible hematoma to prevent recurrent bleeding from a possible cryptic angioma. Surgical evacuation may be life saving in patients with a large hematoma. Smaller hematomas appear to resolve spontaneously, with a relatively good neurologic outcome.

▶ Although the rebleeding rate is unknown, recurrence of lobar hemorrhage from a small AVM certainly can occur. When angiographic study demonstrates an AVM, there is no hesitancy in recommending surgery.

When the hematoma is large (greater than 2 cm), the outcome is worse, as again confirmed by this study. In this group, evacuation of the hematoma may be done to minimize the mortality (and perhaps the morbidity).

However, there is no real evidence that small lobar hematomas harbor angiographically occult AVMs that threaten recurrent bleeding. It is difficult to justify exploration of such cases, even in the young. A more prudent approach is repeat study after 3 months, when mass effect has abated, with the use of CT, without and with contrast as well as angiography. Magnetic resonance imaging may also be helpful in such cases.—Robert M. Crowell, M.D.

Notes on Spontaneous Hemorrhage

▶ Transcranial Doppler can be used to evaluate cerebrovascular vasospasm (Aaslid et al.: *Neuroradiology* 28:1–16, 1986).

External pneumatic calf compression reduces deep venous thrombosis in patients with ruptured intracranial aneurysms (Black et al.: *Neurosurgery* 18:25–28, 1986).

Occult arteriovenous malformations can be detected on magnetic resonance when computed tomography (CT) scans are often normal (Gomori et al.: *Radiology* 158:707–713, 1986).

High-resolution CT can diagnose almost all temporal bone fractures, especially when coronal views are added to axial (Schubiger et al.: *Neuroradiology* 28:93–99, 1986). Metrizamide with CT almost always can localize cerebrospinal fluid leakage sites.

Traumatic basal ganglia hematomas carry a worse prognosis than other intracranial hematomas; these patients behave like patients with diffuse white matter injury (MacPherson et al.: *J. Neurol. Neurosurg. Psychiatry* 49:29–34, 1986).

Home observation of victims of mild head injury may be unreliable (Saunders et al.: *Ann. Emerg. Med.* 15:160–163, 1986).

The Queen Square group reports that sequential changes in brain stem auditory evoked responses denote transtentorial herniation in primate experiments (Tsutsui et al.: *Acta Neurochir.* 79:132–138, 1986).

In yet another controlled study, steroids had no beneficial effect on outcome in severe head injury (Dearden et al.: *J. Neurosurg.* 64:81–88, 1986).

Phenylpropanolamine, as found in "diet pills," has been associated with cerebral hemorrhage in 3 cases (McDowell and Lablanc: *West. J. Med.* 142:688–691, 1985).

Among 26 cases of pontine hemorrhage, a good prognosis was found when the transverse diameter of the hematoma was 20 mm or less (*J. Neurol. Neurosurg. Psychiatry* 48:658–662, 1985).

Brain stem hematoma confirmed by CT scanning can be associated with complete recovery (Cappa et al.: *J. Neurol.* 232:352–353, 1985).—Robert M. Crowell, M.D.

24 Trauma

Introduction

Several publications centered on the question of deployment of personnel for the care of head-injured patients. Miller and Jones (Digest 24–1) noted a change in the policy of admission such that temporary loss of consciousness was not grounds for admission led to a reduction in admissions of 24%. Gorman (Digest 24–2) suggests that data indicate that this policy is safe and results in great lessening of cost for care of these patients. Review of experience with acute head injuries in American Samoa is interpreted to suggest that general surgeons can provide effective energy care in rural settings (Digest 24–3). This concept is bound to cause great discussion in the neurosurgical community.

As regards management of head injury cases, magnetic resonance imaging may show pathology when computed tomography (CT) does not (Digest 24–4). Dynamic CT scanning may help discriminate hyperemia from ischemia in severe head injuries (Digest 24–5). Positive and expiratory pressure up to 10 cm can be tolerated without increasing intracranial pressure in patients with head injury (Digest 24–6). Nonoperative management of traumatic facial nerve palsy leads to good results in many cases (Digest 24–7).

In studies of spinal injury, fractures of the dens of type III are found to lead to nonunion in a large proportion of the cases (Digest 24–8). Duff reports good results with stabilization of the cervical spine with methyl methacrylate (Digest 24–9). In patients with T1–T10 injuries, laminectomy was associated with poor results, whereas anterior transthoracic deocompression led to improvement (Digest 24–10). Interoperative spinal sonography can be helpful in the evaluation of Harrington rod instrumentation for thoracic and lumbar fractures (Digest 24–11). A large cooperative study indicates that high-dose methylprednisolone treatment has no advantage over low-dose treatment in terms of neurologic function one year after spinal cord injury (Digest 24–12).

Robert M. Crowell, M.D.

Head Injury

The Work of a Regional Head Injury Service
J. Douglas Miller and P. A. Jones (Univ. of Edinburgh)
Lancet 1:1141–1144, May 18, 1985   24–1

In Edinburgh, all head-injured patients requiring admission are referred to a single head and spinal injury unit staffed by neurosurgeons, and patients from southeast Scotland with moderate and severe head injury are also referred. The workload was examined for 1981, when 1,959 patients were admitted to the unit, and 1,919 were assessable. Ninety-three patients were classified as comatose and 210 as moderately affected; the other 1,616 patients were fully conscious or merely confused at admission.

Intracranial hematoma, life-threatening complications, and deaths were most frequent in the severe cases, but a comparable amount of work was involved in caring for moderately and minimally injured patients, with respect to the number of studies performed, operations, complications, hospital stay, and morbidity. Five percent of all patients had cranial surgery. Reduction and fixation of unstable spinal fractures was performed mostly in patients with minor head injuries.

The policy was subsequently altered so that temporary loss of consciousness no longer led to admission. Admissions declined 24% as a result. Seat belt legislation was associated with a further 21% reduction in admissions. Many patients are adequately managed on an overnight casualty admission ward, with a decision about admission or discharge made next morning by the neurosurgical team.

▶ Miller and Jones found that, on their unit, as in many others, management of patients with minor head injuries requires a great deal of time and effort. By simply not admitting patients with brief loss of consciousness, admissions declined by 24%. The authors maintain that patients are safely managed on an overnight casualty admission ward that is evidently not staffed by neurosurgeons, but data to support the effectiveness of this policy are not presented. Implementation of such a program in the United States, where malpractice is a much more prevalent problem, could be difficult in the absence of substantial data. This article should be compared with the following presentation by Gorman, which advocates the same policy.—Robert M. Crowell, M.D.

Were You Knocked Out?—Yes, But I Wasn't Admitted

D. F. Gorman (Chester Royal Infirmary, England)
Arch. Emerg. Med 2:121 129, September 1985   24–2

A recent policy for admitting adult accident and emergency patients omitted initial unconsciousness and amnesia as absolute indications for admission. This policy was evaluated in a prospective series of 6,685 head-injured patients seen at the accident and emergency department who were managed according to the new policy, and 5,768 others managed on a conventional admission policy. The latter group was studied retrospectively. Both posttraumatic intracranial hematoma and death were more frequent in the later prospective series.

The more selective admission policy was no worse than current practice with regard to immediate morbidity and mortality. Survival of patients with posttraumatic intracranial hematoma was greater in the prospective series, and more such lesions were diagnosed and treated in this group. The number of admissions for head injury alone was reduced to one third of the expected number. Rates of admission after returning following an initial assessment were 0.1% in the retrospective series and 0.3% in the prospective series.

Adoption of a more selective admission policy for head-injured patients could lead to substantial cost savings. Such a policy appears to be safe and is common practice in the United States, despite a litigious atmosphere.

▶ In this important article, it is suggested that data from a controlled study indicate no adverse effects from not admitting patients on the basis of loss of consciousness following head trauma. A very substantial savings on the basis of this policy could be realized. However, the accuracy of follow-up for the patients not admitted has not been adequately addressed. Did the patients go home to slip into coma undetected by the study? This circumstance seems not entirely unlikely in the setting of an urban head trauma unit in the United States. Were there criteria relative to the length of duration of loss of consciousness? The data are interesting and suggestive; however, it remains premature to adopt such a policy in an urban setting in the United States, where accuracy of follow-up and patient compliance may be more difficult than in Britain. Moreover, our British colleagues do not have to deal with the malpractice situation facing the American neurosurgeon.—Robert M. Cromwell, M.D.

Can General Surgery Improve the Outcome of the Head Injury Victim in Rural America? A Review of the Experience in American Samoa
William P. Schechter, Eric Peper, and Vaiula Tuatoo (Univ. of California at San Francisco and Pago Pago, Lyndon Baines Johnson Tropical Med. Ctr., American Samoa)
Arch. Surg. 120:1163–1166, October 1985   24–3

General surgery programs in the United States do not train residents in the operative management of head injuries. Since the interval to decompression of subdural hematoma is critical in survival, general surgeons in rural areas should be adequately trained in emergency aspects of head injury management. Records of 50 head-injured patients (mean age, 23 years) who had burr hole procedures by general surgeons in American Samoa between 1974 and 1981 were reviewed. Twenty-three patients were alert at presentation, 7 were obtunded, and 20 were comatose. Indications for surgery included a compound, depressed skull fracture; localizing neurologic signs or neurologic deterioration; failure of the obtunded state to improve after 24–48 hours; and coma. Comatose patients received mannitol and dexamethasone perioperatively.

Six cases of extradural hematomas and one of subdural hematoma were found in the alert group. Five of the obtunded patients had an intracranial hematoma, as did 18 of the 20 comatose patients. Three of 9 deaths were directly attributable to delay in diagnosis of an intracranial hematoma.

Nearly all unconscious patients in this series had an intracranial hematoma amenable to drainage. Patients with head trauma can be effectively and safely treated by general surgeons in remote areas. Burr holes should be made in obtunded patients with localizing signs and in unconscious patients. General surgery residents should be trained in all aspects of head injury management, including the placement of diagnostic burr holes.

▶ This report is bound to cause controversy. The data indicate that patients in remote settings with head trauma can be treated by general surgeons who utilize burr holes to evacuate intracranial hematomas. The presentation raises the specter of general surgeons supplanting more broadly trained neurosurgeons in the area of head injury management.

This study presents unusual circumstances. Pago Pago, 5 hours by air from the nearest neurosurgical facility, is unlike any community in the continental United States. Moreover, the complex approach used by the general surgeons in this report included more than just burr holes—trephine craniotomies were performed in some cases. The utilization of a new classification of head injuries, exclusive of the Glasgow Coma Scale, may not be an advance in the description of groups of head injury patients.

Neurosurgeons may feel uncomfortable with the idea of general surgeons treating head injury. However, reports such as this suggest that pressure along these lines is likely to mount. Another building pressure is the need for personnel to man Trauma I facilities in urban centers in the United States. Difficulty in staffing with neurosurgeons has led to request for trained general surgeons to fulfill these functions. Education for general surgeons is raised in the discussion of providing head injury care. Provision of emergency head injury care on a timely basis by the neurosurgical community could go far toward alleviating these pressures. Neurosurgeons must address these issues or prepare for directives from others.—Robert M. Crowell, M.D.

Comparison of Magnetic Resonance Imaging and Computed Tomography in the Evaluation of Head Injury
Robert B. Snow, Robert D. Zimmerman, Samuel E. Gandy, and Michael D. F. Deck (Cornell Univ.)
Neurosurgery 18:45–52, January 1986   24–4

Computed tomography (CT) may fail to identify parenchymal or extraparenchymal intracranial abnormalities. Computed tomography and magnetic resonance (MR) imaging were compared in 35 patients with head trauma varying from mild concussion to severe neurologic dysfunction. The patients were evaluated 1 day to 10 years after injury. Magnetic resonance imaging was performed with two spin-echo sequences. Five case histories are presented.

CASE 1.—Boy, aged 10 years, in the final stage of renal disease secondary to congenital hypoplastic kidneys, was struck by an automobile. Soon thereafter, he complained of headaches and was admitted to hospital. Slight lethargy and a mild left hemiparesis were noted. Computed tomography revealed a right frontoparietal epidural hematoma with minimal mass effect and a subarachnoid hemorrhage in the contralateral suprasellar cistern and sylvian fissure. Bilateral lucent extracerebral fluid collections were present as well (Fig 24–1). The patient was monitored in the intensive care unit and treated with corticosteroids with resolution of the

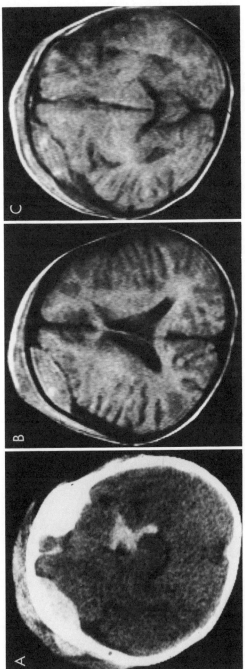

Fig 24–1.—Computed tomography scan without contrast agent demonstrates a right frontal epidural hematoma and subarachnoid hemorrhage in the left suprasellar cistern (**A**). T_1-weighted MR imaging scans reveal the epidural hematoma and bilateral subdural fluid collections but do not demonstrate the acute subarachnoid hemorrhage (**B** and **C**). (Courtesy of Snow, R.B., et al.: Neurosurgery 18:45–52, January 1986.)

headaches, lethargy, and hemiparesis by the next day. Magnetic resonance imaging revealed the epidural hematoma and identified the bilateral extracerebral collections as subdural, but did not show the subarachnoid hemorrhage (Fig 24–1). The dosage of the corticosteroids was tapered off, and the patient recovered without surgical intervention.

In 22 patients with 41 extracerebral lesions seen on MR imaging, all major lesions seen on CT scans were visualized by MR images, but additional subarachnoid clot was seen only on CT in two instances. Eleven small extracerebral collections were seen only in MR images. In most of the 21 patients with intracerebral lesions, the extent of edema and non-hemorrhagic contusion was better appreciated on MR images. Acute non-hemorrhagic contusions were seen only on MR imaging in five instances. Both MR and CT were unremarkable in 7 patients. One of these patients was comatose and had mild cortical atrophy but recovered significantly.

Magnetic resonance imaging appears to be superior to CT in imaging some extracerebral fluid collections and also in visualizing traumatic non-hemorrhagic contusions. Computed tomography remains the procedure of choice for diagnosing head injuries less than 72 hours old, partly because of the shorter examination time and the relative ease of monitoring patients with CT. Acute subarachnoid or parenchymal hemorrhage may be missed on MR. Magnetic resonance imaging is carried out if CT scans are normal or if the abnormalities cannot explain the clinical findings. Magnetic resonance imaging is superior to CT in the detection of all intracerebral and extracerebral traumatic lesions after 3 days.

▶ Magnetic resonance demonstrates lesions in head injury cases in which CT scans are normal. Eisenberg and colleagues from Galveston have shown that such MR-imaged lesions, often seen in deep white matter, resolve on serial studies in temporal correlation with improvement in neuropsychologic test scores. The neuropathology of the lesions is not known (edema vs. petechiae vs. axonal shear injury, etc.), but such structural changes provide the likely basis for "postconcussion syndrome" and other behavioral disorders that follow head trauma. Magnetic resonance is the study of choice in such cases when CT is negative.

The exact interpretation of MR imaging after injuries may be difficult in that resolving injury gives rise to a potpourri of signal generators (hemoglobin, methemaglobin, hemosiderin) and a consequently complex mixture of signals. Autopsy and experimental studies are needed to correlate MR images and pathology.—Robert M. Crowell, M.D.

Acute Brain Edema in Fatal Head Injury: Analysis by Dynamic CT Scanning

Eiji Yoshino, Tarumi Yamaki, Toshihiro Higuchi, Yoshiharu Horikawa, and Kimiyoshi Hirakawa (Kyoto Prefectural Univ. of Medicine and Saiseikai Shigaken Hosp., Shiga, Japan)

J. Neurosurg. 63:830–839, December 1985   24–5

Brain bulk enlargement can result from an increase in brain tissue water content and/or an increase in cerebral blood volume in patients with acute head injury. Dynamic computed tomography (CT) was carried out in 42 such patients seen between 1981 to 1983 to delineate the nature of fatal diffuse brain bulk enlargement. Seventeen surviving patients included 8 with acute epidural hematoma and 9 with acute subdural hematoma. Twenty-five fatally injured patients included 16 with acute subdural hematoma and 9 with bilateral brain bulk enlargement. The patients were previously well and had no other severe injuries. Dynamic CT was performed with bolus intravenous injection of 65% amidotrizoate meglumine. Follow-up conventional CT was done within 12 hours of initial examination.

Marked brain bulk enlargement was seen in all fatally injured patients with acute subdural hematoma. Dynamic CT suggested a hyperemic state in survivors with brain bulk enlargement but a severely ischemic state in

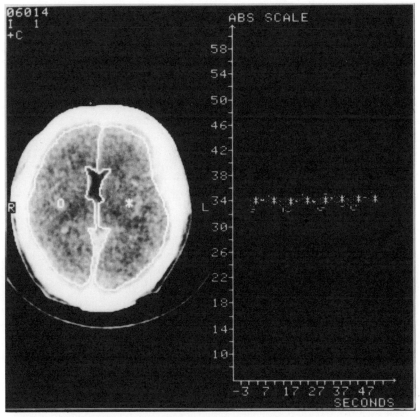

Fig 24–2.—Time-density curves of a fatally injured patient with bilateral brain bulk enlargement. Curves are identically flat on both sides. ABS scale is in Hounsfield units. (Courtesy of Yoshino, E., et al.: J. Neurosurg. 63:830–839, December 1985.)

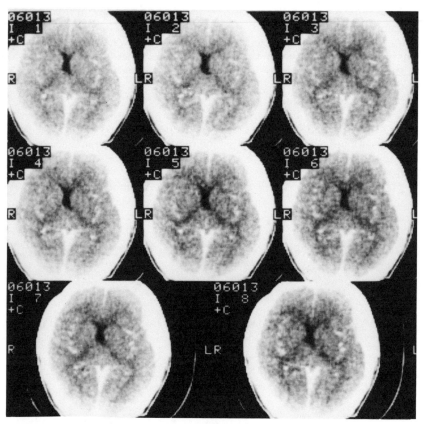

Fig 24–3.—Eight serial dynamic CT images in the same patient; no vascular enhancement can be seen on either side. The high-density area is the subarachnoid hemorrhage. (Courtesy of Yoshino, E., et al.: J. Neurosurg. 63:830–839, December 1985.)

two thirds of the patients who died (Figs 24–2 and 24–3). Most follow-up scans in fatally injured patients showed severe contusional hemorrhage, ventricular bleeding, or hemorrhage of the corpus callosum as a new lesion. Computed tomographic numbers on the side of hematoma were significantly lower than those on the opposite side.

Acute brain edema is the most common cause of fatal brain bulk enlargement in acutely head-injured patients. It is present within a few hours after impact. Dynamic CT is a useful means of evaluating cerebral hemodynamics in this setting. Positron emission tomography and magnetic resonance imaging also may help elucidate the pathophysiologic nature of fatal brain bulk enlargement.

▶ Because dynamic (CT) scanning is readily available in many centers, it could be applied in widespread fashion for the management of head injury. The authors show that this may be worthwhile to identify hyperemia with swelling and ischemia. These conditions might be treated differently. We need further data to know whether dynamic CT can be a useful clinical tool in treating severe brain injury.

In a related study, Powell and Crockard (*J. Neurosurg.* 63:745–749, 1985) report on correlations of intraventricular pressure and extradural pressure in patients with increased intracranial pressure. In the acute group, there was no predictable relation between extradural intraventricular pressure, with pressures varying as much as 30 mm of mercury. Extradural pressure monitoring can be misleading.—Robert M. Crowell, M.D.

Safe Use of PEEP in Patients With Severe Head Injury
Kevin R. Cooper, Peter A. Boswell, and Sung C. Choi (Med. College of Virginia)
J. Neurosurg. 63:552–555, October 1985   24–6

Positive end-expiratory pressure (PEEP) can improve abnormal oxygenation due to reduced lung volume in patients with severe head injury, but its safety remains uncertain. The effects of PEEP on intracranial pressure were examined in 33 patients seen between 1980 and 1984 with severe head injury causing loss of consciousness, but who retained some neurologic function. The intracranial pressure (ICP) was continuously monitored before and after the addition of 5–15 cm water of PEEP to the base-line level of pressure. The mean addition was 10 cm H_2O PEEP.

A statistically significant but clinically insignificant rise of 1.3 mm Hg

EFFECT OF PEEP ON PHYSIOLOGICAL VARIABLES IN
PATIENTS WITH HEAD INJURY*

Variable	Without PEEP	With PEEP	p Value
blood pressure (mm Hg)	101 ± 20	100 ± 24	NS
cardiac output (liter/min): n = 29	7.7 ± 2.3	7.0 ± 2.5	< 0.02
central venous pressure (mm Hg): n = 30	6.6 ± 4.8	9.5 ± 4.5	< 0.0005
static respiratory compliance (ml/cm H_2O): n = 30	48 ± 20	51 ± 25	NS
peak inspiratory pressure (cm H_2O)	28 ± 7	37 ± 9	< 0.0001
pCO_2 (mm Hg)	29.8 ± 5.2	30.6 ± 5.4	< 0.05
functional residual capacity (% predicted): n = 27	68 ± 19	95 ± 22	< 0.0001
venous admixture (%)	21 ± 12	16 ± 10	< 0.001
intracranial pressure (mm Hg)	13.2 ± 7.7	14.5 ± 7.5	< 0.005
cerebral perfusion pressure (mm Hg)	88 ± 22	86 ± 25	NS

*Positive end-expiratory pressure (PEEP) was applied at a mean of 10 cm H_2O. Data are expressed as means ± SD for 33 patients unless otherwise noted. NS, not significant.
(Courtesy of Cooper, K.R., et al.: J. Neurosurg. 63:552–555, October 1985.)

in mean ICP accompanied PEEP application (table). The mean ICP was unchanged in 8 patients with base-line pressures of 20 mm Hg or higher. The mean blood pressure and cerebral perfusion pressure did not change significantly with PEEP. The arterial pCO_2 and functional residual capacity increased significantly. No patient had evidence of neurologic deterioration in conjunction with the addition of PEEP.

A slight increase in intracranial pressure accompanies the addition of 10 cm water of PEEP in patients with severe head trauma. The change appears to be clinically insignificant. This degree of PEEP therefore can be used to prevent or treat hypoxemia in head-injured patients. Larger increases in ICP have been described, as has clinical deterioration, making it wise to monitor the ICP when possible.

▶ This carefully done study provides good evidence that positive and expiratory pressure up to 10 cm. of water does not cause deterious clinical or ICP effects in head injury patients. This is valuable information in that PEEP is frequently important in the care of these multiple injury patients. Caution is advised, however, with utilization of ICP monitoring devices to assure that intracranial pressure is not deleteriously affected.

Atracurium causes less increase in intracranial pressure in neurosurgical patients than other neuromuscular blocking agents (Minton et al.: Anesth. Analg. 64:1113–1116, 1985).

In dogs and cats subjected to expansion of an extradural supratentorial balloon, respiratory arrest occurred in inflation volumes that increased in relation to increasing blood pressure (Schrader et al.: *Acta Neurol. Scand.* 71:114–126, 1985).—Robert M. Crowell, M.D.

Nonoperative Management of Traumatic Facial Nerve Palsy
Dennis J. Maiman, Joseph F. Cusick, Alfred J. Anderson, and Sanford J. Larson (Med. College of Wisconsin and Wood VA Med. Ctr.)
J. Trauma 25:644–648, July 1985   24–7

The long-term results of nonoperative management were examined in a retrospective series of 45 patients (median patient age, 31 years) seen between 1975 and 1981 with head injury and facial nerve palsy. Management was expectant in 44 cases and included eye care and, in some cases, transcutaneous electric stimulation of the facial muscles. Corticosteroids were not used. Polytomography yielded abnormal results in all but 2 of 31 patients. Eight patients had comminuted petrous bone fractures. All patients had associated injuries. Hearing loss was documented in 8 patients.

Eight of the 10 patients who underwent electromyography after 2–4 weeks had evidence of denervation. The ultimate functional grade could not be related to the time of onset of facial paralysis. The type of fracture was not important in the final outcome (table). Most patients reached their final status within 6 months of injury. One patient with complete facial paralysis had a dry eye and poor facial function 1 year after injury. One

PRE- AND POSTRECOVERY GRADES BY FRACTURE TYPE*

	Initial Grade	Ultimate Grade				Per Cent with No Function on Admission	Per Cent Ultimately Becoming Intact
		2	3	4	Totals		
Overall	0	1	9	11	21		
	1	0	4	9	13		
	2	0	1	8	9		
	Totals	1	14	28	43†	49%	65%
Longitudinal	0	0	3	4	7		
	1	0	2	6	8		
	2	0	1	1	2		
	Totals	0	6	11	17	41%	65%
Transverse	0	0	1	2	3		
	1	0	0	0	0		
	2	0	0	1	1		
	Totals	0	1	3	4	75%	75%
Comminuted	0	1	2	4	7		
	1	0	0	0	0		
	2	0	0	1	1		
	Totals	1	2	5	8	88%	63%
No tomography	0	0	3	1	4		
	1	0	2	3	5		
	2	0	0	5	5		
	Totals	0	5	9	14	29%	64%

*$P < .02$ (Fisher's exact test): comminuted and transverse groups compared with longitudinal and no tomography groups.
†Patients with normal polytomographic findings not included.
(Courtesy of Maiman, D.J., et al.: J. Trauma 25:644–648, July 1985. Copyright by Williams and Wilkins, 1985.)

patient had late surgery for removal of a spicule from the facial canal; motor function improved after facial nerve decompression.

Most patients with traumatic facial nerve palsy recover substantial function with supportive management and do as well as they would with operation. The use of surgery for facial nerve palsy due to head trauma should be reassessed. Improvement may relate to resolution of edema or hematoma when the facial canal and nerve are intact. Some patients with transverse fracture who recover slowly may have nerve transection, followed by successful regeneration of the nerve within the facial canal.

▶ For a number of years, there has been controversy about the role of operative decompression for traumatic facial nerve palsy. Some ear, nose, and throat surgeons have recommended this procedure. Often neurosurgeons are reluctant to recommend this form of treatment in patients who may have other substantial head injuries. This contribution from the Medical College of Wisconsin is useful in that it indicates, in a series of 44 cases, that recovery of substantial function with supportive management occurred in most of the cases. Further data are needed to establish the role of operative intervention in such cases.—Robert M. Crowell, M.D.

Spinal Injuries

Fractures of the Dens: A Multicenter Study

Charles R. Clark and Augustus A. White, III (Univ. of Iowa Hosps., Beth Israel Hosp., and Harvard Univ.)
J. Bone Joint Surg. [Am.] 67-A:1340–1348, December 1985   24–8

The best means of treating dens fractures remains uncertain. Fractures managed by 27 different surgeons in 4 countries were classified by the Anderson-d'Alonzo scheme. Type II fractures involve the junction of the dens with the vertebral body, while type III injuries extend into the vertebral body.

Ninety-six cases of type II injury were assessable. Initial management with a halo device succeeded in only 68% of the cases, but posterior cervical fusion was successful in 96% of the cases. One fourth of cases of type II fracture with significant anterior or posterior displacement failed to unite. Forty-eight cases of type III fracture involving the second cervical vertebral body were reviewed. Malunion and nonunion occurred in patients treated with an orthosis alone. More than half the type III fractures were displaced. Eight injuries were managed by skeletal traction, 16 with a halo device, and 6 by anterior or posterior fusion. Ten patients required further treatment. All fractures were stable after secondary treatment. Complications included cardiopulmonary arrest in a patient who died 24 hours after injury. Four patients treated with an orthosis went on to malunion, and one had nonunion.

Dens fractures are serious injuries. Surgical stabilization should be considered in type II cases in which significant displacement and/or angulation is present. Most surgeons have preferred posterior fusion. Type III fractures may malunite after treatment with an orthosis alone. The halo device appears to be the safest and most reliable approach, but surgery may be necessary for very unstable fractures. A high index of suspicion is the key to diagnosis and proper treatment of dens fractures.

▶ This substantial study provides new data on dens fractures, and in general the results correspond with previously held conclusions. A surprise, however, has to do with type III fractures which, in this study, often progressed to malunion or nonunion when treated with an orthosis. It is hard to reconcile these results with previously published data, but the substantial number of cases (48) commands attention. On the basis of the presented data, halo fixation appears to be the best treatment for these type III fractures. Neurosurgeons must be fully aware of the details of modern studies on cervical spine fractures to maintain management of this important category of injury.—Robert M. Crowell, M.D.

Surgical Stabilization of Traumatic Cervical Spine Dislocation Using Methyl Methacrylate: Long-Term Results in 26 Patients
Thomas A. Duff (Univ. of Wisconsin)
J. Neurosurg. 64:39–44, January 1986   24–9

An acrylic inlay was used as the primary stabilizing element in 26 consecutive patients with acute fracture-dislocation of the cervical spine. For the 23 male and 3 female patients (age range, 17–53 years), 78% of whom were younger than 25 years, all fractures were below the C2 level. Representative radiographs are shown in Figure 24–4. Evidence of instability

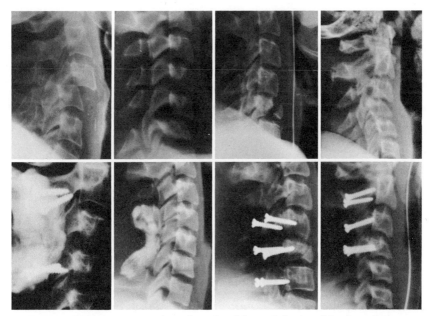

Fig 24–4.—Upper row, preoperative radiographs of the cervical spine of 4 patients. Lower row, postoperative radiographs for each patient, obtained 6 months or more after surgery. Radiolucent methyl methacrylate was used in the 2 patients whose radiographs are to the right. (Courtesy of Duff, T.A.: J. Neurosurg. 64:39–444, January 1986.)

was present on neutral neck radiographs in 17 cases, and on flexion-extension views in 9 cases. Fourteen patients were neurologically impaired, 3 of whom were paraplegic but had evidence of residual cord function at the level of dislocation. Traction was initially used in all cases.

A steel screw usually was inserted into the articular pillars of the fractured vertebra and the adjacent vertebrae before an oblong mold of acrylic was applied over the screw heads. No patient had a worsening of neurologic impairment after surgery. The vertebral elements remained aligned in all but two cases during the follow-up of 6 months to 7 years. All patients recovered to the extent of their physical ability. Two patients had breakage of acrylic side struts, one of whom required reoperation. These failures may have been due to the use of insufficient material.

A large proportion of patients with fracture-dislocation in the lower cervical spine can be stabilized by use of an acrylic implant without bone grafting, but more needs to be learned about the long-term durability of these materials. The mold takes up more space than does wire, and failure can occur if insufficient material is applied. The procedure is, however, a relatively simple and safe one, and provides immediate and long-term stabilization.

▶ Duff provides evidence that posterior cervical spine fusion with screws in facet joints and acrylic provides good stabilization in almost all patients (24 of

26 for 6 months to 7 years). Because of the simplicity and availability of this technique, it deserves further evaluation in the treatment of these common injuries.—Robert M. Crowell, M.D.

The Results of Treatment of Acute Injuries of the Upper Thoracic Spine With Paralysis

Henry H. Bohlman, Alvin Freehafer, and John Dejak (VA Med. Ctr. and High-land View Hosp. and Case Western Reserve Univ.)
J. Bone Joint Surg. [Am.] 67-A:360–369, March 1985   24–10

Of 218 patients seen in 1950–1978 with injury to the spine at the T1–T10 levels, paralysis was complete in 84%; the other 16% had an incomplete lesion. Three fourths of the patients were aged 20–45 years. Sixty patients with a complete cord lesion were managed nonoperatively, as were 5 with an incomplete lesion. A right transthoracic approach was used for decompression of the spinal cord and fusion of the spine. A bed for an iliac bone graft was prepared by removing the end-plates of the adjacent vertebrae. The cortical part of the graft was countersunk into the vertebral bodies, and gelatin foam was placed over the dura. A molded spinal orthosis was applied a few days after surgery and left on until bone union was documented, usually at 3 months.

None of the patients with a complete cord lesion, including 149 who were followed for 2 years or longer, regained motor function or more than two levels of intercostal sensation. None became functional walkers with long braces. Two of 5 patients who were not operated on recovered from incomplete cord injury. The condition of four of 17 patients who underwent laminectomy improved, but 8 lost neurologic function or became totally paraplegic after laminectomy. Five of 8 patients who had anterior transthoracic decompression and spinal fusion recovered. Numerous medical complications were seen, especially in patients with complete cord injury.

Patients with incomplete paralysis after fracture of the upper thoracic spine should have appropriate diagnostic studies and may undergo anterior transthoracic decompression if cord impingement is present. Laminectomy is contraindicated in this setting. Anterior bone or disk fragments cannot be reached without damaging the cord, and removal of the stabilizing elements produces further kyphotic deformity and cord compression.

▶ This is an important contribution that presents a large experience with injury to the thoracic spine. Among 60 patients with complete lesions, none regained significant motor function. Among incomplete lesions, twice as many patients undergoing laminectomy deteriorated as improved. Five of eight patients with anterior decompression recovered. The data strongly indicate that nonoperative therapy is best for patients with complete lesions, while anterior decompression gives the best results for incomplete lesions with compression. Laminectomy appears to have no role. A team effort is best here: the neurosurgeon can provide optimum neurologic assessment and, when indicated, anterior decompression; the orthopedist can effect stabilization. Neurosurgeons must develop their knowledge and skills in this area to maintain a role in the therapy for these injury cases.

A 10-year experience in Canada describes unstable fractures of the thoracolumbar spine (Jodoin et al.: J Trauma 25:197–202, 1985). One-hundred eight unstable fractures were treated. Laminectomy was performed in 30 with Harrington fusion in 71, and 16 without surgery. 75 complications were recorded; complications were more common in the laminectomy group. The group with instrumentation was ambulated earlier. Neurologic recovery in laminectomy and nonlaminectomy groups was not different. Spinal realignment was better in the group with instrumentation and worse when laminectomy was performed.—Robert M. Crowell, M.D.

Intraoperative Spinal Sonography in Thoracic and Lumbar Fractures: Evaluation of Harrington Rod Instrumentation
Robert M. Quencer, Berta M. Montalvo, Frank J. Eismont, and Barth A. Green (Univ. of Miami)
AJR 145:343–349, August 1985   24–11

Intraoperative spinal sonography (IOSS) provides a means of accurately and immediately determining the efficacy of Harrington rod instrumentation for fracture or fracture-dislocation of the thoracolumbar spine. This study was performed in 37 patients with unstable thoracolumbar fractures who underwent rod instrumentation. Spinal computed tomography also was carried out in 35 cases. A laminotomy measuring at least 1.0 × 1.5 cm generally was required for adequate sonographic assessment; spinal instability does not result.

All fractures in these cases were considered potentially unstable and were associated with displaced bone fragments in the spinal canal. Twenty-two patients had significant neurologic deficits. Base-line IOSS showed vertebral malalignment and bone fragments compressing the thecal sac in all cases but 1. Harrington rod instrumentation resulted in adequate spinal decompression in 14 cases (Fig 24–5). Further maneuvers or surgical procedures were performed in 15 patients with inadequate decompression; adequate spinal decompression resulted in 11 instances. In 6 cases, bone fragments were removed or impacted before rod placement. Five of these patients then had adequate decompression, while 1 required additional bone impaction.

Routine use of IOSS can reduce the occurrence of inadequate decompression in patients who undergo Harrington rod instrumentation for thoracolumbar fracture or fracture-dislocation. Spinal malalignment and displaced bone fragments are immediately demonstrated by IOSS, allowing measures to be taken to improve spinal alignment and reduce bone fragments from the canal.

▶ Serial radiographic study of patients with unstable thoracolumbar fractures showed stabilization with Harrington instrumentation and progressive angula-

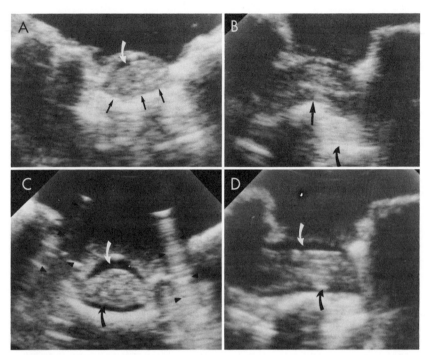

Fig 24–5.—Cauda equina before and after Harrington rod instrumentation. **A,** transverse intraoperative sonogram before Harrington rod instrumentation shows compression of cauda equina by displaced bone fragment *(arrows)*, more marked on right. A small amount of cerebrospinal fluid (CSF) *(curved arrow)* is seen beneath dorsal dura. **B,** longitudinal sonogram shows displaced bone fragment *(straight arrow)* from dorsal part of adjacent vertebral body *(curved arrow)*. **C,** transverse sonogram after bilateral Harrington rod instrumentation shows adequate decompression of spinal canal, with CSF *(arrows)* seen around entire cauda equina. Typical sonographic appearance of Harrington rods *(arrowheads)* is seen. **D,** longitudinal sonogram after bilateral Harrington rod instrumentation also slows adequate decompression of spinal canal, with CSF *(arrows)* seen around entire cauda equina. (Courtesy of Quencer, R.M., et al.: AJR 145:343–349, August 1985. Copyright 1985, by the American Roentgen Ray Society.)

tion in patients treated conservatively (Lindahl et al.: *Acta Radiol.* [*Diagn.*] *(Stockh)* 26:67–77, 1985).—Robert M. Crowell, M.D.

Methylprednisolone and Neurological Function 1 Year After Spinal Cord Injury: Results of the National Acute Spinal Cord Injury Study
Michael B. Bracken, Mary Jo Shepard, Karen G. Hellenbrand, William F. Collins, Linda S. Leo, Daniel F. Freeman, Franklin C. Wagner, Eugene S. Flamm, Howard M. Eisenberg, Joseph H. Goodman, Phanor L. Perot, Jr., Barth A. Green, Robert G. Grossman, John N. Meagher, Wise Young, Boguslav Fischer, Guy L. Clifton, William E. Hunt, and Nathan Rifkinson (Yale Univ.)
J. Neurosurg. 63:704–713, November 1985   24–12

A multicenter trial was carried out to compare the efficacy of a high dose of methylprednisolone sodium succinate (MPSS; 1-gm bolus and 1 gm daily thereafter for 10 days) with that of a standard dose (0.1-gm and

0.1-gm daily) bolus in patients with acute spinal cord trauma. Previous evaluation indicated no effect on high-dose MPSS on neurologic function 6 weeks or 6 months after injury. Patients younger than age 13 years and those with severe comorbidity were excluded. All patients were admitted within 48 hours of injury. The 256 patients followed up for 1 year represented 89.5% of the series. The two treatment groups had similar neurologic findings at admission to the study.

There were no significant differences in recovery of motor function, pinprick response, or touch sensation in the two treatment groups 1 year following injury, after adjustment for possibly confounding factors. Analyses taking total corticosteroid dose and relative weight into account confirmed the lack of a corticosteroid treatment effect. The case-fatality rate was not associated with the treatment protocol, but mortality was related to age and to more severe injury.

Treatment with MPSS after acute spinal cord injury has not promoted neurologic recovery 1 year after injury. The case-fatality rate of 11% suggests that the likelihood of death within a year after hospital discharge is low.

▶ To establish the efficacy of any therapy, controlled trials of treatment with the use of modern techniques are highly desirable. Confounding variables, even those that have not been identified, may be obviated and equally distributed between treatment and control groups.

There are a rationale and supporting data from animal experiments to suggest that high-dose steroid therapy is effective in the treatment of spinal cord injury. There is also a strong acceptance of this concept among clinicians to the point that the withholding of steroid treatment is believed to be risky from the malpractice standpoint. Therefore, the results of a controlled study of high-dose steroid treatment are especially welcome at this time.

The results indicate that high-dose steroid therapy is not more effective than low-dose steroid therapy in the treatment of patients with spinal cord injury. Thus, there is no reason to continue high-dose steroid therapy for such patients. With the background of this study, the National Spinal Cord Injury Study Group may now proceed to add a placebo arm and the more fundamental question of whether steroid therapy at any dose is helpful in the treatment of these patients.

There are some minor problems with this study, for instance, exclusion of certain patients at the discretion of the local center, but fundamentally the study is sound and puts treatment in this particular area on solid scientific ground.

Steroids may, of course, *cause* problems, e.g., septic complications are more common in patients with CNS trauma who are treated with corticosteroids, according to De Marin et al. (*Ann. Surg.* 202:248–252, 1985). Furthermore, a recent court decision held that sustained steroid therapy for spinal cord injury, which caused aseptic necrosis of the femoral head, constituted malpractice.

In another drug treatment regimen, a Phase I trial of naloxone treatment in acute spinal cord injury showed minimal side effects and encouraging improvement in clinical status, according to Flamm et al. (*J. Neurosurg.* 63:390–397, 1985).—Robert M. Crowell, M.D.

Long-term Follow-up of Renal Function After Spinal Cord Injury
K. V. Kuhlemeier, L. K. Lloyd, and S. L. Stover (Univ. of Alabama)
J. Urol. 134:510–513, September 1985   24–13

Urologic complications secondary to neurogenic bladder continue to compromise the long-term outlook for patients with spinal cord injury. The extent of renal functional deterioration was determined in 519 patients with cord dysfunction of rapid onset and usually of traumatic origin. Function was assessed by measuring effective renal plasma flow (ERPF) by renal scintigraphy. The mean age at injury was 31 years, and that at evaluation 34 years. Forty-three percent of the patients were quadriplegics. About half the patients had complete cord injuries.

Renal function tended to decline over time after injury. Some reduction in ERPF was evident 9–10 years after injury. The mean reduction in ERPF associated with renal stone disease was 51 ml per minute, but fortunately only 4% of patients had a history of renal stones. Quadriplegia was associated with a greater reduction in ERPF than was paraplegia. A history of chills and fever was also associated with a significant decrease in ERPF. Renal function was less in older patients, but the difference between older and younger patients was stable in time after cord injury. Effective renal plasma flow to the lower functioning kidney was unrelated to bladder stones, the completeness of cord injury, or concurrent bacteriuria.

Cord-injured patients generally maintain acceptable or good renal function for at least 10 years after injury, if treatable risk factors are properly managed. Treatment of renal stones is most important, and extracorporeal shock wave lithotripsy should be useful in this setting. The pathophysiologic state of the entire urinary tract after cord injury is primarily related to the state of the bladder.

Notes on Spinal Injury

▶ The National Football Head and Neck Injury Registry indicates a drop in the number of cases of permanent cervical quadriplegia from 34 in 1976 to 5 in 1984. This is probably due to rule changes banning "spearing," the practice of using the top of the helmet as the initial point of contact in making a tackle. Implementation of appropriate changes in sports such as diving, rugby, and ice hockey might lead to reduction of cervical spine injuries in these activities (Torg et al.: *JAMA* 254:3439–3443, 1985).

In a group of 105 patients with cervical spine injuries, twenty-four percent showed evidence of injuries of multiple levels (Hadden and Gillespie: *Injury* 16:628–633, 1985).

In the treatment of unstable spines with Luque rods, postoperative brace protection is necessary to obtain successful stabilization (Nasca: *S. Med. J.* 78:303–309, 1985).

Use of cadaver bone graft in children for treatment of posterior cervical fusion leads to pseudarthrosis (Stabler et al.: *J. Bone Joint Surg.* [Am] 67A:370–375, 1985).

After high cervical cord injury, home ventilator support is economically desirable and technically feasible (Gower and Davis: *S. Med. J.* 78:1010–1011, 1985).

High-resolution computed tomography scanning can detect with surety uncal vertebral and facet joint dislocations and cervical articular pillar fractures (Yetkin et al.: *AJNR* 6:633–637, 1985).

Patients with cervical cord lesions have an increased susceptibility to peptic gastrointestinal complication (Soderstrom and Ducker: *J. Trauma* 25:1030–1038, 1985).

An impalement injury of the abdomen and spine may be effectively treated by simultaneous laminectomy and laparotomy with careful preplanning of removal of the impaling object. (Horowitz et al.: *J. Trauma* 25:914–916, 1985).—Robert M. Crowell, M.D.

Other Injuries

Subclavian-Axillary Vascular Trauma

Robert A. McCready, C. Daniel Procter, and Gordon L. Hyde (Univ. of Kentucky)

J. Vasc. Surg. 3:24–31, January 1986   24–14

The records of 40 patients seen from 1963 to 1984 with traumatic injury to the subclavian and axillary vessels were reviewed. All patients with iatrogenic injuries were excluded. One patient had isolated subclavian vein injury, 18 patients had subclavian artery trauma, and 21 had axillary artery trauma. Concomitant venous injuries were frequent. Thirty-five patients were male and 5 were female, with an average age of 30 years. Gunshot injuries predominated. Three patients with subclavian vascular injuries died. Eighty-two percent of the patients had signs of distal ischemia. Five patients with subclavian artery injuries, including 4 with pseudoaneurysms, had delayed treatment, as did 2 with axillary artery trauma. An infraclavicular approach was used in most cases of axillary artery injury. The most frequent approach to subclavian artery injuries was clavicular resection.

Thirty-three patients were followed up for an average of 34 months. Axillary artery repairs in two of the patients failed. Thrombosis of an axillary venous repair was suspected but not proved in 2 patients. No subclavian artery repairs failed. Venous repairs were patent in all instances. Two patients had subclavian vein ligation and tolerated it well.

Hemodynamically stable patients with signs of arterial insufficiency should have angiography. The extent of injury to the subclavian or axillary artery dictates the method of repair to be used. Primary repair by lateral arteriorrhaphy or resection with end-to-end anastomosis is preferred whenever feasible. Otherwise, an interposition graft must be used, or the vessels ligated. It seems reasonable to attempt venous repair in patients with stable vital signs. Permanent disability often results from associated neurologic injury in these cases.

▶ In subclavian-axillary artery trauma, associated injury to brachial plexus is the most important determinant of eventual outcome. Neurosurgery, therefore, ought to be involved early in the care of such patients. The use of electrodiagnostic studies may have prognostic value (Digest 28–1). Early vascular repair is recommended by the present report, and primary suture can be recommended for sharply divided plexus elements. When the patient is unstable or neural elements are ragged, cut ends should be tagged for secondary reconstruction.—Robert M. Crowell, M.D.

25 Spine

Introduction

Cervicomedullary junction pathology was mentioned in several reports. Crockard et al. (Digest 25–1) describe transoral decompression of the cervicomedullary junction for rheumatoid arthritis, and results were encouraging. In patients with rheumatoid arthritis and "cranial settling," Menezes et al. (Digest 25–2) obtained good results with cranial traction in a number of cases but resorted to transoral decompression in some. Transoral decompression can also be effective when compression is caused by an enlarged odontoid process (Digest 25–3).

Regarding cervical pathology, posttraumatic progressive myelopathy is well imaged by magnetic resonance, and intraoperative sonography can help with cyst drainage (Digest 25–4). Senagas et al. recommend treatment of cervical spondylotic myelopathy by extensive anterior decompression and report good results with this approach (Digest 25–5).

In the area of lumbar pathology, intact-arch spondylolisthesis can be recognized on computed tomography and treated by open surgery with good results (Digest 25–6). Review of the available randomized clinical trials suggest a significant effect of chymopapain injection in the treatment of lumbar disk herniation (Digest 25–7); good results without controls continue to be reported (Digest 25–8). Surgical findings after failure of chemonucleolysis suggest that free fragments and lateral recess stenosis are important causes of failure of injection (Digest 25–9). A recent review of lateral mass fusion shows that there are many poor results, especially in patients with previous surgery (Digest 25–10).

Syringomyelia is beautifully demonstrated by magnetic resonance (Digests 25–11 and 25–12). Postoperative metrizamide computed tomography studies are helpful; reduction in cyst size can be demonstrated (Digest 25–13). Syringoperitoneal shunting leads to clinical improvement in the great majority of patients (Digest 25–14).

In the area of spinal tumors, neoplastic cord compression may be treated by vertebral body resection and stabilization with good palliative short-term results (Digest 25–15). Myelography is recommended for spinal cord compression in breast cancer (Digest 25–17). Laminectomy and anterolateral approach for the vertebral artery dissection can produce total resections of cervical neurinomas with excellent results (Digest 25–18). Myxopapillary ependymoma remains a challenge for the neurosurgeon; there are substantial neurologic deficits after tumor removal with significant numbers of recurrence, findings that lead to the idea that radiation therapy may be offered after subtotal removal (Digest 25–19). Cooper and Epstein report good results with radical resection of intramedullary spinal cord tumors in adults (Digest 25–20).

Robert M. Crowell, M.D.

Cervicomedullary Junction

Surgical Treatment of Cervical Cord Compression in Rheumatoid Arthritis
H. A. Crockard, W. K. Essigman, J. M. Stevens, J. L. Pozo, A. O. Ransford,
and B. E. Kendall (Natl. Hosps. for Nervous Diseases and Univ. College Hosp.,
London, and Lister Hosp., Stevenager, England)
Ann. Rheum. Dis. 44:809–816, December 1985   25–1

Cervical myelopathy is a rare but serious complication of rheumatoid arthritis. Conservative management carries a high mortality, but reduction of subluxation and posterior fusion may require prolonged bed rest and traction, and prolonged immobilization and external fixation have been problems when anterior decompression has been attempted. Twenty-three rheumatoid patients with cervical myelopathy were treated since 1979. Twenty patients had atlantoaxial subluxation. Sensory symptoms were frequent and varied. Motor weakness usually was spastic in nature. Seventeen patients underwent anterior decompression, 14 with transoral removal of the odontoid peg and pannus and posterior occipitocervical fusion at the same session.

None of the patients died after transoral surgery, but 1 patient had bleeding from a displaced vertebral artery during odontoid removal. No embolism occurred after external splintage was abandoned. All patients but one improved after anterior cord decompression, but 2 have deteriorated since surgery. Quadriparetic patients became able to walk and recovered sphincter function. Paresthesias also improved, and the Lhermitte's sign consistently disappeared.

Early diagnosis of cervical myelopathy by computed myelotomography in patients with rheumatoid disease will maximize the chances of a good surgical outcome. Single-stage anterior decompression and posterior internal fixation are well tolerated and produce clinical improvement. This approach is less dangerous than conventional treatment. Use of the anterior route is especially necessary if there is compression by rheumatoid pannus.

▶ Crockard and colleagues present an extensive experience with this relatively uncommon entity. In 14 cases of transoral removal of the odontoid peg and pannus followed by posterior fusion, excellent results have been documented, with quadriparetic patients becoming able to walk and recovering sphincter function. On the basis of personal experience with 5 cases, I am convinced that the transoral route to the dens provides an excellent route for decompression in this area. Dr. Crockard's addition of the fibrin glue method for sealing cerebrospinal fluid leaks is especially welcome. The results reported by Crockard excite enthusiasm about this approach for rheumatoid disease. I believe that as neurosurgeons become more familiar with this approach the results are likely to establish this approach for the treatment of a number of lesions in this area.

The transoral-transclival approach to the base of the brain and upper cervical cord is safe and effective for a variety of pathologies, according to Crockard (*Ann. R. Coll. Surg. Engl.* 67:321–325, 1985). Division of the soft palate is recommended, permitting exposure down to the fourth cervical vertebra. Closure of the dura is carried out by use of a fibrin glue. Posterior fixation with bone grafting permits immediate postoperative mobilization. Indications include C1–2 fracture dislocation, basilar impression, rheumatoid arthritis, extradural masses, and intradural mass lesions.

For thoracic kyphosis in ankylosing spondylitis, compensatory lumbar lordosis may be achieved by lumbar osteotomies with internal fixation. Among 22 patients undergoing such a procedure all patients reported subjective respiratory improvement (Styblo et al.: *Acta Orthop. Scand.* 56:294–297, 1985).

Good results are reported among 14 cases treated with spinal osteotomy for ankylosing spondylitis (McMaster: *Ball and Joint Surgery* 67B:204–210, 1985).—Robert M. Crowell, M.D.

Odontoid Upward Migration in Rheumatoid Arthritis: An Analysis of 45 Patients With "Cranial Settling"
Arnold H. Menezes, John C. VanGilder, Charles R. Clark, and George El-Khoury (Univ. of Iowa)
J. Neurosurg. 63:500–509, October 1985   25–2

Forty-five rheumatoid arthritis patients were seen between 1978 and 1984 with evidence of "cranial settling," or vertical penetration of the odontoid process through the foramen magnum. All had symptoms from compression of the cervicomedullary junction. The anterior arch of the atlas was telescoped onto the body of the axis, and its posterior arch was displaced rostrally and ventrally, reducing the anteroposterior diameter of the spinal canal. Atlantoaxial instability was demonstrated in all cases. Degenerative erosive changes were seen in the atlas lateral masses and correlated with the degree of odontoid invagination. Occipital headache was a constant feature. A majority of patients had limb paresthesias, and most had progressive trouble walking. Four had acute onset of quadriparesis. About half the patients had vertigo, diplopia, and transient blackouts. Ten patients had evidence of cranial nerve dysfunction.

Cervical traction was applied with Gardner-Wells tongs or the halo ring apparatus. Traction for 1 to 2 weeks was necessary in severe cases. Thirty-six patients had acceptable reduction and underwent posterior occipito-cervical fusion with wire and bone grafting and including C1 decompression if necessary. Acrylic fixation has also been used in recent years. Seven patients with irreducible compression had transoral resection of the lesion and subsequent posterior occiput-C2 fusion. Two severely debilitated patients refused surgery. All patients improved neurologically. Bone union occurred in all cases, and there were no infections. Cranial settling did not recur during the 1- to 6-year follow-up.

Cranial settling is a potentially life-threatening complication of rheumatoid arthritis. Catastrophic sequelae are possible even without gross neurologic abnormality. Even severely incapacitated patients can recover neurologically after appropriate surgery.

▶ This fine contribution is likely to be the key reference for "cranial settling" for years to come. The authors describe in detail the pathophysiology, pathoanatomy, and clinical presentation of this rheumatoid condition, which evidently is more common than generally thought, in view of the 45 cases collected by the authors in a 6-year period.

Undoubtedly, magnetic resonance imaging will add significantly to the depiction of pathologic anatomy and perhaps replace other studies. Results of management are most impressive. All treated patients improved neurologically (by at least two functional grades). In the great majority, prolonged skull retraction followed by posterior fusion (with bone and acrylic fixation, followed by immobilization in a sterno-occipitomandibular immobilizer [SOMI] brace) was highly effective treatment. In 7 patients, transoral removal of the dens was required to decompress the craniovertebral junction. The authors have substantial experience with this latter procedure for basilar invagination of other cause. Those unfamiliar with the method should know that the technical challenge is formidable: the approach is aided by an experienced ear, nose, and throat surgeon; removal of the dens requires patience and care to avoid a cerebrospinal fluid leak; and management of rhinorrhea can be difficult. Nonetheless, in experienced hands, as in the present report, the method can be highly effective in providing definitive decompression of the cervicomedullary junction.—Robert M. Crowell, M.D.

Foramen Magnum Syndrome Caused by a Dolichoodontoid Process

Yoshimi Yanai, Reizoh Tsuji, Shigehiro Ohmori, Satoru Kubota, and Chikao Nagashima (Chikamori Hosp., Kohchin, and Saitama Med. School, Japan)
Surg. Neurol. 24:95–100, July 1985   25–3

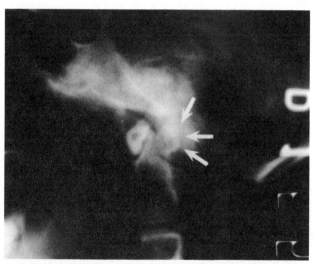

Fig 25–1.—Sagittal tomogram of the region of the foramen magnum. The *arrows* point to the posterior margin of the odontoid tip. The odontoid peg and the atlantoaxial joint are located much higher than normal, and the odontoid tip protrudes dorsally. (Courtesy of Yanai, Y., et al.: Surg. Neurol. 24:95–100, July 1985. Reprinted by permission of the publisher, Copyright 1985, Elsevier Science Publishing Co., Inc.)

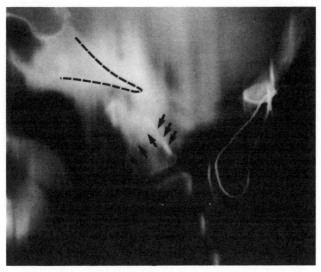

Fig 25–2.—Sagittal tomogram of the region of the foramen magnum 7 days after the operation. The *arrows* point to the residue of the body of the axis. The odontoid tip, the anterior arch of the atlas, and the posterior border of the foramen magnum have been drilled away sufficiently. Twisted wires used for occipito–C 3 fixation are seen. (Courtesy of Yanai, Y., et al.: Surg. Neurol. 24:95–100, July 1985. Reprinted by permission of the publisher, Copyright 1985, Elsevier Science Publishing Co., Inc.)

Congenital basilar impression may be associated with a wide range of vertebral anomalies and brain or spinal cord anomalies. The present patient had an anomalous configuration of the odontoid tip and several other vertebral anomalies. Marked improvement followed transoral removal of the odontoid tip and the anterior arch of the atlas with posterior fixation of the occipital squama to the lamina of C3.

Man, 21 years old, presented with difficulty swallowing and dysarthria 7 years after the onset of swallowing problems and intermittent amaurosis. A short neck and low hairline were noted. Bilateral horizontal nystagmus was present, as was dysarthria with paresis of the pharyngeal constrictor muscles on the left and of the left side of the soft palate. Static ataxia of both legs also was noted. The basiocciput was shorter than normal. The odontoid tip protruded dorsally, and the posterior lip of the foramen magnum was infolded. Tomography scans showed a ball-like odontoid tip that protruded dorsally (Fig 25–1). Hypoplasia of the posterior vertebral arches and absence of the spinous process of the axis were observed, as well as bilateral cervical ribs and eight cervical vertebrae. Metrizamide myelography showed arrest of dye flow at the C3 level.

Dentectomy was performed transorally, with decompression of the foramen magnum and posterior fixation at the same session. The occipital squama and the lamina of C3 were joined using wire and acrylic. Postoperative tomography confirmed adequate removal of the infolded odontoid tip and the posterior border of the foramen magnum (Fig 25–2). There was no instability at the occipitoatlantal or atlantoaxial joint. The patient swallowed and spoke normally at discharge from the hospital and has remained asymptomatic.

Posterior decompression usually suffices when basilar impression causes myelopathy, but a mass anterior to the upper portion of the spinal cord or medulla may necessitate a transoral procedure, as in the present case. Either improvement or arrest of the clinical disorder can be expected.

Cervical Pathology

Posttraumatic Progressive Myelopathy: Clinical and Radiologic Correlation Employing MR Imaging, Delayed CT Metrizamide Myelography, and Intraoperative Sonography
Stephen S. Gebarski, Fredrick W. Maynard, Irygve O. Gabrielsen, James E. Knake, Joseph T. Latack, and Julian T. Hoff (Univ. of Michigan)
Radiology 157:379–385, November 1985   25–4

Various diagnostic modalities were compared in nine patients seen in a 9-month period with posttraumatic progressive myelopathy (PTPM). A motor vehicle accident was the most frequent cause of injury. The time from injury to presentation with new neurologic disorder was 9 months to 16 years. Both magnetic resonance imaging and delayed computed tomography metrizamide myelography correlated with the findings at intraoperative sonography and the pathologic findings in the demonstration of myelomalacia, small cysts (Fig 25–3), or large cysts. Sonography was best at detecting septations and small additional cysts.

Five patients had shunt placement, and one underwent hemilaminectomy and foraminotomy. Shunt placement consistently was followed by stabilization or a decrease in signs and symptoms, except in one patient who had increased spasticity. Sonography proved useful in myelotomy positioning, shunt placement, and verification of cyst decompression.

Magnetic resonance imaging alone may adequately assess patients with PTPM and myelopathy as the dominant feature. Intraoperative sonography then can be used to improve spatial resolution, define septation and web formation, and guide shunt placement with minimal trauma. Cyst decompression can be visualized sonographically and intraoperative complications ruled out. Large cysts are effectively treated by decompression.

▶ The Ann Arbor Group present in fine detail results in nine patients with PTPM. The good results support their contention that evaluation is best served by magnetic resonance imaging, operative decompression directed by intraoperative sonography, with decompression of large cysts by shunting. Further experience will be needed to confirm this approach and indicate appropriate exceptions.—Robert M. Crowell, M.D.

The Treatment of Myelopathy in Cervical Spondylosis by Extensive Anterior Decompression of the Cord
J. Senegas, J. Guérin, J. M. Vital, B. Duplan, and J. M. Dols (Groupe Hospitalier Pellegrin-Tripode, Bordeaux, France)
Rev. Chir. Orthop. 71:291–300, 1985   25–5

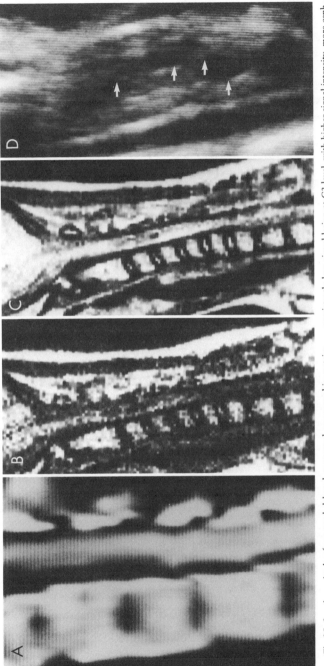

Fig 25–3.—**A,** sagittal reformatted delayed computed tomographic metrizamide myelography (DCTM) image. Extensive high attenuation is seen throughout the upper cervical spinal cord substance. With DCTM alone, large-cyst PTPM would be suspected. **B,** sagittal magnetic resonance (MR) image (Repetition time [TR], 500 msec; echo time [TE], 56 msec); with body coil shows complex, apparently multicystic appearance of cervical spinal cord. Coarse image results from use of a rapid imaging mode, with an average of half the usual number of repeated acquisitions. **C,** sagittal MR image (TR, 1,500 msec; TE, 56 msec) with body coil shows persistent complex appearance of the spinal medullary lesion. There is a persistently low-signal lesion at C3 level, with higher signal intensity, more cephalad. The MR imaging study correctly classified this lesion as small-cyst PTPM. **D,** sagittal intraoperative sonography image provides fine detail showing multiple small cystic lesions within the spinal medullary substance (*arrowheads*). Scattered areas of increased echogenicity are intermixed with these lesions. This increased echogenicity corresponds to the regions of increased MR signal intensity and is not simply increased by through transmission. These findings may represent edema and/or gliosis. (Courtesy of Gebarski, S.S., et al.: Radiology 157:379–385, November 1985. Reproduced with permission of the Radiological Society of North America.)

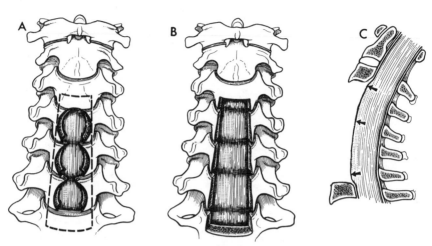

Fig 25–4.—Longitudinal anterior resection permits trephination of vertebral bodies up to the common posterior vertebral ligament (**A**), followed by enlargement of the trench by drilling to a depth of 2 cm (**B**). After resection of the ligament, the dura mater bulges outward over the entire length of the decompression (**C**). (Courtesy of Senegas, J., et al.: Rev. Chir. Orthop. 71:291–300, 1985.)

Myelopathy is undoubtedly the most severe complication of cervical arthrosis. Compression of the medulla or its vessels is indeed the major cause of this condition. The authors' original technique of anterior decompression, which consists of a median resection involving the entire expanse of the stenosis, was introduced. A total of 45 patients suffering from severe myelopathy due to cervical spondylosis associated with extended congenital or acquired stenosis of the spinal canal were treated by this method after having failed to respond to immobilization by cervical collar. In 37 instances a complementary bone graft was carried out. In 30 patients the surgical procedure extended over three levels, in 14 over four, and in 1 case over five levels; and decompression was achieved in a two-

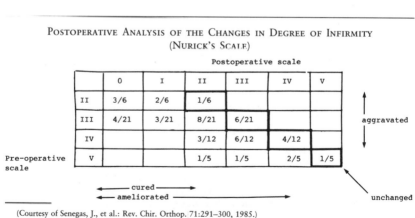

POSTOPERATIVE ANALYSIS OF THE CHANGES IN DEGREE OF INFIRMITY
(NURICK'S SCALE)

Postoperative scale

		0	I	II	III	IV	V	
	II	3/6	2/6	1/6				
	III	4/21	3/21	8/21	6/21			aggravated
	IV			3/12	6/12	4/12		
Pre-operative scale	V			1/5	1/5	2/5	1/5	

← cured →
← ameliorated →   unchanged

(Courtesy of Senegas, J., et al.: Rev. Chir. Orthop. 71:291–300, 1985.)

step procedure (Fig 25–4). An iliac bone graft is required in cases in which flexion-extension radiographs reveal instability. Postoperative care includes the use of a cervical collar for 3 months, radiologic follow-up through dynamic radiographs in flexion-extension at 3 and 6 months, and yearly monitoring by complete clinical and radiologic assessment. Postoperative results in relation to preoperative degree of infirmity are given in the table. In 12 patients unequivocal cure was achieved; 21 were clearly improved; and only 12 remained unchanged. No severe complications were encountered. In all, good results were obtained for 73.5% of the patients, and no aggravation was noted. Anterior resection of the vertebral bodies is thought to be a more reliable procedure than extensive laminectomy.

▶ The authors report relatively good results with radical anterior decompression for the treatment of myelopathy followed by cervical spondylosis. That this approach is more effective than extensive laminectomy is not proved by the uncontrolled results reported here; that demonstration could be achieved only by a controlled study, which seems very difficult to mount. Moreover, the risk of such extensive anterior decompressive surgery in the hands of most neurosurgeons would, I believe, be substantial. The more familiar extensive posterior laminectomy without opening of the dura carries relatively restricted risk and is effective in many cases. At the moment, I recommend extensive cervical laminectomy for decompression in cases of multilevel compressive myelopathy from cervical spondylosis.

Analysis of 25 patients followed up for as long as 12 years showed improved results by spondylectomy and fusion as compared with laminectomy or standard anterior interbody fusion (Yonenobu et al.: *Spine* 10:710–716, 1985).

In 191 cases followed for 12 years after surgical treatment of cervical spondylotic myelopathy, posterior operations gave better results than anterior ones for more advanced myelopathies, but brachialgia and the central cord syndrome were satisfactorily treated by anterior operations (Hukuda et al.: *J. Bone Joint Surg.* [*Br*] 67B:609–615, 1985).

Five of 6 patients with pathologic fractures of the cervical spine were effectively treated by internal stabilization with halo brace support (Fiedler et al.: *J. Bone Joint Surg.* 67B:352–357, 1985).—Robert M. Crowell, M.D.

Lumbar Pathology

Intact Arch Spondylolisthesis: A Review of 50 Cases and Description of Surgical Treatment
Eben Alexander, Jr., David L. Kelly, Jr., Courtland H. Davis, Jr., Joe M. McWhorter, and William Brown (Wake Forest Univ.)
J. Neurosurg. 63:840–844, December 1985   25–6

Fifty patients with intact arch spondylolisthesis were treated between 1972 and 1983. The 38 women and 12 men had an average age of 66 years. Nearly all the patients had marked low back pain, which was made worse by standing or walking. Leg pain was present in all but 7 patients, usually unilaterally, and was often accompanied by numbness or weakness.

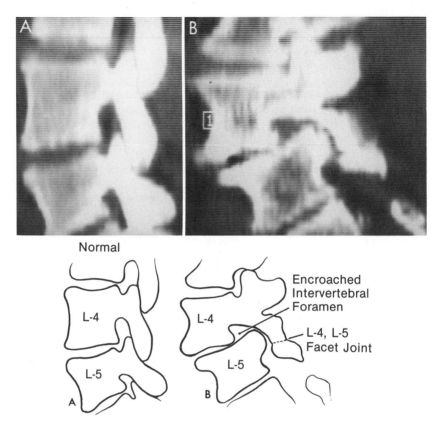

Fig 25–5.—Top, reconstructed sagittal lateral computed tomographic scans through the L4-L5 joints show normal joints (A) and intact arch spondylolisthesis (B). Bottom, corresponding line drawings show the normal joints (A) and encroachment on the intervertebral foramen (B). (Courtesy of Alexander, E., Jr., et al.: J. Neurosurg. 63:840–844, December 1985.)

Mild cauda equina compression was evident in some cases, but severe compression with paraparesis and incontinence was rare. Myelography almost always showed significant extradural compression, constriction of the dural sac, dorsal compression, and a waist deformity. Block was complete in 12 cases. Subluxation ranged from 6 to 10 mm in extent.

Wide decompression and laminectomy were performed on all patients, with a medial facetectomy of the inferior and superior facets. Four patients also had spinal fusion. A protruded or bulging disk was found in 11 patients and an extruded disk in 7. Twenty-six of 41 patients followed up for an average of 3 years were essentially free from pain, and 11 others had much less pain. One patient had another operation for pseudospondylolisthesis one level above the initial operation. Another has had slight further slippage of the spinal deformity.

Removal of the arthrotic facets decompresses the nerve root in these cases (Fig 25–5). There is controversy over whether these defects should be fused. Many patients have significant disorders other than the spinal deformity, but if these can be managed, surgery may give gratifying results.

▶ Neurosurgeons need to know about this relatively common, treatable spinal disorder. The authors provide a lucid, well-illustrated overview of intact arch spondylolisthesis. The clinical signature is low back pain exacerbated by standing, usually accompanied by leg pain. Sagittal computed tomography depicts encroachment on foramina; myelography shows constriction of the dural sac. Laminectomy decompresses the dural sac. Removal of the facets decompresses the nerve roots. Fusion is not needed unless the segments are unstable. With this approach, relief of pain occurs in the great majority of patients.—Robert M. Crowell, M.D.

The Chymopapain Clinical Trials
Stephen J. Haines (Univ. of Minnesota)
Neurosurgery 17:107–110, July 1985   25–7

The controversy over the usefulness of chymopapain in the treatment of lumbar disk herniation continues. Three published, randomized clinical trials comparing chymopapain and placebo injections are available for review. The study methods, techniques, and selection criteria are similar enough that the results of the studies—the Walter Reed study, the Australian study, and the Smith Laboratories study—can be pooled. A total of more than 200 patients participated in the three studies. Pooled results indicated that some symptomatic improvement was 2.6-fold more likely with chymopapain injection than with placebo injection. The probability of success was 50% greater with chymopapain injection, and the number of patients successfully treated was increased 23% compared with placebo injection.

The overall results of these studies suggest that chymopapain injection has a significant effect in the treatment of lumbar disk herniation. The failure of the Walter Reed study to confirm a significant difference may be related to its relatively small sample size. The studies are not considered definitive because they are not large enough and are methodologically flawed. Properly conducted clinical trials comparing surgery and chymopapain injection might help resolve the question. Outcomes should be independently evaluated by blinded observers, and the final results assessed no sooner than 6 months after intervention. Complications and technical failures should be analyzed separately from the results of technically successful procedures. Randomized clinical trials can be informative when uncontrolled studies of much larger numbers of patients are not.

▶ In the literature and at meetings, the controversy continues. In general, critics of chymopapain predominate in our specialty, while orthopedic proponents of the method remain vocal, with a few outspoken neurosurgical supporters. In this arena, only scientific evaluation of appropriate data can resolve the issue. Haines points out that the use of a relatively small number of patients in an adequately controlled randomized trial could go far toward resolving the issue. Such a trial would require substantial effort and support, but surely the result would justify this effort because of the enormous medical, economical, and ethical importance of the issue.—Robert M. Crowell, M.D.

Efficacy of Chymopapain Chemonucleolysis: A Long-Term Review of 105 Patients
Manucher J. Javid (Univ. of Wisconsin)
J. Neurosurg. 62:662–666, May 1985   25–8

Between 1972 and 1975, 124 patients with herniated nucleus pulposus producing sciatica were treated by intradiskal chymopapain injection, and 105 were followed up for 9 to 12 years. The 77 men and 47 women had an average age of 42 years. Sciatica had failed to respond to conservative measures. Fourteen patients had had laminectomy, including 12 of those followed. Eighteen of the follow-up group received workers' compensation.

Seventy-nine (75.2%) of the 105 patients, including 4 of those who had laminectomy, were markedly improved (table). About one fifth of the patients were unimproved. The rates of marked improvement were 80.5% in noncompensation cases and 50% in compensation cases. Seventeen patients underwent laminectomy after failed chemonucleolysis; 11 were markedly and 2 were slightly improved. Fifty-eight percent of all patients were working full time at follow-up, and another 12% had retired. Fifteen patients had to change their work to a less physically demanding type.

Strict criteria are needed in selecting patients for chemonucleolysis. All such patients are also candidates for surgery, but the reverse is not the case. The results can be improved by using computed tomography to exclude patients who are not candidates for chemonucleolysis but who can be operated on, such as those with spinal stenosis, facet arthropathy,

OUTCOME IN 105 PATIENTS ASSESSED 9 TO 12 YEARS
AFTER CHEMONUCLEOLYSIS

Outcome	Overall		Noncompensation		Compensation	
	No.	%	No.	%	No.	%
marked improvement	79	75.2	70	80.5	9	50.0
pain-free	53	50.5	48	55.2	5	27.8
excellent (> 85%)	14	13.3	12	12.6	2	11.1
good (50%–85%)	12	11.4	10	11.5	2	11.1
slight improvement	6	5.7	4	4.6	2	11.1
no improvement	20	19.0	13	14.9	7	38.9
total cases	105	100.0	87	100.0	18	100.0

(Courtesy of Javid, M.J.: J. Neurosurg. 62:662–666, May 1985.)

or lateral recess syndrome. Patients with back pain but without sciatica are not candidates for chemonucleolysis. For such patients, only the lateral injection approach should be used; intrathecal needle insertion is not permissible. Results comparable with those obtained surgically are achieved in properly selected patients.

▶ Dr. Javid presents a noncontrolled, long-term review of 105 patients treated with chymopapain. Beneficial results are suggested, and methods for selection, including computed tomography analysis, are emphasized. These results should be compared with controlled randomized studies, as discussed in Haines' recent article (Digest 25–7).—Robert M. Crowell, M.D.

Surgical Findings and Results of Surgery After Failure of Chemonucleolysis
A. Deburge, J. Rocolle, and M. Benoist (Hôpital Beaujon, Paris)
Spine 10:812–815, 1985   25–9

Chemonucleolysis gives good results in 70%–80% of cases; treatment failures usually are managed surgically. Surgical findings were reviewed in a series of 350 patients treated by chemonucleolysis in 1978–1984. Thirty-eight patients, 21 of whom were male and 17 female (mean age, 38 years; range, 13–63 years) had surgery following chemonucleolysis. The interval to surgery was at least 40 days in all cases but one. Most patients had obtained no relief from chemonucleolysis, but 5 patients had recurrent sciatica after recovering completely. Follow-up after surgery ranged from 3 to 36 months.

The most frequent findings at surgery were lateral stenosis and subligamentous herniation. Bony entrapment of the nerve root was seen at the injected level in all but one of the cases of lateral recess stenosis. Four patients with subligamentous herniation had a sequestrated disk herniation, and 4 had recurrent disk herniation at another level. Fourteen patients had excellent, and 11, good, results from surgery. Results were fair in six other cases and poor in five. Three of 16 patients with lateral stenosis and 2 of 6 with subligamentous herniation had a successful outcome.

Three-fourths of the patients in this series with classical symptoms of lumbar disc herniation responded to chymopapain injection. About 15% of the patients required surgery for persistent sciatica. The most frequent cause of failure was lateral recess stenosis. The results of surgery following chemonucleolysis are similar to those obtained at primary diskectomy. Better results are obtained when a sequestrated disk or lateral stenosis is present than where there is a protruded or extruded disk, or no abnormality.

▶ In 38 patients after chemonucleolysis, laminectomy was performed. The most frequent findings were lateral stenosis and subligamentous herniation. Twenty-five patients had good or excellent results, while results of surgery seemed similar to those performed in patients without chemonucleolysis. The results suggest that, if lateral stenosis or subligamentus herniation can be identified preoperatively, open surgery may be preferred.

Computed tomography after chemonucleolysis showed decreased disk height and increased attenuation (Brown et al.: *AJNR* 144:667–670, 1985).

Onik and colleagues have described a percutaneous lumbar diskectomy method using a new aspiration probe (*Radiology* 155:251–252, 1985). Under fluroscopic control, this probe can be inserted into a lumbar disk with removal of substantial amounts of nucleus pulposus. The technique appears to be an effective alternative to chemonucleolysis and diskectomy.—Robert M. Crowell, M.D.

Lateral Mass Fusion: A Prospective Study of a Consecutive Series With Long-Term Follow-Up
R. K. Jackson, D. A. Boston, and A. J. Edge (Southampton Gen. Hosp., England)
Spine 10:828–832, 1985   25–10

Lateral mass fusion was performed on 144 patients in 1972–1982, and 129, 66 male and 63 female patients with an average age of 37 years, were available for follow-up. The average period of observation was 6 years. Surgery was done chiefly for persistent back pain related to spondylolisthesis, localized degenerative disease of the lumbar spine, and previous laminectomy with disk excision. Single-level fusion was done where possible, usually between L5 and the sacrum. If the transverse process of L5 was below the sacral ala or degenerative disease was present at L4–5, the fourth lumbar segment was included in the fusion.

There were no serious permanent complications of surgery. Results were good in 64% of cases, fair in 16%, and poor in 20%. The best results were obtained in cases of spondylolisthesis (table), and the poorest in patients with previous surgery. Pain usually subsided fairly rapidly in pa-

ANALYSIS OF RESULTS

Operative indication	Good (No.)	Fair (No.)	Poor (No.)
Spondylolisthesis			
Dysplastic	14	2	0
Isthmic	40	8	4
Total	54 (79%)	10 (15%)	4 (6%)
Degenerative disease			
Intervertebral disc	20	7	6
Facet joint	3	1	2
After decompression			
for stenosis	2	0	2
Total	25 (58%)	8 (19%)	10 (23%)
Postdiscectomy			
Syndrome	3 (17%)	3 (17%)	12 (66%)

(Courtesy of Jackson, R.K., et al.: Spine 10:828–832, 1985.)

tients with a good result, but recovery of function took longer. Manual labor usually was resumed after 6–12 months. Seventeen patients developed pseudarthrosis, which correlated with poorer clinical results. Fifteen patients had further surgery, 12 because of poor results and 3 for root symptoms.

Relatively good results have been obtained with lateral mass fusion in cases of spondylolisthesis, but results have been poorer in patients having previous laminectomy and disk excision. Postlaminectomy patients have a high rate of pseudarthrosis, possibly because of greater instability from previous surgery. Patients with degenerative disease frequently do well after lateral mass fusion.

▶ Lateral mass fusion for spondylolisthesis, localized degenerative disease, and previous laminectomy with persistent back pain resulted in good outcome in 64% of patients, with fair and poor results in 36%. Fusion may be helpful to some patients with persistent low back pain, and selection criteria may pinpoint those cases that have a high likelihood of successful outcome, including patients with pain related to mechanical deformation. The precise indications for lateral mass fusion remain to be established. The prospective controlled study remains the most powerful tool for the establishment of indications for various forms of management.

Posterior spinal fusion without blood replacement was carried out successfully in 19 Jehovah's Witnesses. There were no major complications reported by this experienced spinal surgical team (Bowen et al.: *Clin. Orthop.* 198:284–288, 1985).

Arteriovenous fistulas after lumbar laminectomy are rare, but knowledge of the anatomy of the relevant vessels is helpful in their repair (Quigley and Stoney: *General Vascular Surgery* 2:828–833, 1985). At L3–4, the aorta is bifurcating into the iliac arteries on the left and the vena cava is on the right; at L4–5, the common femoral veins are just posterior to the iliac arteries on the lateral aspects of the disc, and this situation persists at L5–S1, even further laterally.

Positioning in the knee-chest position for lumbar laminectomy may obstruct an aortocoronary bypass graft and lead to myocardial ischemia (Weinlander et al.: *Anesth. Analg.* 64:933–936, 1985).—Robert M. Crowell, M.D.

Syringomyelia

Magnetic Resonance Imaging in Syringomyelia
E. Kokmen, W. R. Marsh, and H. L. Baker, Jr. (Mayo Clinic)
Neurosurgery 17:267–270, August 1985   25–11

Myelographic methods have drawbacks in the evaluation of syringomyelia. Sagittal magnetic resonance (MR) imaging of the brain and cervical spinal cord offers a means of visualizing cavities inside the cord and determining their relation to other structures. This MR imaging was performed in 15 patients with typical clinical signs and symptoms of syringomyelia. Images 10 mm thick were obtained in four contiguous slices

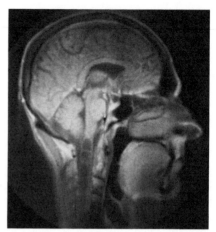

Fig 25–6.—Sagittal cut shows pronounced cystic dilatation in the cervical spinal cord. (Courtesy of Kokmen, E., et al.: Neurosurgery 17:267–270, August 1985.)

over 6 minutes. Free induction-decay and inversion-recovery sequences proved more useful than spin-echo sequences. The patients, who were 9–68 years of age, had had symptoms for periods ranging from a few months to 14 years.

All patients had definite clinical evidence of central cord dysfunction. In 11 patients, cavitation of the spinal cord was confirmed operatively. The MR findings in a patient with remote posttraumatic syringomyelia are shown in Figure 25–6. A syringostomy was carried out at the C2 dorsal root entry zone; repeat MR imaging a month after drainage showed no cavity and an atrophic cord. Nine patients had syringomyelia with Chiari's malformation. One patient had hydrocephalus as well. Four cases were idiopathic.

Magnetic resonance imaging holds promise for studying syringomyelia through visualization of the sagittal plane of the cervical spinal cord. The syrinx cavity is shown in its relation to the cerebellar tonsils, fourth ventricle, and related structures. Surgical planning is aided by MR imaging. Where MR is used, most patients may not require invasive neurologic imaging procedures such as myelography. However, MR imaging might miss some collapsed intramedullary cavitary lesions.

▶ The authors add to a growing literature indicating excellent depiction of syringomyelia by MR imaging. The authors state that a collapsed intramedullary cavitary lesion might be missed by this approach. It seems likely that MR imaging will become the procedure of choice for initial evaluation of these patients. In cases with normal studies, myelographic study with postmyelographic computed tomography is probably indicated.

Magnetic resonance imaging may become the method of choice in the diagnosis of structural spinal cord diseases. It already provides additional diagnostic information for cases of syringomyelia, intraspinal tumor, and multiple sclerosis (Aichner et al.: *J. Neurol. Neurosurg. Psychiatry* 48:1220–1229, 1985).—Robert M. Crowell, M.D.

Hydromyelia and Syringomyelia: Use of C.T. Scan and Magnetic Resonance Imaging: Syringoperitoneal Shunt

H. Petit, D. Leys, F. Lesoin, C. Viaud, F. Dubois, Y. Gaudet, D. Baleriaux, and J. Clarisse (Centre Hospitalier Universitaire Lille, France, and Université libre de Bruxelles)

Rev. Neurol. 141:644–654, 1985   25–12

A review of 21 patients with a spinal cord cavity showed 14 with syringomyelia at presentation and 3 with a syringomyelic syndrome of other etiology. Four other patients had clinical features not usually associated with cord cavities. Computed tomography (CT) was carried out after cervical myelography with metrizamide or iopamiron in 20 cases. The findings in some cases were consistent with Gardner's theory, but a majority of patients had findings consistent with Aboulker's theory. Findings at magnetic resonance imaging in 9 cases included a spinal cord cavity (Fig 25–7), Chiari malformation, and hydrocephalus.

Eleven patients had a syringoperitoneal shunt operation. The results after a brief follow-up are favorable, especially with respect to sensation and trophic changes. Decisions on surgery should be based on the course of the disorder and on the presence or absence of hydrocephalus.

▶ In studies of 21 patients with spinal cord cavitation, CT scanning with cer-

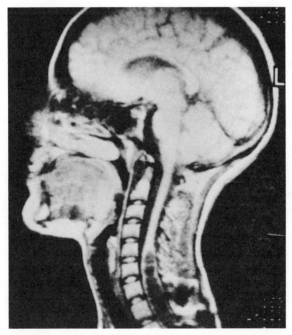

Fig 25–7.—Magnetic resonance image of cervical spinal cord cavity. Spin echo: slices of 5 mm. Echo time, 50 msec; repetition time, 500 msec. (Courtesy of Petit, H., et al.: Rev. Neurol. 141:644–654, 1985.)

vical myelography was helpful in demonstrating spinal cord cyst. Eleven patients had decompressive shunting procedures with favorable follow-up.

Although experience with CT has been favorable, studies with magnetic resonance appear just as good without spinal puncture, and this modality will probably supplant CT.

Over an 11-year study, 30 (3.2%) of 951 patients with spinal cord injury developed cervical syringomyelia, as did 8% of patients with complete tetraplegia. Rarer clinical manifestations included autonomic dysfunction, alterations in sensory level with postural changes, early occurrence of tendon arreflexia, and painless motor deterioration. Prolonged F-wave latencies were present with all patients with a demonstrable syrinx. There was no benefit in operating on a patient with a small syrinx. Most of the patients who underwent surgery for progressive motor weakness or severe pain had good postoperative results (Rossier et al.: *Brain* 108:439–461, 1985).

Anderson et al. describe the natural history and operative results in syringomyelia (*Acta Neurol. Scand.* 71:472–479, 1985). Of 20 patients without surgery, 7 had no further progression in symptoms after presentation. Four of 12 patients with laminectomy and syringostomy, and 7 of 15 patients with decompression of the cervicomedullary junction, showed sustained improvement or stabilization of their neurologic status.

Ultrasonography during spinal operations can check the effectiveness of shunt placement in syringomyelia and the completeness of tumor or disk removal. Precise locations for biopsy of intramedullary lesions can also be made (Rubin and Dohrmann: *Radiology* 155:197–200, 1985).

Intraoperative ultrasound played a useful role in 53% of 191 operative cases. The main utility was in locating subcortical masses, but it was also useful to identify residual tumor after resection, locate cysts within tumors, delineate nearby vascular structures, and locate other subcortical pathology (Rubin and Dohrmann: *Radiology* 157:509–511, 1985).—Robert M. Crowell, M.D.

Delayed Metrizamide CT Enhancement of Syringomyelia: Postoperative Observations
Shinichi Kan, Allan J. Fox, and Fernando Vinuela (Univ. of Western Ontario)
AJNR 6:613–616, July–Aug. 1985   25–13

Both the specific causes of syringomyelia and its proper surgical management remain controversial. Eleven patients with syringomyelia underwent metrizamide myelography with delayed computed tomography (CT) before and after surgical intervention. All patients had syrinx cavities involving both the cervical and the thoracic spinal cord. CT was done 6–12 hours after complete myelography. Postoperative studies were done 1 to 10 months after surgery; the mean follow-up was 4½ months. Patients with Chiari malformation underwent foramen magnum decompression with plugging of the obex, while others had direct drainage to the syringomyelic cavity.

Four of 5 patients with Chiari I malformations improved after foramen magnum decompression and obex plugging. The syrinx was reduced in

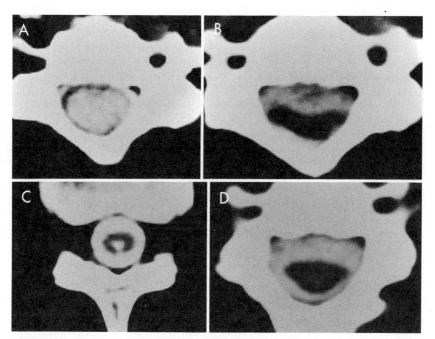

Fig 25–8.—Obex plugging. **A,** preoperative metrizamide CT scan; large syrinx in cervical cord is evident. **B,** 2 months after obex plugging. Marked diminution of cervical cord and nonfilling of syrinx can be seen. **C,** filling of syrinx cavity in lower thoracic cord can be seen. **D,** 5 months after surgery. Enlargement of cord and filling of syrinx cavity in cervical region are evident. (Courtesy of Kan, S., et al.: AJNR 6:613–616, July–Aug. 1985.)

size in three cases, and follow-up of 1 of these patients showed a marked reduction in cervical cord size and partial nonfilling of the cavity (Fig 25–8); subsequently, a large syrinx was present. Three patients had a reduction in size of the syrinx cavity after direct drainage. Both groups of patients improved clinically when the syrinx cavity was unchanged or became smaller on follow-up CT. No patient became clinically worse after surgery.

Follow-up CT studies suggest that persistently abnormal fluid circulation that maintains a syringomyelic cavity represents more than merely flow through the obex to the central canal. Fluid passage through the cord substance may also be a factor. Delayed metrizamide CT can be a useful postoperative study, especially if the clinical outcome is disappointing.

▶ Many surgeons believe that subarachnoid shunting of a syrinx is the best treatment, and all 3 patients treated in this fashion at the University of Western Ontario had reduction in size of their syrinx. Obex plugging, the Gardner procedure, is not widely advocated today; it is therefore all the more interesting that in this series 4 of 5 patients with Chiari I malformations improved after foramen magnum decompression and obex plugging. The role of this type of therapy will require further experience to reach a conclusion. Delayed metrizamide CT myelography to demonstrate the syrinx is recommended, especially when postoperative results are disappointing.

In the diagnosis of posttraumatic syrinx, the most reliable CT scan varies in cord size with position (Stevens et al.: *Neuroradiology* 27:48–56, 1985). Penetration of contrast medium within the spinal cord may be seen when surgery reveals no cyst, though this sign is usually a reliable diagnostic indicator.— Robert M. Crowell, M.D.

Syringoperitoneal Shunt for Treatment of Cord Cavitation

Mikio Suzuki, Charles Davis, Lindsay Symon, and F. Gentili (Inst. of Neurology, London)
J. Neurol. Neurosurg. Psychiatry 48:620–627, July 1985   25–14

Microsurgical methods and improved shunt devices have made shunting an alternative to conventional surgical treatment of cord cavitation. Twenty-nine such patients were managed by syringoperitoneal shunting between 1980 and 1983. The 24 men and 5 women had a mean age of 39 years (range, 18–63 years). Seventeen patients had posttraumatic cord cavitation, while 7 had idiopathic syringomyelia. Three cases were secondary to meningitis and 2 to spinal tumor removal with irradiation. Nine patients had had surgery. Neck and upper limb pain, spinothalamic sensory disturbance, and motor weakness were the common presenting features. A 2- or 3-level laminectomy generally was performed. Microsurgical dissection was used to place the Pudenz ventricular catheter. A connecting catheter was passed subcutaneously from a flank incision to the laminectomy site and attached to the effluent catheter from the syrinx. A low-pressure Raimondi peritoneal catheter then was placed and connected to the flank-site catheter.

The results on an average follow-up of 1 year are given in the table. Twenty-two of the 29 patients were improved symptomatically, while 2 deteriorated. All but 3 of the 17 posttraumatic patients improved, and none deteriorated. Pain responded the best, disappearing in 4 of 20 patients. Six patients who improved had had previous surgery. Three shunt revisions have been carried out; an expanded cyst was confirmed in these cases.

Syringoperitoneal shunting is a reasonably effective approach to cord cavitation of any etiology. It is a technically simple procedure. The upper

SUMMARY OF RESULTS IN 29 CASES

Result	Types of syringomyelia									
	Traumatic		Idiopathic		Meningitic		Spinal tumour		Total	
	No	%	No	%	No	%	No	%	No	%
Improved	14	82	4	57	2	67	2	100	22	76
Unchanged	3	18	2	29	0	0	0	0	5	17
Worse	0	0	1	14	1	33	0	0	2	7
Total	17		7		3		2		29	

(Courtesy of Suzuki, M., et al.: J. Neurol. Neurosurg. Psychiatry 48:620–627, July 1985.)

dorsal spine is the best site for cyst drainage. Syringoperitoneal shunting may become the initial treatment of choice for idiopathic syringomyelia with ectopia cerebelli when there is no radiologic evidence of foramen magnum compression.

Spinal Tumors

Treatment of Neoplastic Epidural Cord Compression by Vertebral Body Resection and Stabilization

Narayan Sundaresan, Joseph H. Galicich, Joseph M. Lane, Manjit S. Bains, and Patricia McCormack (St. Luke's-Roosevelt Hosp. Ctr. and Memorial Sloan-Kettering Cancer Ctr., New York)
J. Neurosurg. 63:676–684, November 1985   25–15

Neoplastic epidural cord compression was managed by vertebral body resection and tumor excision, followed by immediate stabilization with methyl methacrylate, in 101 consecutive patients seen between 1979 and 1984. The 52 male and 49 female patients had a median age of 51 years (range, 9–80 years). The lung, kidney, and breast were the most frequent sites of primary cancer. Indications for surgery included a pathologic compression fracture, a solitary site of relapse, spinal destruction by a

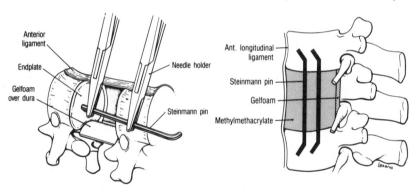

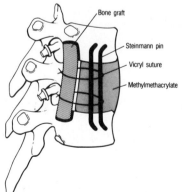

Fig 25–9.—**Above left,** after tumor resection, Steinmann pins are introduced into the healthy vertebrae above and below. Two pins are generally used. All disk tissue above and below must be completely removed to provide a broad base for acrylic. The dura is protected with Gelfoam. **Above,** molded methyl methacrylate is shown filling resected vertebral body space. It can be noted that the end-plates above and below are left intact, including the anterior longitudinal ligament if it is not involved. **Left,** in some patients, the removed portion of the rib is used as a lateral rib graft and held in position with Vicryl sutures tied around Steinmann pins before methyl methacrylate is poured into the defect. (Courtesy of Sundaresan, N., et al.: J. Neurosurg. 63:676–684, November 1985.)

paraspinal tumor, a radioresistant tumor, and segmental instability after radiotherapy. Nine patients had primary osseous tumors of the spine. Nearly all patients had severe, constant neck or back pain. The surgical technique is illustrated in Figure 25–9.

Of 32 ambulatory patients with radicular deficit or plexopathy, 22 had restoration of normal motor strength after surgery. Thirty-two of 46 non-ambulatory patients were considered to be improved. Improvement in neurologic grade paralleled the preoperative deficit. No patient had a worse deficit unless part of the brachial plexus had been deliberately sectioned. Seventy-eight percent of all patients were ambulatory at discharge, and significant back or radicular pain was relieved in 85% of cases. There were eight postoperative deaths, and another 10% of patients had surgical complications. Of 18 surviving patients followed up for a year or longer, 16 remain ambulatory.

Surgery is indicated before radiotherapy in selected patients with neo-plastic spinal cord compression. Curative resection is possible in cases of solitary osseous spinal metastasis if surgery is done when the tumor is confined to the vertebral body. Embolization should be considered in pa-tients with vascular tumors of the spine.

▶ This is an important contribution. The surgical rationale is sound: the lesion is imaged and then directly removed to decompress the spinal cord, with sub-sequent stabilization. The results appear quite encouraging, with 32 of 46 non-ambulatory patients restored to ambulation (with or without support) by the time of discharge.

Certainly, the approach deserves further careful study, which could best be done in a controlled fashion to establish its superiority over conventional treat-ment. This confirmation would be important before widespread implementation because of the substantial 30-day mortality (8 of 101 cases), major effort and investment, and short life expectancy (median survival, 8 months).—Robert M. Crowell, M.D.

Surgical Treatment of Spinal Cord Compression in Patients With Lung Cancer

Narayan Sundaresan, Manjit Bains, and Patricia McCormack (Memorial Sloan-Kettering Cancer Ctr., New York)
Neurosurgery 16:350–356, March 1985   25–16

Spinal cord compression by vertebral metastasis is a prominent com-plication in cancer patients, especially in those with lung, breast, and prostatic tumors. Twenty-five patients seen between 1980 and 1983 with lung cancer and spinal invasion underwent surgical treatment via an an-terolateral approach. The 15 men and 10 women had a median age of 54 years (range, 37–62 years). Eighteen patients had adenocarcinoma. Twelve patients had spinal involvement at their initial clinical visit. Twelve patients had a Pancoast tumor, 8 had thoracic cord compression from direct in-vasion of the chest wall and spine, and 5 had hematogenous metastases.

Severe back pain was present and was often associated with a radicular component. Eight patients had motor deficit in the upper extremities, and 6 patients had paraparesis. Myelography showed significant block in 76% of the cases. Fifteen patients had two or three contiguous vertebrae that were destroyed by tumor.

An anterolateral exposure was made via formal thoracotomy in 22 cases, while 3 patients had a thoracoabdominal flank approach to lumbar lesions. All gross evidence of tumor was removed from the involved paravertebral tissues, vertebral bodies, and epidural space, and the spine was stabilized with methyl methacrylate. Local brachytherapy with ^{192}Ir implants was used in 19 cases. Twenty-two patients were ambulatory 2 months after the operation. Ninety percent of the patients were relieved of pain, but both pain and weakness recurred in several cases. Overall median survival was 6 months. The operative mortality was 8%. Pleural cerebrospinal fluid leakage was avoided by closing all dural rents about nerve roots.

Most cancer patients tolerate thoracotomy for cord compression well. Surgery should be considered before radiotherapy in selected cases of cord compression caused by neoplastic disease. A reasonable performance status should exist, and extensive visceral metastases should be absent. Surgery is indicated in patients who have pathologic compression fracture as the initial manifestation of malignant neoplasm.

▶ The rationale is sound, the technique direct, and the results encouraging. The question is, is it worth it for patients with a mean survival of 6 months? Surgeon and patient must decide this together. To offer this surgery at all, an experienced, energetic team is needed.—Robert M. Crowell, M.D.

Spinal Cord Compression in Breast Cancer
Kevin M. Harrison, Hyman B. Muss, Marshall R. Ball, Michael McWhorter, and Douglas Case (Wake Forest Univ.)
Cancer 55:2839–2844, June 15, 1985   25–17

Spinal cord compression in women is most often caused by metastatic breast cancer. Epidural cord compression is usually secondary to direct extension of vertebral deposits. Seventy-eight consecutive patients with confirmed breast cancer and signs or symptoms consistent with cord compression underwent myelography between 1977 and 1982. Panmyelography was performed with Pantopaque. Bone scanning was carried out with ^{99m}Tc methylene diphosphonate.

Forty-two (54%) of the 78 patients had abnormal myelograms, all of whom (vs. half of those with normal myelograms) had radiographic or bone scan evidence of bone metastasis. In all patients, the myelographic block invariably corresponded with lesions found on radiographs or bone scans. Twenty-one patients had a complete block. Only paraplegia, paraparesis, and a sensory level reliably predicted cord lesions, but back pain, paresthesias, and bladder or bowel dysfunction were more frequent in patients with abnormal myelograms. The cerebrospinal fluid protein concentration was elevated in almost all patients with abnormal myelograms but also in almost half of those with normal myelograms. Cord involvement was unrelated to the cerebrospinal fluid glucose concentration or cytologic findings. Patients with fewer metastatic sites and a shorter time from diagnosis to treatment had the best response to treatment. There was no substantial difference in survival associated with the myelographic findings.

The prognosis of patients with metastatic breast cancer is poor regardless of whether or not spinal cord compression is present. Panmyelography is the most precise means of making a diagnosis. Cord involvement by metastatic cancer should be considered in all patients with bone lesions and clinical evidence of cord dysfunction.

▶ Complete myelography is recommended in this study to confirm the diagnosis of spinal cord compression. More recently, however, magnetic resonance (MR) imaging has been recommended as a highly sensitive and accurate indicator of bone and cord involvement by a metastatic lesion (Ruth Ramsey, meeting of the Chicago Neurological Society, March, 1986). To obtain the highest sensitivity, surface-coil technology is needed. Because it is noninvasive and avoids spinal puncture, which can cause deterioration in patients with cord compression, MR imaging may eventually replace myelography in the evaluation of these cases. In terms of treatment, metastatic breast carcinoma may respond to irradiation therapy. When signs and symptoms progress despite radiation and steroid therapy, anterior cervical decompression might be considered (Digest 25–15).—Robert M. Crowell, M.D.

Extradural and Hourglass Cervical Neurinomas: The Vertebral Artery Problem
B. George, C. Laurian, Y. Keravel, and J. Cophignon (Hôpital Lariboisiére and Hôpital Saint Joseph, Paris, and Hôpital Henri Mondor, Créteil, France)
Neurosurgery 16:591–594, May 1985   25–18

The vertebral artery poses a challenge in the complete removal of cervical neurinomas that have an extradural component, or "dumbbell" tumors. The authors operated on more than 40 tumors related to the vertebral artery during a period of 4 years, including 7 hourglass neurinomas and 4 extradural neurinomas. Most of these lesions were located between C2 and C6 and were related to the second, or transversary segment, of the vertebral artery. Two tumors were located at the C6–7 level, while two were at the C1–2 level. These were surgically removed by a lateral anterior approach after the vertebral artery was controlled. Removal of hourglass tumors required separate surgical stages, with the use of a posterior route and laminectomy to remove the intradural component. Complete gross removal was achieved in all cases, with no morbidity or mortality.

Man, 39 years old, had neck pain and neuralgia at the C2 level on the left side. This was most marked at night and had been present for 3 years. He had also noted paresthesia in the left C2 territory and weakness in the extremities on the left side for longer than a year. Hodgkin's disease had been treated 10 years earlier.

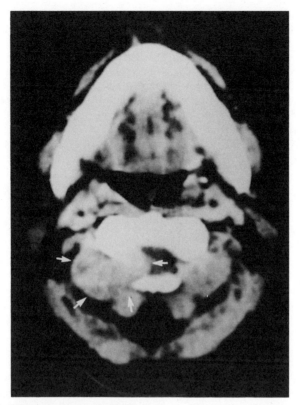

Fig 25–10.—Hourglass neurinoma at C1, C2. (Courtesy of George, B., et al.: Neurosurgery 16:591–594, May 1985.)

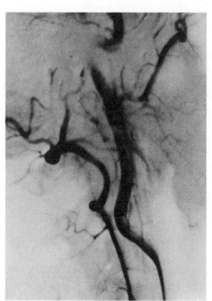

Fig 25–11.—Stretching of the distal vertebral artery by the tumor. (Courtesy of George, B., et al.: Extradural and Hourglass Cervical Neurinomas: The Vertebral Artery Problem, in Neurosurgery 16:591–594, May 1985.)

Increased tendon reflexes and a Babinski sign were noted on the left side. Computed tomography showed an hourglass tumor at C1–2 with a large extravertebral extension (Fig 25–10). Angiography showed elongation of the vertebral artery at C1–2 without tumoral injection (Fig 25–11). The extradural and intra- and extravertebral parts of the tumor were removed via an anterolateral approach after the vertebral artery was controlled, which was markedly shifted externally. Hemilaminectomy by a posterior approach 10 days later allowed for the removal of the intradural part of the tumor. A diagnosis of benign neurinoma was confirmed. The postoperative course was uneventful.

Primary control of the vertebral artery in these cases preserves the vessel and allows for safe, complete tumor removal. The lateral anterior approach provides wide, simple exposure of the artery at any cervical level. Both this and the posterior route may be used at a single sitting, starting with the lateral route.

▶ The authors report superb results with 11 paraspinal neurinomas. Demonstration of the vertebral artery by angiography was important in surgical planning. A two-stage approach utilizing a laminectomy for the intradural component and an anterior lateral approach for the paraspinal component was used. This article sets the standard for surgical management of these lesions. For some cases with tumors at the cervical medullary junction, a transoral approach might be better. For large ventral lesions, especially in older patients, better judgment may dictate a radical subtotal removal.

Correlation with microtomy indicates that current high-resolution computed tomography can resolve detailed anatomy of the cervical neural foramina, including ventral nerve roots, dorsal nerve roots, and ganglion and vertebral artery (Pech et al.: *Radiology* 155:143–146, 1985).—Robert M. Crowell, M.D.

Myxopapillary Ependymoma: A Clinicopathologic and Immunocytochemical Study of 77 Cases
Paula R. L. Sonneland, Bernd W. Scheithauer, and Burton M. Onofrio (Mayo Clinic and Found.)
Cancer 56:883–893, Aug. 15, 1985   25–19

Review was made of 77 cases of myxopapillary ependymoma of the spinal cord that were seen at the Mayo Clinic in 1924–1983. Nearly all lesions involved the filum terminale and/or the conus medullaris. They constituted about one fourth of all spinal ependymomas registered in this 60-year period. Male patients predominated; the mean age at diagnosis was 36 years (range, 6–82 years). The most frequent presenting symptom was low back pain, with or without sciatica. Sensorimotor disorder was present in about half the patients at diagnosis. More than one third were incontinent. Three patients were paraplegic. Two myelograms were falsely normal.

One fourth of the patients had grossly encapsulated tumors that were removed intact. Their mean survival was 19 years; 2 patients had recurrences. One third of the patients had piecemeal gross total tumor removal, while 32 patients had subtotal piecemeal tumor removal. Two thirds of the tumors were limited to the filum, whereas nearly one third involved the conus as well. Four lesions were in the cervicothoracic spinal cord. About one fourth of the patients had significant long-term neurologic deficits after tumor removal. Seventeen percent of the patients had recurrences, and 5 patients died of tumor.

Myxopapillary ependymoma appears to be a low-grade glioma that recapitulates the structure of the filum terminale. Gross total removal is associated with better survival than piecemeal total or subtotal resection. Deaths from disease follow a long course with multiple recurrences. Postoperative radiotherapy appears to be indicated for patients who undergo piecemeal or subtotal tumor removal.

▶ These useful data from the Mayo Clinic confirm the benign course of myxopapillary ependymoma, its surgical curability, and the poor outcome associated with incomplete removal. Since cases in the study stretch back to 1924, many lesions were treated before the modern microsurgical era. With the use of modern diagnostic techniques, including magnetic resonance imaging, it should be possible to diagnose these lesions earlier when total resection is more likely to be achieved. In addition, utilization of the laser and ultrasonic surgical aspirator during surgery seem likely to assist the surgeon in obtaining grossly total removal in these cases. Somatosensory evoked responses may be helpful in monitoring integrity of spinal cord function during surgery.

Among 32 patients with primary tumors of cauda equina, most were initially diagnosed as having prolapsed intervertebral disk and were treated accordingly. Only by obtaining careful myelograms, including that of the cauda equina prior to anticipated disc excision, can such tumors be diagnosed properly (Kerr and Jones: *J. Bone Joint Surg.* [*Br.*] 67B:358–362, 1985).

Among 58 cases with tethered cord and associated lipoma (23 cases), 38 had neurologic symptoms and signs. When surgery released the tether, diminished the volume of lipoma, and reconstructed the posterior dura, 26 patients were cured or improved, 12 stabilized, 19 remained asymptomatic, and only 1 got worse (Lapras et al.: *Rev. Neurol. (Paris)* 141:207–215, 1985).

Intramedullary spinal cord glioma caused intracranial seeding in two documented cases (Hely et al.: *J. Neurol. Neurosurg. Psychiatry* 48:302–309, 1985).

Computed tomography was useful in the evaluation of six sacrococcygeal chordomas for surgical planning and detection of local recurrence (Vanel Rebibo et al.: *Eur. J. Radiol.* 5:87–90, 1985).—Robert M. Crowell, M.D.

Radical Resection of Intramedullary Spinal Cord Tumors in Adults: Recent Experience in 29 Patients

Paul R. Cooper and Fred Epstein (New York Univ.)
J. Neurosurg. 63:492–499, October 1985   25–20

The success of aggressive surgical removal of intramedullary spinal cord tumors in children prompted trial of a similar approach in adults. Twenty-nine consecutive patients—11 men and 18 women with a median age of 37 years (range, 21–74 years)—were operated on between July 1981 and January 1984. The mean duration of symptoms was 9½ years. Twenty-six patients had had previous surgery, and 18 had received radiotherapy. All patients had metrizamide computed tomographic myelography, but magnetic resonance imaging can localize cord widening without the need for contrast. There were 14 ependymomas and 11 astrocytomas in the series. Ultrasonography and the operating microscope were used to control the myelotomy and CO_2 laser destruction of the tumor. Sharp dissection was used when appropriate.

Fourteen tumors were removed completely and 7, virtually completely. Two were only biopsied. There were no surgical deaths, but 6 patients died during follow-up. For 13 (87%) of the patients, upper extremity function had stabilized or improved at the last evaluation. Three patients who did not have closure with muscle flap rotation had wound breakdown and cerebrospinal fluid leakage. Two with upper cervical cord tumors had severe neurologic deterioration immediately after surgery. The condition of three other patients worsened as their corticosteroid dosage was being tapered and have not recovered function. Three patients have had recurrences.

Radical removal of intramedullary spinal cord tumors can be achieved in adults without worsening the neurologic deficit in most instances. Significant neurologic improvement has occurred in many patients and, at the least, radical surgery provides significant palliation.

In an addendum, the authors report having operated on 11 other adults more recently, with comparable results.

▶ The authors present the results of aggressive microsurgical removal of intra-medullary spinal cord tumors in 29 adult patients. Modern technology, including the Cavitron ultrasonic surgical aspirator (CUSA) and CO_2 laser, aided tumor removal, which was complete in 14 patients and virtually so in 7. Clinical results showed lower extremity function of most patients to be unchanged, with that of 8 worse and of 7 improved. Three patients who walked before surgery could not walk after; however, 1 patient regained the ability to walk.

Whether aggressive removal of these tumors clinically benefits patients remains to be established. Because of differences in treatment protocols and limited numbers of patients, it is difficult to compare the results of various forms of therapy. It is rational to expect that application of modern diagnostic and therapeutic methods might be beneficial. Perhaps supravital staining or tracer techniques may help discriminate tumor from normal tissue. No doubt, microsurgical application of CUSA and laser can assist precise removal of tumor.

In the end, only a controlled surgical series will permit the surgeon to demonstrate an advantage in clinical terms after radical surgery. Because of differences in tumor biology, ependymomas and astrocytomas will have to be studied separately. Since the number of tumors is small, such a study would have to be cooperative. A few centers collecting case reports over a few years should be able to answer this important question in neurologic surgery.

In a related report, Reimer and Onofrio (*J. Neurosurg.* 63:669–675, 1985) reviewed 32 case histories of spinal cord astrocytoma in patients younger than 20 years of age at the Mayo Clinic. Although the authors had limited experience with radical removal, follow-up indicated an increased survival time in these patients as opposed to those with biopsy or partial removal. The postlaminectomy spinal deformities were severe in 13 patients. The authors recommend postoperative radiation as an adjunct in therapy.—Robert M. Crowell, M.D.

Notes on Spine

▶ Correlation of computed tomography (CT) myelography and clinical observations in cervical myeloradiculopathy suggest pathophysiologic roles for direct compression, fraction-friction, and vascular compromise (Yu et al.: *Brain* 109:259–278, 1986).

Percutaneous lumbar disk excision was performed with a discoscone and small rongeurs by Schreiber and Suezuwa in Zurich (*Orth. Review* 75:75–78, 1986).

Eighteen of 23 intradural tumors were enhanced on CT study (Lapointe et al.: *AJNR* 146:103–107, 1986).

Regarding spinal diagnosis, Allen et al. (*J. Neurosurg.* 63:510–520, 1985) report on postmetrizamide CT in 46 patients with acute cervical spinal injuries. Despite realignment via traction, 11 patients were found to have significant spinal cord compression, 10 of whom were treated surgically. No long-lasting complications of myelography were noted. The technique seems helpful in evaluating cord compression and the possible need for decompressive surgery.

Computed tomography myelography with gray matter enhancement takes the appearance of "fried eggs" and signifies cystic necrosis, according to Iwasaki et al. (*J. Neurosurg.* 63:363–366, 1985).

Maiman et al. (*Neurosurgery* 17:574–580, 1985) report biomechanical studies of fixation devices in cadaver spines. Luque rods provided the most rigid stabilization, and modified Weiss springs often maintained stability better than Harrington distraction rods. Neurosurgeons who use such stabilization instrumentation should be familiar with these important biomechanical studies.

Koyama and Handa (*Surg. Neurol.* 24:392–394, 1985) describe a conical drill burr with a flat end, the side of which is useful for removal of osteophytes in the spinal canal via an anterior approach. [The Bien-Aire drill manufactured in Geneva, Switzerland, is an otologic high-speed drill, which we have found remarkably smooth and powerful for drilling, particularly on the odontoid process and in the posterior fossa.]

High-resolution CT scanning can detect with surity oncovertebral and facet disk disclocations in cervical articular pillar fractures (Yetkin et al.: *AJNR* 6:633–637, 1985).

Unfused ossicles of the lumbar spine may be diagnosed by CT (Pech and Haughton: *AJNR* 6:629–631, 1985).

Postoperative fracture of the lumbar articular facet is a potential cause of postoperative pain and can be recognized by CT scanning (Rothman et al.: *AJNR* 6:623–628, 1985).

Epidural libomatosis can cause spinal cord compression with resolution after laminectomy (Ferindez et al.: *Sem. Hop. Paris* 61:3327–3328, 1985).—Robert M. Crowell, M.D.

26 Pediatrics

Introduction

Brain tumors in the pediatric age group were considered in several publications. Brain tumors in the first 24 months of life, according to Tomita and McLone (Digest 26–1), have a poor prognosis, but modern technology has been utilized in only a small number of cases yet studied. It is now possible to use ultrasonography to diagnosis intracranial teratoma in utero (Digest 26–2). Good results have been reported with surgery of brain stem tumors in children treated with the Cavitron ultrasonic surgical aspirator (CUSA) and evoked potentials (Digest 26–3). Optic glioma treated by irradiation in children may be associated with eventual development of moyamoya syndrome (Digest 26–4).

As regards congenital malformations, trigonocephaly with fusion of the metopic suture is nicely treated by craniotomy with repair of the fused suture at the age of 4 to 6 weeks (Digest 26–6). Skin expanders may be helpful in achieving tissue coverage after separation of craniopagus twins (Digest 26–7).

Hydrocephalus was the subject of several articles. Torkelson et al. showed that shunting of "arrested" hydrocephalus can lead to psychologic improvement in some cases (Digest 26–8). In the management of fetal hydrocephalus, there is a place for cesarean section and cephalocentesis in certain cases. The role of ventriculoaminiotic shunt placement remains unclear (Digest 26–9). Obliteration of the perimesencephalic cisterns is a computed tomographic sign of life-threatening shunt failure (Digest 26–10). In normal-pressure hydrocephalus in adults, the best diagnostic criteria for satisfactory response to shunt remain the clinical presentation and duration of symptoms (Digest 26–11).

Lansky et al. have developed guidelines toward the development of a play performance scale for children, similar to the Karnofsky scale for adults (Digest 26–12).

Robert M. Crowell, M.D.

Brain Tumors During the First Twenty-Four Months of Life
Tadanori Tomita and David G. McLone (Northwestern Univ.)
Neurosurgery 17:913–919, December 1985   26–1

Review was made of 100 infants treated for intracranial tumors in the first 2 years of life in 1952–1984, representing 16% of all pediatric patients seen in this period. Computed tomography (CT) was used to diagnose brain tumor in the last 36 cases. In the first 24 months of life, the most frequent tumor types were benign astrocytoma, medulloblastoma, and choroid plexus papilloma. A majority of cerebellar-fourth ventricle tumors

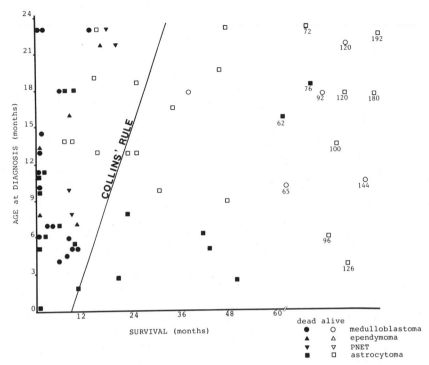

Fig 26–1.—Collins' rule for period of risk for recurrence applied to medulloblastomas, ependymomas, primitive neuroectodermal tumors (PNETs), and astrocytomas during the first 24 months of life. The multiple exceptions to this rule in the astrocytoma group can be noted. (Courtesy of Tomita, T., and McLone, D.G.: Neurosurgery 17:913–919, December 1985.)

were malignant. Half the patients aged 1 year and younger with infratentorial lesions presented with vomiting and increasing sleepiness; subsequently, difficulty walking was prominent. The anterior fontanelle was full or tense in more than two-thirds of patients with either infratentorial or supratentorial tumors.

Fifty-seven of 73 patients with hydrocephalus were shunted before craniotomy. Craniotomy was done in 92 patients. Thirty-two patients had radical tumor resection and 28 others had subtotal resection. The surgical mortality within 1 month was 13%; it was 6% in recent patients diagnosed by CT. About half the patients received radiotherapy. Five-year survival was 41% for the younger patients and 74% for those aged 1–2 years at presentation. Risks of recurrence are shown in Figure 26–1. Patients with cerebral tumor had variable outcomes, but those with medulloblastoma and other infratentorial tumors did poorly.

Total tumor resection was achieved in only about one-fourth of the present patients, but modern techniques such as microsurgery and the surgical laser may result in improved findings. Chemotherapy can be used after complete tumor resection, with radiotherapy reserved for recurrent disease detected by CT. Irradiation adversely affects the developing CNS, and some patients with unresectable benign tumors such as suprasellar astrocytoma may be followed up by CT without radiotherapy in early life.

▶ Tomita and McLone present a substantial experience (100 infants) treated for intracranial tumor in the first 2 years of life. Despite efforts at radical tumor resection, only a quarter underwent total tumor removal. Surgical mortality within one month was 13%, and 5-year survival was 41% for the younger patients.

It is difficult to draw conclusions from the somewhat discouraging results. Modern techniques have been used only in the later portion of the series (microsurgery, laser surgery, chemotherapy). Further data will be needed to establish the best method of treatment for these difficult infantile brain tumors.—Robert M. Crowell, M.D.

Fetal Intracranial Teratoma: US Diagnosis of Three Cases and a Review of the Literature

Steven P. Lipman, Dolores H. Pretorius, Carol M. Rumack, and Michael L. Manco-Johnson (Univ. of Colorado)
Radiology 157:491–494, November 1985   26–2

Seven cases of fetal intracranial teratoma, diagnosed by ultrasonography, have been reported, and three further cases were encountered in the past 4 years.

Pregnant woman, 40 years old, presented at 32 weeks' gestation with an enlarged fetal head. Ultrasonography at 8 weeks had been negative, and the α-fetoprotein at 20 weeks was normal. Ultrasonography showed a biparietal diameter of 12 cm and complete replacement of the brain by a solid mass with multiple cystic areas (Fig 26–2). Calcifications were absent. The fetus was considered to be nonviable, and vaginal delivery of a stillborn male was induced. A 430-gm multicystic, im-

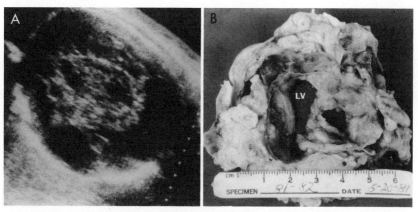

Fig 26–2.—Intracranial teratoma. **A,** a multicystic mass replaces normal brain; no normal parenchyma can be identified. **B,** pathologic section shows dilated lateral ventricle (LV) surrounded by multicystic mass. (Courtesy of Lipman, S.P., et al.: Radiology 157:491–494, November 1985. Reproduced with permission of the Radiological Society of North America.)

mature supratentorial teratoma was present, apparently arising in the pineal region and producing massive obstructive hydrocephalus of the lateral ventricles. Postmortem computed tomography confirmed the ultrasonographic findings.

Most neonatal teratomas are supratentorial, in contrast to the usual infratentorial site of tumors in older children. The usual presentation is that of sudden large-for-date status in an otherwise normal pregnancy. An intrauterine diagnosis of intracranial teratoma has been made by ultrasonography in 10 previous cases. The cerebral architecture is grossly distorted by a multicystic mass, with internal echoes of varying intensity.

Cephalopelvic disproportion is usual in these cases, even in the second trimester. Fetal intracranial teratoma remains a fatal disorder despite advances in neonatal surgery.

▶ Ultrasonographic resolution and sophistication have advanced to the point where the diagnosis of fetal intracranial teratoma is possible in utero. So far, the prognosis for this particular lesion is dismal. However, other lesions with more favorable progress may be encountered by intrauterine ultrasonography. Neurosurgeons will be increasingly requested to comment on management programs for such lesions diagnosed in utero.

Paraplegia in children with malignant teratoma be successfully treated with partial resection and aggressive chemotherapy (Weinblatt and Kenigsberg: *Cancer* 56:2140–2142, 1985).—Robert M. Crowell, M.D.

Use of the Cavitron Ultrasonic Surgical Aspirator and Evoked Potentials for the Treatment of Thalamic and Brain Stem Tumors in Children

A. Leland Albright and Robert J. Sclabassi (Univ. of Pittsburgh)
Neurosurgery 17:564–568, October 1985   26–3

Gliomas in the thalamus and brain stem of children are not often extensively removed because of the risks involved. The Cavitron ultrasonic surgical aspirator (CUSA) was used to remove subtotally 5 brain stem and 4 thalamic gliomas in nine pediatric patients. Evoked potentials were recorded during six operations; four of these patients had no deficit, and two had single cranial nerve palsies. One of the 3 other patients was permanently obtunded, and 1 died of pulmonary embolism 6 weeks after the operation.

Boy, aged 13 months, developed a left hemiparesis and macrocephaly, and computed tomography (CT) showed a large, cystic right hemispheric mass. The cyst was drained at parietal craniectomy, and most of the tumor was removed by standard microsurgical technique. The tumor was an astrocytoma arising in the right side of the thalamus. The hemiparesis was worse after surgery. Computed tomography showed a small crescent of residual tumor, which progressed slowly. The tumor had tripled in size by age 23 months (Fig 26–3). The tumor was removed with the CUSA via the residual cyst cavity, without evoked potential monitoring. Intraoperative CT with contrast enhancement confirmed complete tumor removal. No new deficit was present after surgery. Focal radiotherapy was delivered. Computed tomography 6 months later showed no tumor (Fig 26–4).

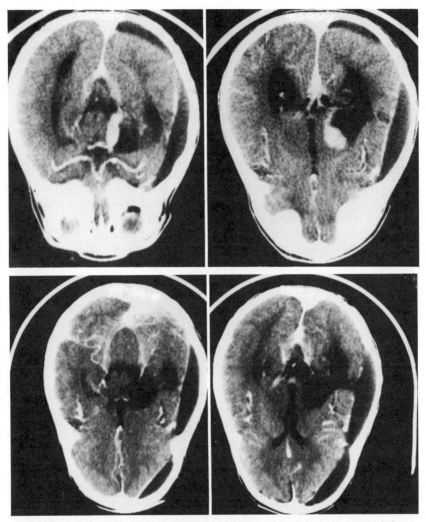

Fig 26–3 (top).—Contrast-enhanced CT of recurrent thalamic-hypothalamic astrocytoma before resection.
Fig 26–4 (bottom).—Postoperative scan.
(Courtesy of Albright, A.L., and Sclabassi, R.J.: Neurosurgery 17:564–568, October 1985.)

Some brain stem and thalamic tumors can be extensively removed with the CUSA. Evoked potential recording is useful in reducing intraoperative morbidity from the resection of central gliomas. Serious morbidity is a possibility but is probably acceptable. Surgery may be especially indicated in children with relatively discrete, enhancing central tumors, since mortality from pediatric astrocytoma appears to correlate with the extent of tumor removal.

▶ In this small series, the results of radical excision were impressive when

CUSA and brain stem evoked potentials were used. Other similar reports have appeared from such major pediatric centers as Salt Lake City and Toronto. This aggressive approach needs further careful evaluation and comparison with conventional therapy before it can be recommended for general use.—Robert M. Crowell, M.D.

The Moyamoya Syndrome Associated With Irradiation of an Optic Glioma in Children: Report of Two Cases and Review of the Literature
Takehito Okuno, Arthur L. Prensky, and Mokhtor Gado (Washington Univ.)
Pediatr. Neurol. 1:311–316, 1985   26–4

Moyamoya disease consists of stenosis or occlusion of the internal carotid and/or proximal parts of the anterior and middle cerebral arteries at the base of the brain. It has been associated with both irradiation in early life and neurofibromatosis. Two children with optic glioma, of whom one had neurofibromatosis, developed moyamoya syndrome after irradiation of the tumor in early life.

Girl, 2 years old, was found to have café-au-lait spots and an enlarged optic foramen. An optic glioma involving the chiasm was irradiated with 4,500 rads. Mild headache and increasing fatigue were present at age 7 years, and seizures occurred on the day of admission, followed by right facial and upper extremity weakness and a partial right hemianopia. Radionuclide scanning showed increased flow in the area of the left middle cerebral artery. A cerebral angiogram showed occlusion of both internal carotid arteries, and leptomeningeal anastomoses with

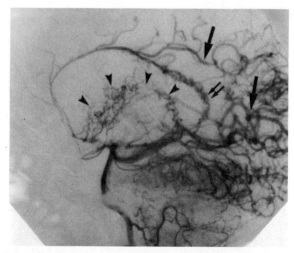

Fig 26–5.—Left vertebral angiogram demonstrating enlargement of the posterior cerebral arteries. There was rich retrograde flow into the anterior and middle cerebral artery branches of the posterior cerebral arteries *(large arrow)*. The flow in the pericallosal arteries was further enhanced by collateral circulation through the hypertrophied dorsal callosal arteries *(double arrows)*. There were telangiectasias involving the lenticulostriate arteries and the posterior choroidal arteries *(arrowheads)*. (Courtesy of Okuno, T., et al.: Pediatr. Neurol. 1:311–316, 1985.)

cortical branches of the posterior cerebral arteries (Fig 26–5). There also were telangiectasias of the lenticulostriate and thalamoperforate arteries and transdural anastomoses with the ophthalmic arteries. Subsequent computed tomography showed left hemispheric atrophy, which progressed. Most recently the patient had episodes of trembling of the left hand and pain in the left arm, inattention in the right visual field, left optic atrophy, mild right hemiparesis, and slurred speech.

Twelve other cases of moyamoya syndrome following irradiation of intracranial tumor have been reported. Most patients were irradiated at ages 5½ months to 12 years and developed manifest disease 6 months to 15 years after. Nine children had optic gliomas, of whom 5 also had neurofibromatosis. All tumors were in the anterior half of the cerebral hemisphere, but there is no evidence that they directly compressed the carotid arteries or their major branches. Irradiation might best be withheld until there is definite growth to adjacent areas of the brain or progressively deteriorating vision.

▶ The authors report two children and review 12 others from the literature, in which moyamoya syndrome followed irradiation of intracranial tumor. The data suggest a causative relationship. The authors suggest withholding irradiation for optic gliomas and neurofibromas until there is definite growth to adjacent areas of brain or progressive deterioration of vision.

This report emphasizes that intracranial irradiation is not without hazard. The precise magnitude of risk, however, remains poorly defined. For patients with slowly progressive intracranial neoplastic conditions, the clinician must weigh against the natural history of the condition the benefits and risks of various forms of therapy, including surgery and radiation. Radiation therapy for optic nerve glioma and neurofibromatosis remains controversial.

Radiation may induce stenosis of the supraclinoid portion of the internal carotid artery with a moyamoya collateral circulatory network (Benoit et al.: *Rev. Neurol. (Paris)* 141:666–668, 1985).—Robert M. Crowell, M.D.

Real Time Ultrasound Diagnosis of Hemorrhagic Pathological Conditions in the Posterior Fossa of Preterm Infants
Raul Bejar, Ronald W. Coen, Ikpe Ekpoudia, Hector E. James, and Louis Gluck (Univ. of California at San Diego)
Neurosurgery 16:281–289, March 1985   26–5

Portable real-time echoencephalography (RTE) was used to study the posterior fossa in newborn infants at the bedside. Infants with a gestational age of less than 34 weeks now are routinely scanned with RTE to rule out intraventricular-subependymal hemorrhage and its complications. A sector scanner with a 5-MHz transducer is used. The posterior fossa is visualized in the coronal, modified coronal, sagittal, and parasagittal planes. The findings were compared with computed tomographic (CT) findings in five patients and with the autopsy findings in 18 infants who died in the first week of life.

Hemorrhagic complications were readily distinguished from normal

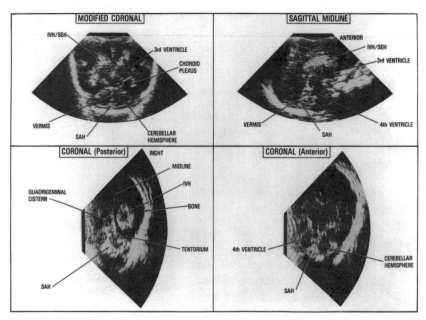

Fig 26–6.—Large subarachnoid hemorrhages *(SAH)* in the cisterna magna, which was confirmed by direct examination of the brain. (Courtesy of Bejar, R., et al.: Neurosurgery 16:281–189, March 1985.)

anatomy, and the RTE diagnosis was confirmed by both CT and autopsy of the brain. Coronal studies were useful in evaluating the size of the fourth ventricle and the absence of blood in the quadrigeminal and supracerebellar cisterns. The appearances in an infant in whom hemorrhage developed on the first day of life are shown in Figure 26–6. Both acute and insidious posthemorrhagic enlargement of the fourth ventricle were visualized.

Hemorrhagic pathologic changes in the posterior fossa can be precisely diagnosed in preterm infants at the bedside by the use of RTE. Modified coronal and sagittal studies have been most useful. The study is helpful in following the course of third and fourth ventricular obstruction and in evaluating the results of shunting.

▶ This report documents that a great deal of anatomic detail may be identified in the posterior fossa of preterm infants by the use of ultrasound diagnosis. The neurosurgeon must become familiar with these foreign-appearing images to gain information important to neurosurgical management. The same kind of information may be obtained in patients of various ages during surgery of the posterior fossa; tiny lesions within the parenchyma may be identified with this technique.

Agenesis of the corpus collosum can be confidently recognized with ultrasonography (Atlas et al.: *AJNR* 145:167–173, 1985).

Neonatal periventricular leukomalacia can be recognized with ultrasonography (Chow et al.: *AJNR* 145:155–160, 1985).

In infants undergoing extracorporeal membrane oxygenation, ultrasonography may show hemorrhages of uncommon extent and location, which are presumably due to required anticoagulation (Bowerman et al.: *AJR* 145:161–166, 1985).—Robert M. Crowell, M.D.

Management of Trigonocephaly
G. Salkind, L. N. Sutton, D. A. Bruce, L. Schut, and A. Schut (Univ. of Pennsylvania)
Surg. Neurol. 25:159–162, February 1986   26–6

Premature fusion of the metopic suture with associated trigonocephaly is an infrequent form of craniosynostosis. The skull base is usually involved. Abnormal psychomotor development can occur in severe cases. Fourteen patients (13 male and 1 female; age range, 9 weeks to 9 months) with isolated metopic synostosis were encountered between 1969 and 1982. All patients were considered neurologically normal. Four had associated abnormalities. Eleven patients were operated on by a simple method in which the metopic suture is not opened. A bicoronal scalp flap was reflected to the glabella and supraorbital ridges, and a "gull-wing" bone flap formed in the frontal region and hinged forward on the metopic ridge. The midline strut in the area of the fused suture was burred down but not removed.

Optimal cosmetic results were obtained in all patients during follow-up from 3 months to 10 years. No patient required reoperation. No cranial defects were noted at last follow-up. The patients tolerated the operation well, with no major postoperative problems.

The best cosmetic results are obtained with this procedure if it is done at ages 4–6 weeks. Early surgery is technically easier and avoids restraint of brain growth. Immediate decompression is warranted if there are signs of increased intracranial pressure at any time. The precise operation should be adjusted to the magnitude of deformity and to any associated anomalies that may be present. This procedure is not indicated for cases of severe hypotelorism in which lateral orbital advancement is required as well.

▶ An individualized approach is needed for management of the varied forms of craniosynostosis. Moss has suggested that cranial growth is stimulated by the "neural mass" (*Childs Brain* 1:22–23, 1975). Cranial sutures thus provide a site for passive cranial expansion. For metopic synostosis, it is therefore enough to provide for lateral expansion by creating a bifrontal bone flap. Experience at Children's Hospital of Philadelphia supports this approach.

Using a multiple fragment reconstruction technique, good results were obtained in the surgical treatment of trigonocephaly in 33 cases (Albin et al.: *Plast. Reconstr. Surg.* 76:202–211, 1985).—Robert M. Crowell, M.D.

Separation of Craniopagus Twins Utilizing Tissue Expanders
Raymond E. Shively, Michael A. Bermant, and Richard D. Bucholz (St. Louis Univ.)
Plast. Reconstr. Surg. 76:765–772, November 1985   26–7

Skin and subcutaneous tissue can be selectively expanded to great pro-portions for coverage of adjacent defects in the head and neck and scalp. Tissue expanders were used to gain extra scalp needed for the closing of defects after the separation of craniopagus twins.

Twins were conjoined at the left parietal region of the heads, facing in opposite directions. One twin also had an imperforate anus, but no other defects were apparent. The conjoined area had a circumference of 34 cm and a surface area of 90 sq cm. It was just superior to folded left ears located slightly low on the heads. A colostomy was performed for the imperforate anus at age 3 days; 6 days later, a coronal scalp flap was elevated on each twin, and initial separation of shared parietal brain was carried out through a superior bone window. An ectopic dural sinus connecting the two sagittal sinuses was divided at age 46 days, and two subgaleal, 200-cc hemispheric tissue expanders were placed over the occiput in each child. Saline was injected in a volume of 50 cc, and starting 2 weeks later, expansion was achieved over 1 month. The separation was completed at age 106 days, with skin flaps raised as shown in Figure 26–7. Rapid closure of the scalp permitted resuscitation of 1 of the infants with bleeding from a large sinus. Several resuturings and revisions of the scalp closures were necessary because of subgaleal cerebrospinal fluid collections. One infant required temporary lumboperitoneal shunting. One infant was discharged at age 8 months with age-appropriate de-velopment; the other remained in the hospital with severe developmental delay.

Hemispheric skin expanders were extremely useful in this case for closing the large scalp defects that remained after separation of craniopagus twins.

▶ Successful separation of craniopagus twins has been rarely achieved. The management of at least one of the major problems, skin coverage, seems to be materially aided by the ingenious use of tissue expanders. Management of sinuses might be assisted by preoperative depiction by magnetic resonance imaging.—Robert M. Crowell, M.D.

Neurological and Neuropsychological Effects of Cerebral Spinal Fluid Shunting in Children With Assumed Arrested ("Normal Pressure") Hydro-cephalus

Richard D. Torkelson, Lyal G. Leibrock, John L. Gustavson, and Robert R. Sundell (Univ. of Nebraska)
J. Neurol. Neurosurg. Psychiatry 48:799–806, August 1985   26–8

The distinction of normal-pressure hydrocephalus from "arrested" hy-drocephalus remains problematic. Four normocephalic children who were found to have ventriculomegaly during assessment for long-standing neu-rologic disorder (4½-8½ years) were tested for academic achievement, IQ, and neuropsychologic functioning. Radioiodinated serum cisternography

---

Fig 26–7.—Top, incision used for final separation. Middle, flaps as raised and twins divided. Bottom, flap 1 covers conjoined defect, flap 2 covers occipital donor site. (Courtesy of Shively, R. E., et al.: Plast. Reconstr. Surg. 76:765–772, November 1985.)

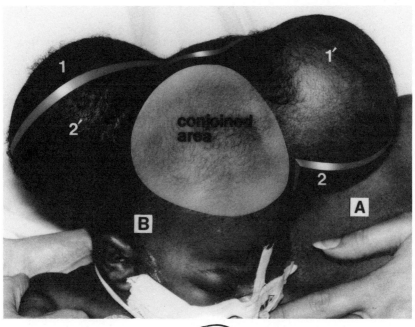

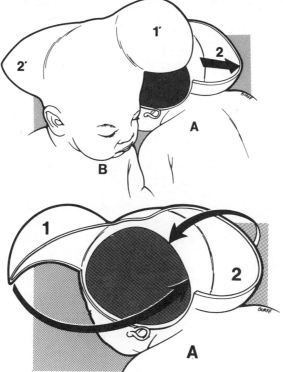

was carried out, and postshunt visual evoked responses, brain stem auditory evoked potentials, and sleep EEGs were recorded.

All four study children were followed up for at least a year after placement of a ventriculoperitoneal shunt. All of them improved psychometrically, and computed tomography and EEG recording also showed improvement. Neuropsychologic performance was the most sensitive initial indicator of improvement. Intelligence scores improved later, but achievement test scores showed no consistent change. Achievement scores did not relate directly to either chronologic age or the improvement noted with other measures.

These preliminary findings suggest that there is a group of asymptomatic children with apparently stable hydrocephalus who have abnormal neuropsychologic test findings, indicating the need for cerebrospinal fluid shunting. The present patients improved after shunt placement. Further longitudinal studies of larger samples should help identify those patients who are likely to benefit from cerebrospinal fluid shunting.

▶ This report draws attention to a common but important syndrome of "asymptomatic" hydrocephalus in children. The only apparent tip-off to the condition is mental retardation, which may be modest in degree. Computed tomographic scanning or magnetic resonance imaging is needed to demonstrate ventriculomegaly. At this point, the only way to distinguish between "arrested" hydrocephalus and symptomatic normal-pressure hydrocephalus in these children is to proceed with the shunt procedure. Neuropsychologic testing is important to document change in mental performance.—Robert M. Crowell, M.D.

The Management of Fetal Hydrocephalus

Frank A. Chervenak, Richard L. Berkowitz, Marge Tortora, and John C. Hobbins (Yale Univ. and Mt. Sinai School of Medicine, New York)
Am. J. Obstet. Gynecol. 151:933–942, Apr. 1, 1985   26–9

The management of 53 consecutive cases of documented fetal hydrocephalus seen between 1977 and 1983 was reviewed. The diagnosis was based on an abnormal lateral ventricle-to-hemisphere width ratio as defined by nomogram or on the presence of marked and obvious dilation of the ventricles. Twenty-seven cases were collected prospectively in 1982 and 1983. Mean gestational ages were 31.5 weeks in the earlier, retrospective series and 28 weeks in the prospective series.

Hydrocephalus was associated with other abnormalities in 83% of the patients, most often with spina bifida. The prenatal diagnosis of isolated hydrocephalus was incorrect in 14 instances. Obstetric management is shown in the table. Ventriculoamniotic shunts were placed in two cases. Cephalocentesis was done in two other cases, besides cesarean section, and 18 section deliveries were carried out without either adjunctive procedure. Fourteen pregnancies were terminated. Spontaneous abortion oc-

MANAGEMENT OF 53 CASES OF DOCUMENTED FETAL HYDROCEPHALUS

	Abortion	Intrapartum death	Postnatal death	Alive	Total
Termination of pregnancy	14	–	–	–	14 (26%)
Cesarean section					
Ventriculoamniotic shunt and cesarean section	–	–	–	2	2 (4%)
Cephalocentesis and cesarean section	–	–	2	–	2 (4%)
Cesarean section (other)	–	–	7	11	18 (34%)
Vaginal delivery					
Cephalocentesis and vaginal delivery	–	6	3	–	9 (17%)
Vaginal delivery (other)	–	2	4	2	8 (15%)
Total	14 (26%)	8 (15%)	16 (30%)	15 (28%)	53 (100%)

(Courtesy of Chervenak, F.A., et al.: Am. J. Obstet. Gynecol. 151:933–942, Apr. 1, 1985.)

curred in 26% of cases, intrapartum death in 15%, and postnatal death in 30%. Fifteen infants were alive at follow-up.

Fetal hydrocephalus is usually associated with other abnormalities. Delivery is recommended once pulmonary maturity is demonstrated. Amniocentesis should be performed weekly from 36 weeks' gestation. The risks of respiratory distress syndrome and delayed ventriculoperitoneal shunt placement must be weighed against the potential effects of progressive ventriculomegaly. Cephalocentesis, when indicated, is facilitated by sonographic guidance. Fetuses with isolated hydrocephalus and macrocephaly are best delivered by cesarean section. If the prognosis is extremely poor, however, cephalocentesis and vaginal delivery may be most appropriate. The role of ventriculoamniotic shunt placement remains uncertain.

▶ With the advent of ultrasonic diagnostic techniques, prenatal diagnosis of fetal hydrocephalus is now a common event. What is the outlook? What should the neurosurgeon do? This useful review shows that the outlook is very poor for these fetuses: of 53 cases, only 15 infants were alive at follow-up. Moreover, no one knows the eventual developmental course of these little babies. Because of the very bad prognosis, it certainly is worthwhile for investigators to attempt to develop new methods for salvage. However, published reports to date, including this one, have not established an important, effective role for intrauterine surgery, despite a small number of cases highlighted in the popular press. Practical guidelines regarding cephalocentesis and timing and route of delivery are given. Neurosurgeons will find this communication helpful as they approach this difficult and ethically disturbing problem.—Robert M. Crowell, M.D.

Perimesencephalic Cistern Obliteration: A CT Sign of Life-Threatening Shunt Failure

Dennis L. Johnson, Charles Fitz, David C. McCullough, and Saul Schwarz (Children's Hosp. Natl. Med. Ctr., Washington, D.C., and Bethesda Naval Hosp., Md.)

J. Neurosurg. 64:386–389, March 1986   26–10

Two deaths of children from shunt malfunction led to a review of the case histories of seven patients with life-threatening shunt malfunction associated with obliteration of the perimesencephalic cistern. All patients were lethargic when admitted, and a precipitous worsening of neurologic status led to emergency shunt revision in each case. The age range was 1–17 years. Spina bifida was diagnosed in three patients. The average duration of symptoms, most prominently headache, was 5 days. Five patients had decerebrate posturing just before surgery. Palpation indicated good shunt function in all but 1 patient. Computed tomography (CT) revealed obliteration of the perimesencephalic cistern. Review of 43 hydrocephalic patients showed the absence of cisterns in four of them, in association with ventriculomegaly. All four patients electively underwent shunt revision, and the cisterns reappeared.

A review of 407 patients followed up for more than 15 years revealed 4 deaths associated with shunt malfunction. Two of the present 7 patients with sudden deterioration died following emergency intervention. It appears that CT findings of obliteration of the perimesencephalic cistern should be taken as a warning of life-threatening shunt failure. Cisternal obliteration in children with lumboperitoneal shunts is a nonspecific find-ing; however, it is more specific in the setting of severe head injury or cerebral anoxia. Immediate shunt revision is indicated if the patient pre-sents with shunt failure and obliteration of the basal cisterns on CT.

▶ The neurosurgeon is often asked to evaluate patients with possible shunt malfunction. A host of methods have been suggested to determine whether the shunt is actually working. Unfortunately, no method short of open revision has proved reliable. When there is a serious question of function, revision is the safest approach.

Johnson and colleagues report that obliteration of the perimesencephalic cis-tern is a sign of life-threatening shunt failure. Recognition of this sign is a clear indication for shunt revision.

Neurosurgeons are becoming aware that obliteration of basal cisterns is an important sign of increased intracranial pressure and impending herniation in a variety of settings (trauma, tumor, subarachnoid hemorrhage).—Robert M. Crowell, M.D.

Surgical Treatment of Idiopathic Hydrocephalus in Elderly Patients
Ronald C. Petersen, Bahran Mokri, and Edward R. Laws, Jr. (Mayo Clinic and Found.)
Neurology 35:307–311, March 1985   26–11

The pathophysiologic features of normal-pressure hydrocephalus are uncertain. The records of 45 adults seen between 1966 and 1981, who underwent a shunting procedure for idiopathic normal-pressure hydro-cephalus, were reviewed. The 24 men and 21 women had a mean age of 68 years (range, 56–84 years). The mean follow-up after shunting was 51 months.

Three fourths of the patients exhibited some improvement after shunt-ing, and 42% had definitive, continuous improvement. The median du-ration of improvement was 2 years. Patients with gait disorder, dementia, and urinary incontinence seemed likeliest to respond to shunting. The course after shunting is related to the computed tomographic (CT) findings in the table. All but 2 of 15 patients with a definitely abnormal result on radionuclide cerebrospinal fluid cisternography responded favorably to shunting. Most complications from shunting were minor, and no deaths resulted directly from the procedure.

Prolonged clinical improvement can follow cerebrospinal fluid shunt operations in patients with idiopathic hydrocephalus. Computed tomog-raphy is a useful means of evaluating these patients, but the CT findings were not closely related to the response to shunting in this series. More than a third of patients can be expected to have a satisfactory and lasting response to shunting. The best diagnostic criteria are the clinical presen-tation and the duration of symptoms.

▶ In the 20 years since normal-pressure hydrocephalus was first described, a

CORRELATION OF CT FINDINGS WITH RESPONSE
TO SHUNTING PROCEDURE

	Pts, no.	Response Improved, no. (%)	Not improved, no.
CT assessment	29	24 (83)	5
Before shunting			
Ventricular dilatation			
Mild	1	1 (100)	0
Moderate	9	8 (89)	1
Severe	19	15 (79)	4
Cortical atrophy			
None	12	10 (83)	2
Mild	13	10 (77)	3
Moderate	4	4 (100)	0
Periventricular lucency*			
Present	10	10 (100)	0
Absent	13	10 (77)	3
After shunting			
Ventricular size			
Decreased	12	10 (83)	2
No change	17	14 (82)	3
Periventricular lucency*			
Decreased	6	6 (100)	0
No change	17	14 (82)	3

*Lack of adequate resolution on early-generation CTs prevented assessment of scans of 6 patients.
(Courtesy of Petersen, R.C., et al.: Neurology 35:307–311, March 1985.)

wide variety of tests have been described for identification of cases likely to respond to surgery. As indicated in this report from the Mayo Clinic, the neurologic presentation—the clinical triad of gait disturbance, dementia, and urinary incontinence—remains the best indicator of a useful neurologic response to shunting. Even CT findings are not an accurate reflection of the postoperative course. Dr. C. Fisher (Lancet 1:37, 1978) has suggested that improvement after removal of 25 cc of cerebrospinal fluid by spinal puncture is a helpful index of response after shunting. He also emphasized that in cases with gait disturbance earlier and disproportionate to other symptoms the chance for improvement is better. When the clinical triad is present and the ventricles are enlarged, the surgeon can proceed to shunting without the need for ancillary tests, which will not further clarify the picture.—Robert M. Crowell, M.D.

Toward the Development of a Play Performance Scale for Children (PPSC)
Lester L. Lansky, Marcy A. List, Shirley B. Lansky, Michael E. Cohen, and Lucius F. Sinks (Univ. of Illinois and Illinois Cancer Ctr., State Univ. of New York at Buffalo and Buffalo Children's Hosp., and Natl. Insts. of Health, Bethesda, Md.)
Cancer 56:1837–1840, Oct. 1, 1985

PLAY/PERFORMANCE STATUS

A. Normal range of play

Able to carry on usual play activities both active and quiet; child initiates play; no special adult assistance or direction needed; participation in interactive play

100 • Fully active
90 • Minor restrictions in physically strenuous play
80 • Restricted in physically strenuous play (*e.g.,* chasing games); may tire more easily, otherwise active

B. Mild to moderate restriction of play

Able to engage in some active play, but spends greater than usual time in quiet play; requires varying degree of assistance in setting up and completing play; restricted in interactive play

70 • Both greater restriction of, and less time spent in, active play
60 • Ambulatory 50% of time; limited active play with adult assistance, supervision
50 • Considerable adult assistance required for any active play; fully able to engage in quiet play (set up games, turn on TV, *etc.*)

C. Moderate to severe restriction of play

No active play; play limited to quiet activities; requires varying degree of assistance for quiet play

40 • Able to initiate most quiet activities
30 • Needs considerable assistance even for quiet activities
20 • Play entirely limited to very passive activities initiated by other (*e.g.,* TV)
10 • Completely disabled, no play
0 • Unresponsive

(Courtesy of Lansky, L.L., et al.: Cancer 56:1837–1840, Oct. 1, 1985.)

No single, easily measurable scale is available for evaluating the performance status of children. Children with cancer, particularly brain tumor, would benefit from a simply administered and rapid assessment method. Any test should be equally valid at all age levels and should be accessible to nonprofessionals. The impact of play behavior on children parallels the parameters measured by the Karnofsky Scale in adults. A performance scale (table) was developed based on play, using the Gesell Scales of child development as a model to describe play patterns at different ages. A spectrum of age-appropriate play is scored from 0 to 100. The age level correlating with the child's play activities is used by the scorer. The level of play at baseline may not be at a child's chronologic age.

Pilot study of this instrument is needed before it can be included in experimental protocols. Actual descriptions of play activities will require continuous updating to keep the test in conformity with current social norms. Multiple regression analysis may be used to learn which types of play are most predictive of performance status. The present scale can be used by nonprofessionals and does not require extensive instrumentation.

It is hoped that it will prove useful in the development of effective rehabilitation programs for children with cancer.

▶ This is a logical approach toward the development of a Karnofsky scale for children. It is hoped that further application of this approach will result in a standardized scale.—Robert M. Crowell, M.D.

Notes on Pediatrics

▶ Metrizamide shuntography usually demonstrates the cause of shunt malfunction (Mirfakhrall et al.: *AJNR* 6:815–822, 1985). However, a normal study does not exclude intermittent malfunction and does not necessarily exclude revision.

According to Naidich et al., chronic cerebral herniation in shunted Dandy-Walker malformation is not uncommon (6,125 cases) and carries a bad prognosis (*Radiology* 158:431–434, 1986).

Dobie and Fisch report satisfactory results in 74% of patients with facial spasms who were treated with selective peripheral neurectomy (*Arch. Otolaryngol. Head Neck Surg.* 112:154–163, 1986).

All 21 patients undergoing posterior fossa exploration for disabling positional vertigo had vascular compression of the 8th cranial nerve (Moller et al.: *J. Neurosurg.* 64:21–28, 1986). Postoperatively, 16 were symptom-free, 3 improved, and 2 unchanged.

Combined percutaneous thermocoagulation of the 5th and 9th cranial nerves can control oral pain from cancer (Solar et al.: *J. Maxillofac. Surg.* 14:1–4, 1986).

All eight children not offered immediate meningomyelocele repair after birth have survived to school entry and are no more handicapped than children offered immediate surgical treatment. The choice at birth is not necessarily an urgent one between life and death (Menzies et al.: *Lancet* 2:993–995, 1985).

Since pediatric patients can have normal interpeduncular distance despite intraspinal pathology and abnormal interpeduncular distance without intraspinal pathology, this measurement is no longer of value in diagnosis (Markound: *Acta Radiol. [Diagn.] (Stockh)* 26:599–602, 1985).

Persuasive data are presented to suggest a dramatic decline in spina bifida births and congenital CNS defects over the past 12 years in Great Britain (Lorber and Ward: *Arch. Dis. Child* 60:1086–1091, 1985).—Robert M. Crowell, M.D.

27 Infection

Introduction

For fungal infections of the CNS, early diagnosis guided by computed tomography (CT), aggressive surgery including placement of Ommaya devices, and appropriate chemotherapy can reduce a high morbidity and mortality (Digest 27–1). Polygloycolic sutures carry no higher risk of infection than do silk ones (Digest 27–2). Studies have not shown a useful effect for antibiotic prophylaxis in shunting for hydrocephalus patients (Digest 27–3). Subdural empyema may be diagnosed on CT scan with contrast material; suboccipital craniectomy is necessary to remove the purulent material (Digest 27–4). Postmastoidectomy cerebrospinal fluid leaks can be cured with a "minicraniotomy" to seal the leak (Digest 27–5).

Robert M. Crowell, M.D.

Surgical Treatment for Fungal Infections in the Central Nervous System
Ronald F. Young, George Gade, and Verity Grinnell (Univ. of California at Los Angeles)
J. Neurosurg. 63:371–381, September 1985   27–1

Intracranial fungal infections are being diagnosed with increasing frequency. Seventy-eight patients had surgical treatment for such infection between 1964 and 1984, 56 males and 22 females with a mean age of 34.6 years (range, birth to 72 years). Approximately two thirds of the infections were due to *Coccidioides immitis* and *Cryptococcus neoformans*. Neurologic symptoms were the first indication of fungal infection in 39% of the cases. Predisposing factors were identified in 29 patients, and 22 others with coccidioidomycosis had traveled to or lived in an endemic region. Forty-seven patients were known to previously have had local or systemic fungal infections. Contrast-enhanced computed tomography was diagnostically helpful (Fig 27–1).

All patients received antifungal chemotherapy, usually intrathecal amphotericin B. A total of 144 surgical procedures were carried out, including lesion biopsy or excisional procedures in 13 patients, primary cerebrospinal fluid (CSF) shunting in 22, and placement of an Ommaya reservoir in 48. The overall mortality was 43.6%. Twenty-four deaths resulted directly from uncontrolled CNS fungal infection. Nine of 14 patients whose diagnosis was delayed died. Only 38.5% of patients could be considered cured of fungal infection. Mortality ranged from 42% in patients with mass lesions to 50% for those with hydrocephalus.

Fungal infection should be suspected in patients with basal meningitis, and the CSF examined in cases of undiagnosed communicating hydrocephalus, before shunting if possible. If recurrent bacterial CSF shunt in-

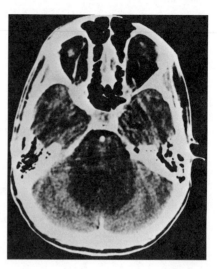

Fig 27–1.—Computerized tomography scan following intravenous infusion of contrast material. A large radiolucent mass, caused by an infection due to *C. neoformans,* is seen in the cerebellum, compressing the fourth ventricle. Hydrocephalus was present. (Courtesy of Young, R.F., et al.: J. Neurosurg. 63:371–381, September 1985.)

fection is found, *Candida albicans* meningitis should be ruled out. Mortality from CNS fungal infection can be reduced by early diagnosis, aggressive surgery, and appropriate chemotherapy.

▶ The mortality of fungal infections in CNS remains very high despite moderate antifungal therapy. Cerebrospinal fluid sampling is essential for specific diagnosis, but fungal infection may be suspected according to the poststatus and clinical presentation, as well as the findings on computed tomography. Nonsurgical intervention and antifungal therapy may be useful, but it is worth noting that the mortality remains staggering despite the availability of the Ommaya device and amphotericin B for almost 20 years.

Actinomycotic infections of the CNS may be treated with antibiotics and surgery (Tvede et al.: *Acta Immunol. Scand.* 93:327–330, 1985).

Intracranial tuberculosis may present as hydrocephalus, exudate in the basal cisterns, tuberulomanous mass lesions, or cerebral infarcts, often multiple (Witoak and Ellis: *South. Med. J.* 78:386–392, 1985).

Chowdhary et al. advocate radical débridement surgery with bone grafting for thoracic and lumbar spinal tuberculosis confirmed by computed tomography scanning (*J. R. Coll. Surg. Edinb.* 30:386–390, 1985).—Robert M. Crowell, M.D.

Infections in Neurosurgery: A Randomized Comparison Between Silk and Polyglycolic Acid
G. C. Blomstedt (Helsinki Univ.)
Acta Neurochir. 76:90–93, 1985   27–2

Polyglycolic acid (PGA) is an alternative to silk for use in buried sutures, since it is fully absorbed in 6 weeks. Silk and PGA suture materials were compared in a randomized study with regard to infectious complications in a series of 1,011 patients who underwent neurosurgical procedures in 1979–1981. In 1 group, all layers were closed with silk; in the other group, the skin was closed with Surgilone (a twisted polyfilament siliconated polyamide), and all other layers were closed with PGA suture material. Shunt tubing was secured with Surgilone.

No significant differences in the risk of serious infection were found between the silk and PGA groups. Superficial wound infections also were similarly frequent in the two groups. Suture fistulas were more prevalent when silk suture material was used, occurring in 3% of cases, compared with 1% in the PGA group. Protruding stitches occurred in the same proportions of cases.

Polyglycolic acid and other absorbable suture materials are recommended for closing the galea, subcutis, fascia, and muscle. Modern suture materials all are relatively reliable and nontraumatic, and selection should be made more on the basis of strength, cosmetic results, ease of handling, and cost than on wound infection rates. Silk is conveniently used for skin suturing, and the breaking strength of 4–0 silk prevents sutures from being pulled too tight.

▶ Silk and absorbable sutures evidently show no major difference in their predilection to wound infection. Previous work has indicated that the likelihood of meningocerebral cicatrix is less when the dura is closed with a PGA suture.— Robert M. Crowell, M.D.

Antibiotic Prophylaxis in Cerebrospinal Fluid Shunting: A Prospective, Randomized Trial in 152 Hydrocephalic Patients
Kaare Schmidt, Flemming Gjerris, Ole Osgaard, Eigill F. Hvidberg, Jette E. Kristiansen, Benedicte Dahlerup, and Christian Kruse-Larsen (Hvidore Hosp., Rigshospitalet, and Univ. of Copenhagen)
Neurosurgery 17:1–5, July 1985   27–3

Shunt infection is reported in an average of 15% of hydrocephalic patients, a finding that suggests the possible value of antibiotic prophylaxis. Prophylaxis for 24 hours was evaluated in 152 hydrocephalic patients referred to two neurosurgical clinics in an 18-month period who underwent clean shunt operations or revisions. Study patients received 200 mg of methicillin/kg in six intravenous doses, starting at induction of anesthesia. Allergic patients received 20 mg of erythromycin/kg divided into three doses. The Hakim shunt was used in 75% of the patients. Seventy-seven patients had ventriculoatrial and 75 ventriculoperitoneal shunts.

The rate of infection was 7.2% overall, 8.9% in antibiotic-treated patients, and 5.5% in control patients. Infection could not be related to age, sex, type of shunt, cause of hydrocephalus, or duration of the procedure. No infected patient had clinical signs of shunt malfunction. Six patients were septicemic. Two of the 4 patients with peritonitis had signs of meningitis. The shunt system was replaced in 10 infected patients; 1 patient recovered with antibiotic therapy alone. No recurrent infection was seen.

Antibiotic prophylaxis failed to reduce the rate of infection associated with cerebrospinal fluid shunt procedures in hydrocephalic patients in this study. The results do not rule out the possibility of reducing the infection rate by using a different prophylactic antibiotic regimen.

▶ Haines has recently reviewed a variety of studies of prophylactic antibiotics for cerebrospinal fluid shunting (Meeting of the American Association of Neurological Surgeons, Denver, 1986). He noted methodologic flaws and low statistical power in many of the studies, including the present study. He concluded that prophylactic antibiotics can be recommended in especially high-risk situations, but that routine prophylactic antibiotic therapy in neurosurgery is not warranted.—Robert M. Crowell, M.D.

Posterior Fossa Subdural Empyema
David W. Morgan and Bernard Williams (Midland Centre for Neurosurgery and Neurology, Warley, England)
Brain 108:983–992, December 1985   27–4

Posterior fossa subdural empyema is a rare form of intracranial sepsis that can complicate otogenic infection and whose diagnosis is often delayed. Mortality is high unless early, aggressive surgery is undertaken. Of seven patients encountered between 1955 and 1984, three survived.

Man, 17 years old, was admitted to the hospital after a week of postnasal discharge with fever and right retro-orbital pain, with weakness of the left leg for two days. He was drowsy and disoriented and had marked neck stiffness, papilloedema, and gross left leg weakness. The white blood cell count was 17,000/cu mm, with 80% polymorphs. A computed tomographic (CT) scan showed a parasagittal subdural empyema with pus beside the falx, and extensive ethmoid and

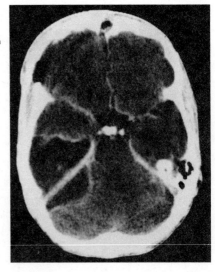

Fig 27–2.—Computed tomography scan with contrast. Extensive subtentorial pus, of which there is more on the right side than the left and which extends toward the midline, can be seen. Supratentorial pus is also present under the temporal and occipital lobes on the right. Enhancement of the tentorium can be noted. (Courtesy of Morgan, D.W. and Williams, B.: Brain 108:983–992, December 1985.)

maxillary sinusitis. A double right craniotomy revealed much pus coating the brain surface. Benzyl penicillin and chloramphenicol were given intravenously; culture yielded group C β-hemolytic streptococci. Seizures and a squint occurred transiently after surgery. Symptoms recurred 3 weeks later after an antral washout, and CT showed reaccumulation of pus below the tentorium (Fig 27–2) with obstructive hydrocephalus. Widespread posterior fossa decompression was carried out. The arachnoid was intact. A complete neurologic recovery followed.

All patients were male, aged 15–44 years. Five patients had otogenic infection, while two had spread of pus from subdural empyema secondary to acute frontal sinusitis. Two of the former patients had recently had mastoid surgery. Marked neck stiffness and papilloedema were usual findings. Four patients had localizing posterior fossa signs. Initial CT scans sometimes were not diagnostic, and exploration may be indicated to make a definitive diagnosis.

Posterior fossa craniectomy is the procedure of choice in these cases. All patients treated only by posterior fossa burr holes died. Timely and adequate surgery can be expected to produce good results with minimal morbidity.

▶ Subdural empyema is too often overlooked, especially in the posterior fossa. As indicated in this article, diagnosis can be difficult and can be missed by CT scanning. Early experience with magnetic resonance imaging indicates that this method may be more sensitive in detecting such empyemas. Posterior fossa evacuation of infected material can be curative. The neurosurgeon must be alert to this possible diagnosis and aggressive in advancing operative invention.—Robert M. Crowell, M.D.

Diagnosis and Treatment of Iatrogenic Cerebrospinal Fluid Leak and Brain Herniation During or Following Mastoidectomy
J. Gail Neely and John R. Kuhn (Univ. of Oklahoma)
Laryngoscope 95:1299–1300, November 1985   27–5

Iatrogenic brain herniation with (meningoencephalocele) or without meninges (encephalocele) is a rare complication of mastoidectomy. Six patients sustaining small iatrogenic dural injuries during mastoidectomy in a 11½-year-period were reviewed. An intact canal wall technique was used in all cases to perform tympanoplasty and mastoidectomy for chronic suppurative otitis media, with or without cholesteatoma. Injury occurred at the tegmen of the mastoid just above the squamous bone contribution of the external meatus. Two patients with three spontaneous meningoencephaloceles and one patient with a large encephalocele also were studied.

No herniation occurred in association with a bony defect alone, without dural injury, and the dura was abruptly defective in areas of herniation. Areas with defective dura but intact arachnoid exhibited herniation of the arachnoid, filled with cerebrospinal fluid (CSF) and a small protrusion of brain. Symptoms did not occur until sudden rupture of the arachnoid produced a CSF-filled middle ear and conductive hearing loss. Leakage in areas in which the dura and arachnoid were defective stopped when protruding brain obstructed the flow of fluid. All defects were successfully repaired with cartilage-perichondrial grafts placed through the tegmen via a mastoid approach into a space created extradurally in the middle fossa.

The integrity of the arachnoid determines whether encephalocele or meningoencephalocele will develop in these cases. Repair probably should be done if there is any doubt about the integrity of the dura. The tegmental defect may be repaired with fascia or muscle, but this may not be adequate for large defects. A composite cartilage-perichondrial graft can be placed via a "mini-craniotomy."

▶ When CSF or an encephalocele appears in the external auditory canal, there is an indication for repair of the defect. A satisfactory neurosurgical approach to such lesions is through a small craniotomy for excision of the encephalocele and placement of a dural graft. Coronal CT (and in some cases polytomography) can pinpoint the lesion and thus guide the surgery.

We have successfully treated three cases of CSF leakage following mastoid surgery. In each instance, CT scans, especially coronal cuts with bone windows, demonstrated a defect in the tegmen tympani. The defect was definitively closed through a small craniotomy. Excision of a small brain hernia facilitated placement of a dural graft that was sutured in place. There were no complications and the CSF leakage was eliminated in each case. This route may be preferable to operating through the mastoid, which may be infected.—Robert M. Crowell, M.D.

28 Nerve

Introduction

Brachial plexus exploration is indicated for sharp lacerations of plexus with deficit and schwannomas (Digest 28–1). Intraplexal transfer in traumatic avulsions of the brachial plexus are recommended in selected cases (Digest 28–2). Shoulder arthrodesis in cases of brachial plexus injury serves to place the hand in a functional position while useful motion persists at the scapulothoracic joint (Digest 28–3). The diagnosis of thoracic outlet syndrome remains difficult even with physiologic techniques (Digest 28–4).

In the area of direct nerve injury, indications have been developed for early exploration of radial nerve injury complicating fracture of the humerus (Digest 28–5). Microsurgical repair of lower limb nerve injuries with complete lesions can produce good results (Digest 28–6). Several experimental studies suggest that nerve conduits may assist in the repair of peripheral nerves: polytetrafluorinated ethylene (Digest 28–7) and biodegradable polyester tubes have been used with encouraging results.

Robert M. Crowell, M.D.

Surgery for Lesions of the Brachial Plexus
David G. Kline, Earl R. Hackett, and Leo H. Happel (Louisiana State Univ.)
Arch. Neurol. 43:170–181, February 1986   28–1

Electromyography is a useful means of establishing denervation early in the course of brachial plexus disorders. Examination 2–3 weeks after injury is most helpful. Intraoperative nerve action potential recording across plexus lesions can demonstrate the presence or absence of regeneration and distinguish between the lesions affecting each element. Computed tomography (CT) with or without metrizamide can be helpful when a meningocele is present or disk herniation is associated with stretch injury to a root.

The most frequent plexus lesion is caused by stretch contusion, usually secondary to motor vehicle accidents. Various neurotization procedures have been described in which cervical plexus, accessory nerve, or intercostal nerves are used as a proximal outflow to attach to a sural graft; the results have been variable. The best results in stretch contusion injuries have been with the elements C5, C6, and the upper trunk, and with lateral and posterior cord lesions. Many of the elements injured by gunshot wounds require resection and repair. Exploration is indicated for sharp lacerations of the plexus producing a significant distal deficit, especially if loss is complete in the distribution of one or more elements.

Schwannomas can be removed with relatively little added deficit. The management of thoracic outlet syndrome remains uncertain in some instances, but cervical rib excision can give good clinical results. Surgery is not indicated for brachial plexus neuropathy or brachial plexitis.

▶ To recommend surgery for brachial plexus lesions, the surgeon must rely on careful pre- and intraoperative electrodiagnostic studies, as well as operative technique tailor-made to the individual case. The aggressive approach advocated here requires expertise and instrumentation beyond the reach of many institutions. Regionalization of treatment for these lesions seems warranted.— Robert M. Crowell, M.D.

Neuro-Neural Intraplexal Transfers in Traumatic Radicular Avulsions of the Brachial Plexus: Report on Fifteen Cases
A. Narakas and G. Herzberg (Clinique de Longeraie, Lausanne, Switzerland; and Hôpital Edouard Herriot, Lyons, France)
Ann. Chir. Main. 4:211–218, 1985   28–2

The large number of axons present in the severed brachial plexus root and the scarcity of interfascicular connective tissue enhance the chances of reinnervating the postlesional segment of nerve. Intraplexal neuroneural transfer (IPNNT) was carried out in 15 patients, 13 adults and 2 infants, with plexus injury and root avulsions. The stumps of the plexal roots were utilized in IPNNT. A total of 28 procedures were performed. Autografts from the sural nerve or a brachial plexus segment were used in 24 instances. Three injuries were directly sutured, while spontaneous neuroneural adherence occurred in 1 case.

Plexal root-to-plexal root transfer did not provide useful motor benefit, whereas plexal root-to-trunk transfers yielded satisfactory but inconsistent results. Transfers to a plexus branch had worthwhile motor results. All plexal root-to-cord transfers gave useful results, including three C5-to-lateral cord transfers and three C5-to-posterior cord transfers. Only 7 patients made significant use of recovered motor activity in their daily lives. Synkinesia occurred in eight cases.

Intraplexal neuroneural transfer is a sound approach to reinnervation in cases of brachial plexus injury in which a stump of a disrupted plexus root is available. Proximal exploration is necessary to detect available plexus roots. Sutures should be placed distal to the plexus trunk to prevent axonal dispersion. Synkinesia is a significant problem but does not contraindicate this approach.

▶ This report presents one technical approach to brachial plexus repair. Further experience from specially experienced centers will be needed to establish any technical approach for general utilization.—Robert M. Crowell, M.D.

Shoulder Arthrodesis for the Treatment of Brachial Plexus Palsy

Robin R. Richards, James P. Waddell, and Alan R. Hudson (St. Michael's Hosp. and Univ. of Toronto)
Clin. Orthop. 198:250–258, September 1985   28–3

Shoulder arthrodesis in cases of brachial plexus injury serves to place the hand in a functional position, and useful motion persists at the scapulothoracic joint. Subsequent surgical reconstruction can focus on the restoration of elbow flexion and improvement of hand function. Fourteen adults with brachial plexus injuries had shoulder arthrodesis in a position of 30 degrees abduction, 30 degrees flexion, and 30 degrees internal rotation. Internal fixation with a 9- or 10-hole dynamic compression plate was carried out in all cases (Fig 28–1). Three patients with complete paralysis underwent above-elbow amputation at the time the shoulder was fused.

Nine of the 14 patients had had previous operations. All shoulders fused during a mean follow-up of 32 months. Limb function was improved by fusion in all instances. Minimal shoulder motion was 60 degrees of abduction and 50 degrees of flexion. Three procedures failed because of continued pain. Plate removal was necessary in seven cases. Only one of the three amputees became a good prosthesis user. Patients with proximal

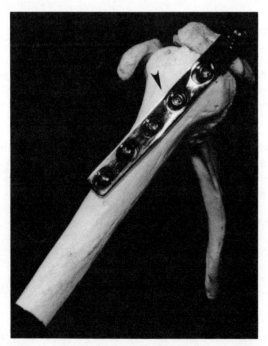

Fig 28–1.—Specimen preparation of a shoulder fusion showing correct application of a DC plate. The plate must be bent as it crosses the acromion and twisted *(arrow)* distal to the bend to closely appose the surface of the humerus. (Courtesy of Richards, R.R., et al.: Clin. Orthop. 198:250–258, September 1985.)

brachial plexus lesions consistently obtained improved arm function after fusion.

Shoulder arthrodesis is a reliable means of improving upper extremity function in adults with brachial plexus injury. The chief cause of failure has been pain. Arthrodesis places the limb in a stable, functional position, and permits the patient both to control and move the extremity. Good motion is possible even with severe paralysis. Fusion is reliably obtained with the use of internal fixation with a dynamic compression plate.

▶ Brachial plexus injuries have incited various degrees of enthusiasm, pessimism, and passivity in neurosurgeons. By and large, conservative therapy has been advocated. A few energetic proponents of exploration, such as Kline, point to neurologic improvement in limited numbers of cases. Richards and collaborators noted improved limb function after shoulder arthrodesis in all 14 patients undergoing this procedure. Complications were attributed to plate removal in seven cases. Only one of three amputees became effective prosthesis users. Because of potential benefit from this procedure, patients with significant deficit after brachial plexus palsy should be considered for arthrodesis.

Among six patients with brachial plexus injuries, early operation disclosed axillary nerve rupture in all six, musculocutaneous nerve rupture in two, and radial rupture in two. The differentiation between branch rupture and a lesion continuity can be made only by surgical exploration, which is recommended as soon as other injuries permit (Burge et al.: *J. Bone Joint Surg.* [*Br*] 67B:630–634, 1985).

Brachial neuritis is characterized by sharp pain, usually in the elbow or shoulder, with weakness in the deltoid spinati biceps and triceps supervening as the pain subsides (Dillin et al.: *J. Bone Joint Surg.* [*Am*] 67A:878–879, 1985). Sensory loss is inconstant.—Robert M. Crowell, M.D.

A Neurophysiologic Investigation of Thoracic Outlet Syndrome
Erik Ryding, Else Ribbe, Ingmar Rosén, and Lars Norgren (Univ. Hosp., Lund, Sweden)
Acta Chir. Scand. 151:327–331, 1985   28–4

There is evidence that compression of the lower brachial plexus is important in thoracic outlet syndrome (TOS). The value of extensive conventional neurophysiologic studies for plexus compression was examined in 41 patients given a clinical diagnosis of TOS in a vascular surgery unit. The mean age was 39 years (range, 18–63 years). The diagnosis was based on the history and clinical findings. Most patients had paresthesia in the ulnar region of the arm and hand, which worsened on elevation of the arm, and a positive "hands up" test.

The neurophysiologic findings in 37 patients without evidence of other nerve disorders are summarized in the table. Neurographic findings were normal apart from the ulnar nerve sensory amplitude, plexus latency, and

SUMMARY OF NEUROPHYSIOLOGIC FINDINGS IN PATIENTS
WITH CLINICAL THORACIC OULET SYNDROME

	No. of Patients
Diagnostic for brachial plexus compression	2 (5%)
Indicating C$_8$ or brachial plexus compression	10 (27%)
Only EMG indications of C$_8$ rhizopathy	4 (11%)
Insufficient for diagnosis	10 (27%)
Normal findings	11 (30%)
Total	37 (100%)

(Courtesy of Ryding E., et al.: Acta Chir. Scand. 151:327–331, 1985.)

F-response latency. There were no significant overall differences in any of these parameters between the symptomatic and nonsymptomatic sides, although a few patients had values outside the normal range. Temperature perception was reduced in the symptomatic hand. Electromyography revealed neurogenic changes in C8-innervated muscles of the symptomatic arm in about one third of the patients.

Fewer than half the patients in this series with clinically diagnosed TOS had pathologic neurophysiologic findings. There is no clinically useful method of detecting pathology in nerve fibers irritated by slight compression in the thoracic outlet. Present study methods are most useful in excluding peripheral nerve compression or a root lesion.

▶ Despite the appearance of reports claiming ease of diagnosis, TOS remains an elusive diagnostic entity to many neurosurgeons. The present report does not clarify that vague situation. The presence of a surgical rib and clear-cut compression of vascular channels, particularly during upper limb movement, remain the best definitive diagnostic aids in this arena.—Robert M. Crowell, M.D.

Immediate Radial Nerve Palsy Complicating Fracture of the Shaft of the Humerus: When is Early Exploration Justified?
O. Böstman, G. Bakalim, S. Vainionpää, E. Wilppula, H. Pätiälä, and P. Rokkanen (Univ. Central Hosp., Helsinki)
Injury 16:499–502, July 1985   28–5

Fifty-nine patients seen in 1960–1969 and 1972–1981 with immediate complete radial nerve palsy complicating humeral shaft fracture were reviewed. The mean age was 36 years (range, 13–79 years). Ten patients had open fractures and 7 had a comminuted fracture. Twenty-seven patients had exploration and internal fixation of the fracture, usually by the AO method, within 3 weeks of injury, 14 on an emergency basis. Twelve others were explored an average of 17 weeks after injury. Twenty patients

RECOVERY OF THE RADIAL NERVE

Treatment	Recovery				Time from accident to complete recovery (mean and range in weeks)
	None		Useful		
	No.	%	No.	%	
Early exploration	8	29·6*	19	70·4*	10 (4–24)
Delayed exploration	5	41·7*	7	58·3*	27 (19–52)
None (spontaneous recovery)	—		20		15 (4–28)
Total	13	22·0	46	78·0	15 (4–52)

*.50 > P > .10.
(Courtesy of Böstman, O., et al.: Injury 16:499–502, July 1985.)

who had signs of recovery within 4 months of injury were managed conservatively. The mean follow-up was 3 years.

A radial nerve laceration was found in 5 patients having early surgery and in 2 having delayed exploration. All but 1 of these patients had neurorrhaphy. Entrapment necessitated neurolysis at delayed surgery in 5 cases. Treatment of the nerve was necessary in 41% of all patients explored. Nerve involvement was more frequent with longitudinal distal-third fractures than with transverse middle-third fractures. Useful nerve recovery was found in two-thirds of the patients explored. Early and delayed exploration yielded comparable results (table).

Early exploration of the radial nerve with internal fixation of a humeral shaft fracture carries a risk of damage when no more than neurapraxia is present. Early surgery is warranted in cases of immediate radial nerve injury complicating a spiral or oblique fracture of the distal third of the humeral shaft.

▶ In this series early and delayed exploration yielded comparable results. Therefore, one may question the recommendation for early surgery in cases of immediate radial nerve injury with spinal or oblique fracture of the distal third of the humerus.

Sural nerve grafting can lead to good results for severe injuries of the radial nerve (Fisher and McGeoch: *Injury* 16:411–412, 1985).

When severance of the thenar branch of the median nerve occurs at carpal tunnel release, repair at reexploration can lead to return of function (Liloy and Magnell: *J. Hand Surg. [Am]* 10A:399–402, 1985).—Robert M. Crowell, M.D.

The Surgical Management of Nerve Lesions in the Lower Limbs: Clinical Evaluation, Surgical Technique and Results
L. Sedel (Hôpital Saint-Louis, Paris)
Int. Orthop. 9:159–170, November 1985   28–6

Microsurgical techniques have given hope of improved results from surgery on nerve lesions in the lower extremities. Such lesions have been operated on in 54 cases since 1974, and nerve grafting done by the use of microsurgical methods in 26 cases. Surgery is not recommended if a lesion is more than 2 years old, some recovery of paralysis has occurred, pain is severe, or a compression lesion is present that recovers spontaneously.

Among seven patients with clean traumatic lesions, all four who were followed up had a good or very good result. One of two partial graft procedures for missile injury gave a good result, and two other patients were partially relieved of persistent pain. Ten traction injuries of the common peroneal or sciatic nerve were treated. Two of six patients had a satisfactory result after nerve grafting, three a fair result, and one a poor result. Nerve compression injuries, when acute, did well when decompressed within 6 or even 12 hours. Compression injuries related to entrapment neuropathy, tumor, and leprosy also were treated.

Since many partial nerve lesions in the lower extremity resolve spontaneously, careful assessment for surgery is necessary. All complete lesions should be repaired by the use of microsurgical techniques. Vascularized sural nerve grafts may be useful. Hematoma compressing a nerve should be evacuated on an emergency basis. Electromyography and radiculography may be helpful in cases of chronic nerve entrapment, upper sciatic nerve lesions, or root lesions following injury to or surgery on the hip.

▶ Data in this report suggest that microsurgical handling of traumatic nerve lesions of the lower extremity may produce good results. However, it is to be emphasized that many partial nerve lesions in the lower limbs resolve spontaneously. Further experience comparing conservative and surgical therapy will be needed to establish a place for microsurgery in the therapy for these lesions.

In 22 patients, neurolysis of the common peroneal nerve in leprosy gave good results (Chaise and Roger: *J. Bone Joint Surg. [Br.]* 67B:426–429, 1985).—Robert M. Crowell, M.D.

Use of Polytetrafluorinated Ethylene Compound in Peripheral Nerve Grafting: Experimental Study
Dale H. Rice, Fernando D. Burstein, and Anita Newman (Univ. of Southern California and Univ. of California at Los Angeles)
Arch. Otolaryngol. 111:259–261, April 1985   28–7

Bridging of nerve gaps remains a problem despite trials with many autogenous and manufactured materials. Polytetrafluorinated ethylene (Gore-tex), a biologically inert material of varying rigidity, has now been evaluated as a nerve conduit. Tubing with an internal diameter of 2 mm and a wall thickness of either 0.36 or 0.17 mm was used in a rat sciatic nerve model involving excision of a 1-cm nerve segment. The nerve ends were secured to the tubing with 10–0 nylon epineural sutures; the operating microscope was employed.

The use of thin-walled tubing led to favorable functional and microscopic results in five of seven rats, and thick-walled tubing was associated with favorable results in three of six. Rats with good leg function and no ulcerations exhibited neural elements in a substantial part of the tube lumen. There was much less inflammatory response and minimal fibrosis in the thin-walled grafts. Distal cross sections in the thin grafts showed fascicle formation as the nerve left the graft lumen; thick grafts showed only small-diameter nerve bundles.

Gore-tex may prove to be useful in bridging nerve gaps, especially when thinner-walled tubing is used. Materials such as this may protect against neuroma formation by shielding the anastomotic site from fibroblast infiltration. Operating time is shortened when nerve harvesting is unnecessary. The grafts, unlike long nerve-nerve cable grafts, are not subject to ischemia or fibrosis.

▶ The use of external sheets for nerve grafting has been suggested before. In the 1970s, experience finally demonstrated that Silastic sheets offered no advantage. More recently, a variety of other materials, including artificial skin, have been recommended for this purpose. Further clinical studies will be required to demonstrate an advantage for any particular nerve grafting technique.—Robert M. Crowell, M.D.

Nerve Regeneration Through Biodegradable Polyester Tubes
Earl Webb Henry, Tin-Ho Chiu, Emery Nyilas, Thomas M. Brushart, Pieter Dikkes, and Richard L. Sidman (Children's Hosp. and Harvard Univ., Boston, and Allied Health and Scientific Products, Andover, Mass.)
Exp. Neurol. 90:652–676, December 1985   28–8

Transected nerves can be approached by attempting extrinsic guidance of axons across the gaps. The proximal and distal stumps of severed sciatic nerves in mice were inserted into the ends of biodegradable polyester tubes and examined for up to 2 years afterward. In each successfully regenerated nerve the myelinated fiber number was estimated and correlated with the residual lumen size. The experimental model is illustrated in Figure 28–2. Most of the tubes were 5 mm long and had initial internal diameters of 0.5 or 0.75 mm. In some studies the nerve ends were joined with a single 10–0 nylon suture.

A nerve regenerated within the tube to bridge the gap between the proximal and distal stumps in more than 50% (34 of 63) of the implants. Regenerated nerves at all ages consisted of multiple small fascicles, each with its own perineurial sheath, and with the whole sheathed in a thick epineurium. Myelinated fibers were more numerous in tubes with larger initial lumens. Axonal areas in regenerated nerves were about half as large as those of normal nerves, although appropriately thick myelin sheaths were observed. Most failures occurred in tubes with an initial luminal diameter of 0.5 mm or less.

New polymers for use in nerve guidance systems are quite inert, and the polymers are biodegradable. Dimensional instability is an undesirable effect of these properties, however. Flexibility is also less than optimal.

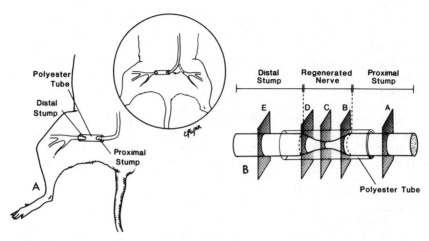

Fig 28–2.—A, a drawing of the experimental paradigm. A mouse's sciatic nerve was severed at midthigh, and a precut polymer tube was used to bridge a gap of the desired length between the proximal stump of this severed nerve and either the distal stump of the same nerve or *(inset)* the distal stump of the severed contralateral sciatic nerve. The nerve was then allowed to regenerate within the tube and to bridge the gap between the proximal and distal stumps. **B,** a schematic drawing of a sciatic nerve with an initial gap of 3 mm that has been bridged by regeneration through a polymer tube. The five levels sampled along this nerve are indicated by A through E. Level A is through the proximal nerve stump; B, C, and D are successively more distal levels along the regenerated nerve within the polymer tube; E is through the distal sciatic stump, into which successfully regenerated nerves grew. (Courtesy of Henry, E.W., et al.: Exp. Neurol. 90:652–676. December 1985.)

With regard to nerve regeneration, an adequate luminal diameter appears to be more important than the composition of the tube.

► Experimental studies are presented which indicate that new guidance systems, which are biodegradable, may be utilized to assist in peripheral nerve regeneration. Other studies by Norregaard et al. indicate that artificial skin may be utilized as a matrix to guide nerve regeneration. In such studies investigators are hopeful that improved nerve regeneration in the clinical setting may be fostered by appropriate surgical invention.—Robert M. Crowell, M.D.

Selected Recent Advances in Peripheral Nerve Injury Research
David G. Kline and Alan R. Hudson (Louisiana State Univ. and Univ. of Toronto)
Surg. Neurol. 24:371–376, October 1985   28–9

The importance of Schwann cells in nerve regeneration has been confirmed in a number of tissue culture and graft transfer studies. The Schwann cells retained and proliferating in the distal stumps of injured nerve apparently provide an as yet unidentified trophic substance to the growing tips of axons. Nerve growth factor stimulates increased myosin production in at least some sympathetic nerves and adrenergic axons arising from sensory ganglion cells. Axonal growth might be accelerated by creating a "conditioning" lesion or second axotomy 2 to 3 weeks after the initial injury. Motility and growth of the neurite are related at least in part to the production of cytoskeletal proteins such as tubulin and neurofilament protein. Studies of myelin degradation and reformation after injury show the importance of the local environment. The peripheral nerves have a rich blood supply, and the "blood-nerve" barrier may be an important aspect of regeneration.

Clinical interest in fascicular repair has increased in recent years. Failure to resect back to healthy neural tissue and distraction of a suture repair are the leading causes of failure after end-to-end nerve repair, and nerve grafting procedures are therefore a welcome addition. Whether optimal graft lengths exist for certain nerves is unclear. The proper timing of repair also remains to be established. A delay of months has been recommended for some lesions produced by contusion and stretching. Interest in the surgical management of brachial plexus lesions is increasing. Neurofibromas of the brachial plexus unassociated with Recklinghausen's disease can sometimes be safely resected by microscopic technique with repeated electrophysiologic assessment.

29 Functional

Introduction

Careful preoperative neuropsychologic testing is an aid to selection of patients for electrode implantation in the treatment of chronic pain (Digest 29–1). Interhemispheric commissurotomy has been recommended for the treatment of congenital hemiplegics with intractable epilepsy (Digest 29–2). Awareness of secondary epileptogenesis can help in the analysis of cases for potential surgical therapy for epilepsy (Digest 29–3). Baclofen may be delivered by a lumbosubarachnoid catheter to improve severe spasticity (Digest 29–4). The second sensory area has been demonstrated by evoked potentials and electrical stimulation studies in patients undergoing surgery (Digest 29–5).

Robert M. Crowell, M.D.

Psychological Factors and Outcome of Electrode Implantation for Chronic Pain
Michael S. Daniel, Charles Long, W. L. Hutcherson, and Samuel Hunter (Memphis State Univ. and Univ. of Tennessee)
Neurosurgery 17:773–777, November 1985   29–1

Surgical implantation of electrodes in the CNS is being increasingly used to relieve chronic pain, but which patients will respond the best is unclear. Psychologic factors have been associated with successful results from other treatments for chronic pain. Two raters independently reviewed functional pain protocols of 35 patients, 22 of whom were men with chronic pain. Thirteen patients were candidates for deep brain and 17 for spinal cord electrode implants. The mean duration of pain was 9 years, and a mean of three operations had been performed unsuccessfully. Eleven patients had a single electrode placed in the periaqueductal gray matter. Four others received two brain electrodes, and 1 patient had a single implant in the thalamus. Most spinal cord implants were between T7 and T11. Two electrodes were used in most of these cases.

Five (38.5%) of the 13 brain implant patients followed up had a good response, as did 4 (23.5%) of 17 with spinal cord implants. The overall rate of good response was 30%. Treatment outcome was accurately predicted for 80% of patients. Assessments were based on a patient interview, a pain questionnaire, the Minnesota Multiphasic Personality Inventory, the Cornell medical index, the Beck depression inventory, a health index, and the McGill pain adjective checklist.

Psychologic factors appear to be related to the outcome of electrode implantation in the CNS to relieve chronic pain. Implant candidates may be carefully screened or the procedure made available to patients with a poor outlook, but functional pain assessment is useful in either instance.

▶ This report underscores the need to take psychologic factors into account when dealing with chronic pain. Dr. William Sweet has long advocated that neuropsychologic evaluation be conducted prior to contemplated pain procedures. The present report indicates that neuropsychologic testing can assist in patient selection for electrode implantation.—Robert M. Crowell, M.D.

Interhemispheric Commissurotomy for Congenital Hemiplegics With Intractable Epilepsy
Robert N. Goodman, Peter D. Williamson, Alexander G. Reeves, Susan S. Spencer, Dennis D. Spencer, Richard H. Mattson, and David W. Roberts (Yale Univ.; VA Med. Ctr., West Haven, Conn.; and Dartmouth Med. School)
Neurology 35:1351–1354, September 1985   29–2

Hemispherectomy carries excessive morbidity and mortality rates in patients with congenital hemiplegia and incapacitating, refractory seizures. Five such patients underwent commissurotomy as an alternative and have been followed up for 2–12 years (mean, 5 years). All would have met criteria for hemispherectomy. Incapacitating seizures resolved in four patients, although some relatively benign seizures persisted. Two patients became able to work and live normally. In one patient, disabling seizures persisted at a reduced frequency. Hemiparesis was no worse after commissurotomy in any patient. Useful vision could be retained bilaterally, in contrast to hemispherectomy. No patient deteriorated intellectually, and one patient appeared to improve. No late complications have occurred.

Commissurotomy appears to be a major improvement on classic hemispherectomy in patients with congenital hemiplegia and incapacitating seizures refractory to medical measures. Anterior callosotomy is performed initially and is followed by a posterior callosotomy after a few months only if this is necessary. Sparing of the most posterior part of the corpus callosum permits the interhemispheric transfer of visual information. If commissurotomy fails, a classic or modified hemispherectomy can still be performed. In all but one of the authors' five patients, intractable seizures were relieved and there were no late complications from commissurotomy. Hemiparesis and intellectual function were not worsened by the procedure. Residual seizures were generally no more than a minor irritant.

▶ This innovative report provides data on five patients treated with commissurotomy for intractable seizures. The results are encouraging. Further data will be needed to establish a role for such surgery in the treatment of congenital hemiplegics with intractable epilepsy.

Corpus callosum section decreased the frequency of bilateral synchronous discharges in 12 patients and abolished such discharges in 1 patient (Spencer et al.: *Neurology* 35:1689–1694, 1985).

Magnetic resonance imaging can be used to assess the completeness of callosal section for epilepsy (Gazzaniga et al.: *Neurology* 35:1763–1766, 1985).

Reformated imaging to define the intercommissural line may be done to assist computed tomography-guided stereotaxic functional neurosurgery (Litchaw et al.: *AJNR* 6:429–433, 1985).

King et al. (*Neuropediatrics* 16:46–55, 1985) suggest that hemimegalencephaly with intractable seizures may be substantially helped by hemispherectomy.—Robert M. Crowell, M.D.

Secondary Epileptogenesis in Man
Frank Morrell (Rush-Presbyterian-St. Luke's Med. Ctr., Chicago, and Marine Biological Lab., Woods Hole, Mass.)
Arch. Neurol. 42:318–335, April 1985   29–3

The concept of secondary epileptogenesis implies that an actively discharging epileptogenic region that has massive neuronal connections with another site may gradually somehow "induce" similar paroxysmal behavior in the latter network. It has been difficult to prove the existence of secondary epileptogenesis in humans. In a majority of cases of focal epilepsy due to traumatic, infectious, or vascular disease, other or new epileptogenic foci are usually ascribed to multiple primary injuries maturing at different rates or to progressive disease. Cerebral tumor is the only common cause in which the likelihood of multiple primary lesions is extremely low.

Thirty-four percent of a series of 47 cerebral tumor patients with epilepsy had evidence of secondary epileptogenesis. Eleven patients had an intermediate stage of secondary epileptogenesis, and 5 had the irreversible (independent) stage. Methohexital suppression testing was able to distinguish between the reversible and irreversible stages of secondary epileptogenesis. The outcome was best predicted by the number of seizures.

If secondary epileptogenesis in nontumor cases operates in a similar manner, a rough correlation might be expected between the incidence of multiple foci and the duration of illness. One third of the patients with tumor in this series exhibited secondary epileptogenesis. Long-term monitoring without medication and pharmacologic study may help detect the onset of ictal episodes and distinguish between the reversible and irreversible phases of secondary epileptogenesis. Bilateral independent discharges do not preclude surgery if evidence indicates which site is the primary lesion.

▶ From the standpoint of surgical management of epilepsy, it is important to recognize that bilateral independent discharges do not preclude surgery when preoperative evaluation can identify the primary lesion. It is clear that such evaluation in surgery should be carried out by a team including the neurosurgeon and neurologic seizure specialist.

Scalp ectal EEG records may be unreliable for accurate localization of epilep-

tic foci for surgical excision (Spencer et al.: *Neurology* 35:1567–1575, 1985).—
Robert M. Crowell, M.D.

Continuous Intrathecal Baclofen for Severe Spasticity

Richard D. Penn and Jeffrey S. Kroin (Rush Med. College, Chicago)
Lancet 2:125–127, July 20, 1985   29–4

Baclofen therapy for spasticity sometimes gives only minor relief, but intrathecal administration may be much more effective. Six patients with severe lower limb rigidity, of whom five had frequent spasms, received long-term intrathecal baclofen therapy via an implanted delivery system after oral baclofen therapy had been ineffective in some patients or had produced unacceptable side effects in others. In a trial of intrathecal baclofen, administration of doses of 5–50 μg reduced muscle tone to normal and eliminated spasms for 2–10 hours when delivered via lumbar subarachnoid catheter. At a second operation the drug delivery system was placed subcutaneously in the abdomen. Baclofen was given either continuously or three or four times a day to reduce muscle tone to normal and stop disabling spasms. Initial dosages were 12–200 μg daily.

The response of rigidity to baclofen therapy is shown in Figure 29–1. Dosages stabilized after 4–7 months. Spasms were controlled in all instances. There was no change in voluntary muscle control. None of the patients had any of the central side effects that they had had while receiving oral baclofen. Bladder function improved, and incontinence ceased in three patients. The drug pump and catheter functioned properly, and there were no surgical problems.

Intrathecal baclofen administration is an effective treatment for rigidity and spasms caused by spinal cord damage. Patients have had less discomfort, and daily activities are more easily carried out with this approach. Rehabilitation efforts have been resumed in many instances. Clinical gain has been greatest in patients with the worst rigidity and spasms. Tolerance has not developed with continuous oral baclofen therapy, but this may not hold for intrathecal treatment.

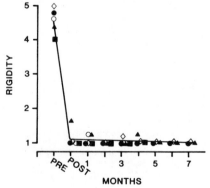

Fig 29–1.—Reduction in rigidity with intraspinal baclofen treatment for five patients evaluated with the Ashworth scale (5, rigid; 1, no increase of tone). (Courtesy of Penn, R.S., and Kroin, J.S.: Lancet 2:125–127, July 20, 1985.)

The Second Sensory Area in Humans: Evoked Potential and Electrical Stimulation Studies

H. Lüders, R. P. Lesser, D. S. Dinner, J. F. Hahn, V. Salanga, and H. H. Morris (Cleveland Clinic Found.)
Ann. Neurol. 17:177–184, February 1985   29–5

The second sensory area (SII) was first described by Penfield and Jasper and Penfield and Rasmussen, who studied stimulation of the perirolandic cortex in connection with the surgical treatment of epilepsy. The existence of SII was demonstrated in an epileptic woman by use of both cortical evoked potential and electric stimulation techniques.

Woman, aged 38 years, with intractable seizures arising from an extensive right frontal focus, had the primary sensory hand area localized by somatosensory evoked potential recording and stimulation of subdural electrodes. Evoked potentials of identical wave form but lower amplitude and longer latency were recorded in the inferior frontal gyrus, just anterior to the face area of the motor strip. Electric stimulation of this area elicited a "paralyzing" feeling in the left arm and face and inhibited rapid alternating movements of the left hand and tongue, strong muscle contractions, and speech.

This is the first documentation of a SII in a human by both electric stimulation and evoked potential recording. The SII appeared to overlap an area of complex motor control, a finding which suggests that it may provide direct sensory feedback information for appropriate motor integration. The SII potentials had a restricted field of distribution. That sensory phenomena were elicited by stimulation of the same prerolandic electrodes from which the highest SII potentials were recorded indicates that the area has a relatively direct somatosensory input. The potentials recorded from SII were not simply volume-conducted from SI.

Notes on Functional Problems

► Payne and Inturrisi report that spinal intrathecal injection of morphine results in detectable drug levels at cisterna magna, whereas methadone does not (*Life Sci.* 37:1137–1144, 1985).

For severe pain due to malignancy, stereotactic pontine spinothalamic tractotomy produces high levels of analgesia with low risk of disorders of respiration and micturition (Hitchcock et al.: *Acta Neurochir.* 77:29–36, 1985).

Ludman and Choa recommend a transtympanic operation for hemifacial spasm that results in improvement or cure in many of the patients (22 of 54 cases). (*J. Laryngol. Otol.* 99:239–245, 1985). Multiple reoperations are possible. The simplicity and lack of complications of this approach make it attractive.—Robert M. Crowell, M.D.

30 Neuroscience

Introduction

Central nervous system neurites grow preferentially on astrocytes and Schwann cells rather on nonglial cells in vitro (Digest 30–1). Some axons derived from the retina in adult rats are capable of regeneration in a suitable milieu (Digest 30–2). Functional synapses between individual neurons may regenerate in the spinal cord in lampreys (Digest 30–3). Levy et al. have developed a model for an in vivo study of individual axons (Digest 30–4). Percutaneous recording of single myelinated nerve fibers in humans has led to an improved understanding of perceived sensation (Digest 30–5). Autoradiographic and localization studies indicate the localization of the substance P in the spinal cord (Digest 30–6). Eicosanoids (including prostaglandins) regulate vascular tone, modulate autonomic transmission, and interact with endogenous opiates systems in the CNS (Digest 30–7).

Robert M. Crowell, M.D.

Preferential Outgrowth of Central Nervous System Neurites on Astrocytes and Schwann Cells as Compared With Nonglial Cells In Vitro

Justin R. Fallon (Univ. College, London)
J. Cell Biol. 100:198–207, January 1985   30–1

Growing axons in both the embryo and regenerating nerves often are closely associated with glial and other nonneuronal cells, which have been implicated in supporting and directing axonal growth, possibly through providing an adherent substrate for the migrating growth cone. Neurite outgrowth in culture was examined using cell type-specific antibodies and highly enriched populations of astrocytes, Schwann cells, and nonglial cells such as fibroblasts. Rat tissues were used and the cell monolayers were more than 95% pure.

Outgrowth of retinal neurites was seen on astrocytes, but not on fibroblasts (table). Scanning electron micrographs showed close adherence of the neurites to the surface of the astrocyte monolayer. Similar findings were obtained with cerebral cortex, but spinal cord showed some neurite growth on fibroblasts. Retinal neurites grew well on monolayers of sciatic-nerve Schwann cells. The latter underwent extensive migration when contacted by growing neurites. In choice studies, retinal neurites grew in a radial, fasciculated manner on the astrocytic side of the monolayer, but stopped or turned when encountering the fibroblast border (Fig 30–1). Studies with conditioned medium confirmed that the influence of astrocytes on growing neurites is localized, rather than due to soluble factors.

Central nervous system neurites grow preferentially on astrocytes and Schwann cells rather than on nonglial cells in vitro. Properties of the glial

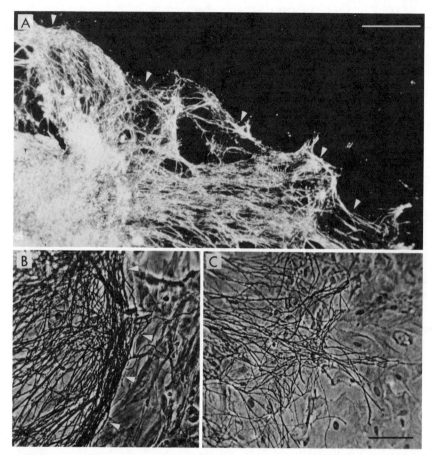

Fig 30–1.—Behavior of retinal neurites confronted with a choice of astrocytes and fibroblasts. Retinal explants were plated on the astrocyte side and the neurites were observed as they encountered the fibroblast frontier. A, low-power, dark-field view of a culture labeled with mouse antibody to neurofilament followed by horseradish peroxidase-coupled goat antibody to mouse Ig. The region of the border between astrocytes *(lower left)* and fibroblasts *(upper right)* is indicated by *arrowheads*. Bar, 0.25 mm. × 93. B and C, phase-contrast images of the outgrowth front of the same explant at border (B) and nonborder (C) regions. It can be noted that the neurites stop or turn at the border *(arrowheads)* between the astrocytes *(left)* and the fibroblasts *(right)* and do not encroach on the fibroblasts. Bar, 100 μm × 140. (Courtesy of Fallon, J.R.: J. Cell Biol. 100:198–207, January 1985.)

cell surface itself appear to be responsible. Peripheral nervous system neurites also have shown a preference for growth on glial cells, although they exhibit differences in response to nonglial cell substrates.

▶ Of particular interest in this study is the use of ingeniously devised tissue culture preparations, particularly the astrocytic monolayer with a fibroglass border. The power of such "choice" studies is demonstrated: CNS neurites grow preferentially on astrocytes rather than on nonglial cells in this preparation.

In mouse studies, autoradiographic and histochemical investigations of cortical trauma indicate that mature oligodendrocytes can proliferate and undergo

RETINAL NEURITE OUTGROWTH ON ASTROCYTES AND
FIBROBLASTS IS UNAFFECTED BY INCUBATION WITH
CONDITIONED MEDIA

Source of media	Monolayer cell type	Growth rate
		$\mu m/h$
Astrocytes	Astrocytes	31 ± 1
Fibroblasts	Astrocytes	33 ± 3
Control	Astrocytes	34 ± 2
Astrocytes	Fibroblasts	<5
Fibroblasts	Fibroblasts	<5
Control	Fibroblasts	<5

Retinal explants were placed on preformed monolayers of 5,000 astrocytes or fibroblasts in 35-mm dishes in the indicated media. The media had been conditioned for 5 to 7 days by more than 100,000 cells. The distance from the explant border to the outgrowth front was measured 24 hours later. The morphology of the neurite outgrowth was not influenced by any of the media tested. Rates are expressed as the mean ± SE for at least 4 explants.
(Courtesy of Fallon, J.R.: J. Cell Biol. 100:198–207, January 1985.)

mitosis in response to nonspecific damage in a manner similar to that seen with other glia (Lundwin: *Lab. Invest.* 52:20–30, 1985).

Rat experiments show that specific cellular terrain is essential for growth of axons into a spinal cord lesion (Guth et al.: *Exp. Neurol.* 88:1–12, 1985).

Topical application of triethnolamine and cytosine arabinoside enhances axonal growth into a spinal lesion in rat experiments (Guth et al.: *Exp. Neurol.* 88:44–55, 1985).

Tissue culture studies of locus coeruleus neurons revealed interesting results. Apparently these neurons can influence cocultured spinal neurons regarding expression of α receptors or induction of innervation of these neurons directly (Bun et al.: *J. Neurosci.* 5:181–191, 1985).—Robert M. Crowell, M.D.

Regeneration of Rat Optic Axons Into Peripheral Nerve Grafts
M. J. Politis and P. S. Spencer (Univ. of Saskatchewan and Bronx, N.Y.)
Exp. Neurol. 91:52–59, January 1986   30–2

The limited regenerative capacity of injured mammalian CNS tissue is ascribed to a posttraumatic environment not conducive to subsequent axonal regeneration. Peripheral nerve grafts were placed in crushed optic nerves in rats, and regeneration was assessed to determine if myelinated CNS axons can regenerate when in a suitable periaxonal milieu and to devise a surgical preparation in which regenerating mammalian CNS axons can be isolated from a single and easily manipulated source (e.g., retina). Part of the intradural tissue of the rat optic nerve was crushed 1 mm distal to the globe, injuring about one third of the cross-sectional area of the nerve. A segment of peroneal nerve was placed in the area of injury, and optic axon regeneration was assessed after 5 weeks.

Regenerating axons grew into graft tissue within 5 weeks of injury and

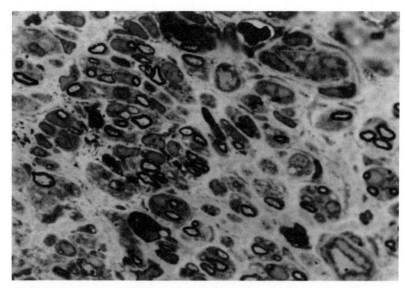

Fig 30–2.—Cross section of a peroneal distal stump graft insert into optic nerve assessed 5 weeks postoperatively. One-micrometer section stained with toluidine blue (×220). (Courtesy of Politis, M.J., and Spencer, P.S.: Exp. Neurol. 91:52–59, January 1986.)

were myelinated by resident Schwann cells. The mean ±SE number of axons in grafts inserted into optic nerves from six animals with intact retinas was 91.0 ± 12.1 (Fig 30–2). Unmyelinated axons were also present when the retinas were intact at the time of killing, but not when enucleation was performed 2 weeks before. Periaxonal Schwann cell cytoplasm was much more evident in peroneal grafts innervated by retinally derived axons than by tibial axons. Horseradish peroxidase studies showed that the retinal ganglion cells were a source for the regeneration of nerve fibers.

Some axons derived from the retinal ganglion cell layer in adult rats are capable of substantial axonal regeneration if a suitable periaxonal milieu is provided. Further experiments using dual-label axonal transport techniques will be required to ascertain if the regenerating axons result from collateral sprouting of intact optic nerve fibers or terminal sprouting of crushed optic axons. The present model offers a source of regenerating CNS axons with a single, readily manipulated source.

▶ The results of this imaginative study suggest that CNS axons can regenerate if local periaxonal conditions are right. Eventually, there could be clinical application; we'll have to await further studies. It is just this kind of basic work that is so needed for the neurosurgery of the future.—Robert M. Crowell, M.D.

Regeneration of Functional Synapses Between Individual Recognizable Neurons in the Lamprey Spinal Cord
Scott A. Mackler and Michael E. Selzer (Univ. of Pennsylvania)
Science 229:774–776, Aug. 23, 1985

30–3

Peripheral nerve grafts and bridges and fetal tissue transplants have produced neurite growth for short distances after injury to the mature spinal cord, but reestablishment of functional synaptic connections across the lesion site has not been demonstrated. It has now been found that giant interneurons can reestablish functional synaptic contacts with other giant interneurons across a healed spinal transection in sea lamprey larvae aged 4 to 5 years.

Cords from larvae that had recovered for at least 7 weeks after spinal transection and from control larvae were studied in a transilluminated perfusion chamber. Microelectrodes containing horseradish peroxidase were used after intracellular stimulation studies at varying frequencies. In four of 30 pairs of giant interneurons, stimulation of the caudal cell elicited a monosynaptic electrochemical excitatory postsynaptic potential (EPSP) in the rostral cell. Fifty percent of such pairs were synaptically linked in control lampreys without cord transection. The amplitude of chemical EPSPs was greater in giant interneurons of spinally transected lampreys, for cell pairs both across and below a healed scar. After recovery from transection, the EPSPs resembled those of normal adult sea lampreys.

These findings indicate regeneration of functional synaptic connections between individual neurons in a vertebrate CNS. Similar connections may well be formed by regenerating axons from mammalian grafts and bridges where the distance of axonal growth is similar to that in the lamprey spinal cord.

▶ This exciting report demonstrates that regeneration of functional connections between neurons is possible in vertebrate CNS. Further basic studies will be required for clarification of mechanisms and investigation of mammalian CNS. This line of inquiry could have profound implications for clinical neurosurgery.—Robert M. Crowell, M.D.

Model for the Study of Individual Mammalian Axons in Vivo, With Anatomical Continuity and Function Maintained
W. J. Levy, R. Rumpf, T. Spagnolia, and D. H. York (Univ. of Missouri at Columbia)
Neurosurgery 17:459–466, September 1985   30–4

A method was developed by which intact axons, with normal proximal and distal connections, can be studied individually in the mammalian nervous system. It is based on enzymatic dissociation of the extracellular matrix and provides a preparation of free axons, with myelination and Schwann cells intact. The surgically isolated sciatic nerve of a rat was passed through a chamber with controlled temperature and flow, and that was placed on an inverted microscope stage, which thereby allows observation of the process. The chamber was perfused with a calcium-free solution, followed by collagenase, trypsin, and hyaluronidase in series. Microelectrode studies and phase-contrast microscopy were performed, and axonal transport was visualized directly with the use of a Nikon Optiphot microscope.

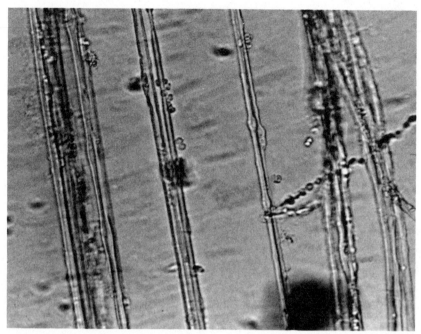

Fig 30–3.—Nerve with all but about one dozen axons severed is shown. The nonsevered axons are still conducting a small nerve signal and producing motor unit potentials on electromyography and are morphologically without sign of damage. (Courtesy of Levy, W.J., et al.: Neurosurgery 17:459–466, September 1985.)

The nerves (Fig 30–3) continued to show action potential conduction and axonal transport. Action potentials were conducted for at least 8 hours. Axonal transport was maintained in more than 90% of the axons that were directly visualized. Phase-contrast microscopy showed intact morphologic features, as did Nomarski microscopy and in situ osmic acid myelin staining. Signs of mechanical damage were less evident than in preparations made by mechanical testing methods.

Properties of axonal transport or active spike propagation can be studied in this in vivo axon model. Such problems as the separation of vascular from mechanical injury and the targeting of treatment to maintain spared motor axons can be approached. Axonal transport now can be studied in vivo without transfer to an in vitro system.

Microneuronography and Its Relation to Perceived Sensation: A Critical Review

P. D. Wall and S. B. McMahon (Univ. College, London)
Pain 21:209–229, March 1985
30–5

Hagbarth and Vallbo, in 1968, described how to record activity in single myelinated nerve fibers by inserting tungsten microelectrodes by hand.

Recordings of single units have now been made through the full diameter range of myelinated A fibers and from single unmyelinated C fibers. A method of "marking" was devised that reportedly identifies the particular fiber closest to the electrode through prolonged tetanus. Low-level stimulation is reported to stimulate selectively the recorded single fiber and evoke the appropriate sensation. Two microelectrodes have been used to record and stimulate the same fiber.

The recording of neuronography provides a means of describing one link in the chain connecting stimulation with sensory experience. Stimulation neuronography allows the introduction of false signals along the chain to determine whether artificially generated afferent impulses evoke the predicted sensation. Neuronography has shown that for suprathreshold stimuli, identification of modality and of intensity is not a property unique to single fibers or single fiber types, but rather depends on the ability of the CNS to extract information from the afferent barrage. Comparison between the time course of the afferent barrage and that of the sensation confirms that the latter is determined by factors other than the stimulus and afferent barrage, factors that can only be located in the CNS.

Neuronographic findings indicate that the brain abstracts the spatial and temporal pattern of the afferent barrage and that the threshold of perceived sensation depends on critical levels of firing. Coactivation of large and small fibers determines the level of pain perceived. Wide spatial gradients of stimulus and afferent activity are processed by the brain to achieve a perception of apparent elementary sensations with a spot location.

Autoradiographic Localization and Characterization of Spinal Cord Substance P Binding Sites: High Densities in Sensory, Autonomic, Phrenic, and Onuf's Motor Nuclei

Clivel G. Charlton and Cinda J. Helke (Uniformed Services Univ. of the Health Sciences, Bethesda, Md.)
J. Neurosci. 5:1653–1661, June 1985   30–6

Substance P (SP) is widely distributed in the spinal cord and has been implicated as a neurotransmitter in several spinal cord neuronal systems. However, SP receptors in the cord are not well characterized. Autoradiography was used to localize and quantify SP receptors in segments of the rat spinal cord. Bolton-Hunter SP labeled with ^{125}I was employed.

Sites of SP binding were found in the dorsal horns, intermediolateral cell column, and lamina X region. In the ventral horns, the phrenic, Onuf, and sacral ventromedial motor nuclei were densely labeled. The distribution of binding sites paralleled that of SP-containing nerve fibers in the spinal cord. Binding sites for SP correlated closely with cholinesterase-stained neurons (Fig 30–4). The density of binding sites in the dorsal horn was highest in the sacral section. In the lamina X region, density was highest in the thoracic section. Differential sensitivity of the SP receptors to unlabeled SP was noted at various sites, a finding that suggests the presence of heterogeneous receptors for SP in the spinal cord.

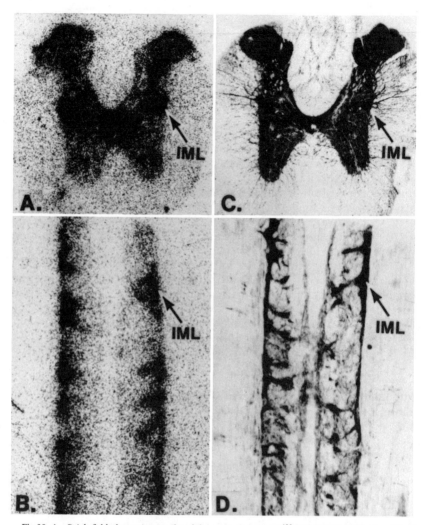

Fig 30–4.—Brightfield photomicrographs of the autoradiogram of ^{125}I-labeled BH-SP binding sites *(A and B)* and matched cholinesterase-stained slices *(C and D)* from the thoracic section of the spinal cord. *A* and *C* are horizontal, and *B* and *D* are longitudinal sections through the intermediolateral cell column (IML). (Courtesy of Charlton, C.G., and Helke, C.J.: J. Neurosci. 5:1653–1661, June 1985.)

The distribution of SP receptors in the spinal cord correlates with the localization of SP-containing nerve terminals. It is similar to the distribution of cholinesterase-stained neurons, except in the ventral horn, where high-density SP binding sites appear to occur only in nuclei that innervate specialized striated muscles.

▶ Neuroscience continues a detailed characterization of neuropeptides in the CNS. The accumulating data supports the concept of specialized systems such as SP, dopamine, and norepinephrine. Though the picture is not yet clear, there are clues that suggest a role for the SP system in nociception. Neurosurgeons should remain abreast of this work to develop clinical utilization of this burgeoning field of knowledge.—Robert M. Crowell, M.D.

Eicosanoids in the Central Nervous System
John B. Leslie and W. David Watkins (Duke Univ.)
J. Neurosurg. 63:659–668, November 1985   30–7

All mammalian tissues studied are capable of the biosynthesis of eicosanoids, compounds that are important modulators of many cellular and organ system functions. The eicosanoids comprise several groups of biologically active unsaturated fatty acids, including the "primary" prostaglandins, the cyclic endoperoxides, the prostanoids, the leukotrienes, and other acid lipids. Biosynthetic pathways of prostaglandin production are shown in Figure 30–5. The presence or absence and relative activity of certain enzymes determine the ultimate metabolite profile produced by the various pathways of cyclic endoperoxides in a given tissue.

The prostaglandins, including prostacyclin and thromboxane A_2, appear to contribute to the regulation of cerebrovascular tone and circulation. The prostagnoids are important mediators in cerebral vasospasm following subarachnoid hemorrhage. Prostacyclin has reversed acute vasospasm in vitro. Elevated levels of prostaglandin E_2 have been described in women during migraine. The eicosanoids are involved in hypothalamic function. The E prostaglandins and cyclic endoperoxides have been shown in vitro to inhibit the stimulated release of norepinephrine from prejunctional nerve

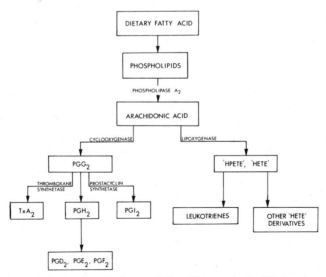

Fig 30–5.—Arachidonic acid intermediary metabolism. PG, prostaglandin; TX, thromboxane; HPETE, hydroperoxyeicosatetraenoic derivative; and HEPE, hydroxyeicosatetraenoic derivative. (Courtesy of Leslie, J.B., and Watkins, W.D.: J. Neurosurg. 63:659–668, November 1985.)

endings and may have a role in the modulation of autonomic transmission. Both direct and indirect interactions are evident between eicosanoid metabolites and endogenous opiate systems.

Further knowledge about prostaglandins in neurobiology may contribute to the understanding of many neurologic disorders.

31 Miscellaneous Topics

Surgonomics: The Identifier Concept—Hospital Charges in General Surgery and Surgical Specialties Under Prospective Payment Systems
Eric Muñoz, David M. Regan, Irving B. Margolis, and Leslie Wise (Long Island Jewish-Hillside Med. Ctr. and State Univ. of New York at Stony Brook)
Ann. Surg. 202:119–125, July 1985   31–1

The DRG (diagnostic related group) mechanism is coming into use in payment for in-hospital surgical care, but a majority of surgical DRGs at the authors' hospital were unprofitable under this scheme. An attempt therefore was made to group patients within each DRG on the basis of identifiers—mode of admission (emergency vs. nonemergency) and presence or absence of blood transfusion—to determine whether meaningful differences in mean hospital charges exclusive of physican fees could be found. Charges for 905 patients seen in 1983 at Long Island Jewish-Hillside Medical Center, in nine DRGs, were analyzed.

The areas of concern included general surgery, thoracic surgery, cardiac surgery, neurosurgery, orthopedics, urology, and head and neck surgery. A greater than 20% difference in charges was found with respect to the emergency-room identifier in eight of nine of the DRGs, and all 9 DRGs were positive for the transfusion identifier. Major chest procedures were most strongly positive for both identifiers.

The use of identifiers such as mode of admission and presence or absence of transfusion may allow teaching institutions to disaggregate each DRG so as to obtain more equitable reimbursement rates. Cost differences within DRGs could be used to propose mechanisms for cost control or negotiate alternate payment rates for teaching hospitals. Surgeons must become actively involved in the financial implications of what they do.

▶ This important article indicates how surgeons may be actively involved in the financial implications of surgery. The authors document that "identifiers," such as emergency admission and blood transfusion, pinpoint specific patients within a particular DRG whose hospital costs will be significantly higher. Accrual of such data by surgeons should be useful in efforts to negotiate more equitable reimbursement for these special high-expense patients.—Robert M. Crowell, M.D.

The Histotoxicity of Cyanoacrylates: A Selective Review
H. V. Vinters, K. A. Galil, M. J. Lundie, and J. C. E. Kaufmann (Univ. of Western Ontario)
Neuroradiology 27:279–291, July 1985   31–2

The alkyl 2-cyanoacrylates are widely used as rapidly polymerized adhesives in oral and general surgery and recently have been used for the embolotherapy of complex cerebral and extracerebral vascular anomalies. Alkyl cyanoacrylate polymerization involves an exothermic reaction. Soluble degradation products of cyanoacrylate adhesives have been implicated in cell death in mouse fibroblast tissue cultures. Extensive experience with ethyl 2-cyanoacrylate has indicated minimal overt vascular histotoxicity. Methyl 2-cyanoacrylate has been associated with neuronal necrosis and gliosis in the CNS as well as with perineural inflammation and neurilemmal damage in the peripheral nervous system. Few studies have been done on the effects of isobutyl cyanoacrylate on human tissues (Fig 31–1).

Every opportunity should be taken to assess the effects of all the cyanoacrylates on human tissues. Present patients will harbor isobutyl cyanoacrylate fragments within embolized lesions or adjacent normal tissues for months or years, and the possible long-term effects of the polymer must be appreciated. There is no evidence that isobutyl cyanoacrylate is carcinogenic. When the material is used for embolization, the potential for embolization of the lungs after passage through an arteriovenous fistula must be recognized. Pulmonary hypertension is a theoretical complication.

▶ A variety of animal studies have indicated that methyl 2-cyanoacrylite does not adhere well to arteries unless they are prepared with special drying techniques. In addition, substantial histotoxicity with gliosis and hemorrhage has been noted. The agent cannot be recommended for the external reinforcement of intracranial aneurysms because of poor adherence and histotoxicity. Muslin reinforcement, as described by Mount and colleagues years ago, is probably a safer method of treatment for unclippable aneurysms.

Preformed polymethylmethacrylate may be used for cranioplasties (Vangool: *J. Maxillofac. Surg.* 13:2–8, 1985). After the head is shaved, an impression of the defect is made, and a positive cast is made in dental cement. The cranioplasty is made from this and then heat-cured for sterility. The only infections occurred in 2 of 45 patients, both of whom had had chronic bone infections before the cranioplasty.

In rat sciatic nerve section, intraneural injection of tissue adhesive resulted in neuromas in only three of 28 experiments (Martini: *Handchir. Mikrochir. Plast. Chir.* 17:78–80, 1985).—Robert M. Crowell, M.D.

Miscellaneous Notes

▶ Ruge et al. (*J. Neurosurg.* 63:532–536, 1985) reviewed nine case histories from the literature and added two case reports of their own patients in whom pneumocephalus complicated CSF shunts. Mental changes and headache were the most common symptoms. Aqueductal stenosis was present in six of the patients, a group for which temporary external ventricular drainage was effective therapy.

Central nervous system fungal infection carries a mortality rate of up to 64%. A high index of suspicion, aggressive efforts at diagnosis (including biopsy), and early therapy (often with an Ommaya device) may improve outcome (Young et al.: *J. Neurosurg.* 63:371–381, 1985).

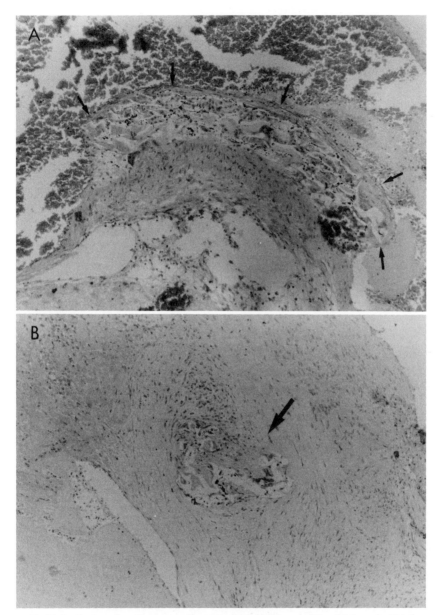

Fig 31–1.—Sections of arteriovenous malformations embolized 2 weeks (**A**) and 4.5 months (**B**) before resection. In **A**, isobutyl 2-cyanoacrylate (IBC) is noted to be adherent to the luminal surface of a vascular channel and is lined by endothelium *(arrows)*. Red blood cells in the lumen can be seen at top. In **B**, IBC-tantalum mixture *(arrow)* is embedded in the fibromuscular cushion of a thickened channel wall. Hematoxylin and eosin; A × 110, B × 130. (Courtesy of Vinters, H.V., et al.: Neuroradiology 27:279–291, July 1985. Berlin-Heidelberg-New York; Springer.)

Genetic studies suggest that neural tube defects are associated with particular combinations of maternal and fetal genes on chromosomes 3 and 6 (Weitkamp and Schachter: *N. Engl. J. Med.* 313:925–932, 1985).

Serious intracranial complications may follow submucous resection of the nasal septum (Haddad et al.: *Am. J. Otolaryngol.* 6:443–447, 1985). Complications include anosmia, visual disturbance, cavernous sinus thrombosis, cerebrospinal fluid rhinorrhea, pneumocephalus, subarachnoid hemorrhage, subdural empyema, and brain abscess.

Spinal cord ischemia can result from ligation of both internal iliac arteries (Kaisaly and Smith: *Urology* 25:395–397, 1985).

Low-dose isoflurane may increase intracranial pressure in patients with known intracranial tumor despite prior hyperventilation (Grosslight et al.: *Anesthesiology* 63:533–536, 1985).—Robert M. Crowell, M.D.

Subject Index

A

Acetazolamide
in hydrocephalus in infancy, 87
Acetylcholine
-receptor antibody, myasthenia gravis
without, 161
Acoustic neuroma
management of, 292
Acquired immunodeficiency syndrome (*see*
AIDS)
Acromegaly
SMS 201–995 in, 276
Acyclovir
in encephalitis, herpes simplex, 135
Adenoma (*see* Pituitary, adenoma)
Adhesive
system, fibrin, for closure of carotid-
cavernous fistula, 252
Aerocele
after posterior fossa and upper cervical
cord surgery, effects of patient
position on, 258
Age
at injury, relation to aphasia and
handedness, 49
Agnosia
environmental, loss of topographic
familiarity as, 43
AIDS, 33 ff.
central nervous system in, 33
HTLV-III in cerebrospinal fluid and
neural tissues in, 34
sequelae of, psychosocial and
neuropsychiatric, 35
Alcohol
polyvinyl, embolization, of cranial
lesions, 355
Alcoholism
epilepsy and, 99
Alexander's disease, 81
Alzheimer's disease
survival in, 81
Alzheimer type dementia (*see* Dementia,
Alzheimer type)
Amitriptyline
in laughing and weeping, pathologic,
191
Amnesia
thalamic, anatomical basis of, 44
Amyotrophic lateral sclerosis (*see*
Sclerosis, amyotrophic lateral)
Amyotrophy
microinfarcts, visual deficits, and
progressive dementia, 89

Anesthetic
abortive agents, local, in cluster
headache, 124
Aneurysm, 55 ff., 347 ff.
basilar, balloon embolization in, 348
carotid artery, extracranial, 330 ff.
case review, 332
surgical management, 330
intracranial, ruptured, volume depletion
and natriuresis in, 55
ruptured, delayed referral to
neurosurgical attention, 347
subarachnoid hemorrhage due to (*see*
Hemorrhage, subarachnoid,
aneurysmal)
vertebral artery, extracranial, dissecting,
311
Angiographically
occult angiomas, 353
Angiography
digital subtraction
current clinical applications, 67
intravenous, for carotid evaluation,
comparison to ultrasound, 318
intravenous, complications of, 76
isotope, portable, for confirmation of
brain death, 226
Angioma
angiographically occult, 353
Angioplasty
in "pre" subclavian steal syndromes,
252
Anhidrosis
chronic idiopathic, 192
Anomalies
arteriovenous (*see* Arteriovenous
malformation)
cortical, in developmental dyslexia, 45
Antiacetylcholine
receptor antibodies in myasthenia
gravis, 162
Antibiotic
prophylaxis in cerebrospinal fluid
shunting, 433
Antibody(ies), 161 ff, 265 ff.
acetylcholine-receptor, myasthenia
gravis without, 161
antiacetylcholine receptor, in
myasthenia gravis, 162
-guided irradiation of brain glioma, 266
to HTLV-I in tropical spastic
paraparesis, 136
monoclonal, in brain tumors, for
diagnosis and treatment, 265
Anticholinergics
high-dose, in adult dystonia, 117

Author Index

TO ORDER: DETACH AND MAIL

Please enter my subscription to the journal(s) and/or Year Book(s) checked below:
(To order by phone, call **toll-free 800-621-5410**. In IL, call **collect 312-726-9746**.)

	Practitioner (approx.)	Resident	Institution
Current Problems in Surgery® (1 yr.)	____$55.00	____$29.95	____$72.00
Current Problems in Pediatrics® (1 yr.)	____$39.95	____$29.95	____$65.00
Current Problems in Cancer® (1 yr.)	____$49.95	____$29.95	____$65.00
Current Problems in Cardiology® (1 yr.)	____$49.95	____$29.95	____$65.00
Current Problems in Obstetrics, Gynecology, and Fertility® (1 yr.)	____$49.95	____$29.95	____$65.00
Current Problems in Diag. Radiology® (1 yr.)	____$49.95	____$29.95	____$72.00
Disease-A-Month® (1 yr.)	____$39.95	____$29.95	____$65.00

Binder____$14.95 (each year)

	Practitioner	Resident
1987 Year Book of Anesthesia® (AN-87)	____$44.95	____$29.95
1987 Year Book of Cancer® (CA-87)	____$44.95	____$29.95
1987 Year Book of Cardiology® (CV-87)	____$44.95	____$29.95
1987 Year Book of Critical Care Medicine® (16-87)	____$44.95	____$29.95
1987 Year Book of Dentistry® (D-87)	____$45.95	____$29.95
1987 Year Book of Dermatology® (10-87)	____$45.95	____$29.95
1987 Year Book of Diagnostic Radiology® (9-87)	____$44.95	____$29.95
1987 Year Book of Digestive Diseases (13-87)	____$42.95	____$29.95
1987 Year Book of Drug Therapy® (6-87)	____$44.95	____$29.95
1987 Year Book of Emergency Medicine® (15-87)	____$44.95	____$29.95
1987 Year Book of Endocrinology® (EM-87)	____$45.95	____$29.95
1987 Year Book of Family Practice® (FY-87)	____$42.95	____$29.95
1987 Year Book of Hand Surgery® (17-87)	____$42.95	____$29.95
1987 Year Book of Hematology (24-87)	____$39.95	____$29.95
1987 Year Book of Infectious Diseases (19-87)	____$39.95	____$29.95
1987 Year Book of Medicine® (1-87)	____$44.95	____$29.95
1987 Year Book of Neonatal-Perinatal Medicine (23-87)	____$39.95	____$29.95
1987 Year Book of Neurology and Neurosurgery® (8-87)	____$44.95	____$29.95
1987 Year Book of Nuclear Medicine® (NM-87)	____$44.95	____$29.95
1987 Year Book of Obstetrics and Gynecology® (5-87)	____$42.95	____$29.95
1987 Year Book of Ophthalmology® (EY-87)	____$44.95	____$29.95
1987 Year Book of Orthopedics® (OR-87)	____$44.95	____$29.95
1987 Year Book of Otolaryngology-Head and Neck Surgery (3-87)	____$44.95	____$29.95
1987 Year Book of Pathology and Clinical Pathology® (PI-87)	____$44.95	____$29.95
1987 Year Book of Pediatrics® (4-87)	____$42.95	____$29.95
1987 Year Book of Plastic and Reconstructive Surgery® (12-87)	____$46.95	____$29.95
1987 Year Book of Podiatric Medicine and Surgery (18-87)	____$39.95	____$29.95
1987 Year Book of Psychiatry and Applied Mental Health® (11-87)	____$42.95	____$29.95
1987 Year Book of Pulmonary Disease (21-87)	____$39.95	____$29.95
1987 Year Book of Rehabilitation (22-87)	____$39.95	____$29.95
1987 Year Book of Sports Medicine® (SM-87)	____$42.95	____$29.95
1987 Year Book of Surgery® (2-87)	____$47.95	____$29.95
1987 Year Book of Urology® (7-87)	____$44.95	____$29.95
1987 Year Book of Vascular Surgery (20-87)	____$39.95	____$29.95

---

*The above Year Books are published annually. For the convenience of its customers, Year Book enters each purchaser as a subscriber to future volumes and sends annual announcements of each volume approximately 2 months before publication. The new volume will be shipped upon publication unless you complete and return the cancellation notice attached to the announcement and it is received by Year Book within the time indicated (approximately 20 days after your receipt of the announcement). You may cancel your subscription at any time. The new volume may be examined on approval for 30 days, may be returned for full credit, and if returned Year Book will then remove your name as a subscriber. Return postage is guaranteed by Year Book to the Postal Service.

Prices quoted are in U.S. dollars. Canadian orders will be billed in Canadian funds at the approximate current exchange rate.
A small additional charge will be made for postage and handling. Illinois and Tennessee residents will be billed appropriate sales tax. **All prices quoted subject to change.**

NAME_____ACCT. NO._____

ADDRESS_____

CITY_____STATE_____ZIP_____

Printed in U.S.A. ZAI

YEAR BOOK MEDICAL PUBLISHERS
35 EAST WACKER DRIVE   CHICAGO, ILLINOIS 60601